NURSING KEY TOPICS REVIEW

Pathophysiology

NURSING KEY TOPICS REVIEW

Pathophysiology

ELSEVIER

ELSEVIER

3251 Riverport Lane
St. Louis, Missouri 63043

Notice

Practitioners and researchers must always rely on their own experience and knowledge in evaluating and using any information, methods, compounds or experiments described herein. Because of rapid advances in the medical sciences, in particular, independent verification of diagnoses and drug dosages should be made. To the fullest extent of the law, no responsibility is assumed by Elsevier, authors, editors or contributors for any injury and/or damage to persons or property as a matter of products liability, negligence or otherwise, or from any use or operation of any methods, products, instructions, or ideas contained in the material herein.

PCN: 2018961458

Senior Content Strategist: Jamie Blum
Senior Content Development Specialist: Heather Bays
Publishing Services Manager: Shereen Jameel
Senior Project Manager: Kamatchi Madhavan
Design Direction: Margaret Reid

Printed in the United States of America

Last digit is the print number: 9 8 7 6 5 4 3 2 1

Melissa Bear, RN
Staff Nurse
DePaul Hospital
St. Louis, Missouri

Michelle Bonnheim
Nursing Student
California State University, Fresno
Fresno, California

Joanna Cain, BSN, BA, RN
President and Founder
Auctorial Pursuits, Inc.
Austin, Texas

Beth Cofini, MANE, RN
Associate Professor School of Nursing
Jersey College
Teterboro, New Jersey

Crystal Gallardo
CNA Nursing Assistant
Cypress College
Cypress, California

Katelynn Landers
Nursing Student
Brockton Hospital School of Nursing
Brockton, Massachusetts

Angela Lanzoni
Nursing Student
Brockton Hospital School of Nursing
Brockton, Massachusetts

Reagan Lizardi
Nursing Student
Polk State College
Lakeland, Florida

Michelle Luckett
Nursing Student
Polk State College
Winter Haven, Florida

Karla Psaros
Nursing Student
Brockton Hospital School of Nursing
Brockton, Massachusetts

Gina Rena
Nursing Student
Polk State College
Lakeland, Florida

Elizabeth Rudshteyn, MSN, RN
RN Program Chair
School of Nursing
Jersey College
Teterboro, New Jersey

Cianna Simpson
Nursing Student
Brockton Hospital School of Nursing
Brockton, Massachusetts

Briana Sundlie
Nursing Student
Cypress College
Cypress, California

Jo A. Voss, PhD, RN, CNS
Associate Professor
South Dakota State University
College of Nursing
Rapid City, South Dakota

Preface

The *Nursing Key Topics Review* book series was developed and designed with you, **the nursing student**, in mind. We know how difficult nursing school can be! How do you focus your study? How can you learn in the most time-efficient way possible? Where do you go when you need help?

We asked YOU and this is what we learned:

- you think textbooks are useful, but they can be overwhelming (also . . . heavy)
- you want quick and easy access to manageable levels of nursing information
- you like questions and rationales to challenge you and make sure you know what you need to know

Nursing Key Topics Review is your solution, whether you're looking for a textbook supplement or NCLEX® examination study aid. Review questions interspersed throughout the text make it easy to test your knowledge. The bulleted outline format allows for quick comprehension. A mobile app with key points lets you take your review with you anywhere you go!

In short, *Nursing Key Topics Review* helps you narrow down what's important and tells you what to focus on. Be sure to look for all the titles in the series to make your studies more effective . . . and your journey a little bit lighter!

Contents

Cells and Tissues 1

PATHOPHYSIOLOGY AND PATHOLOGY

- Pathophysiology is the study of how disease processes or injury cause physiologic changes in the body.
- Pathophysiology includes pathology, which is the laboratory study of cells and tissues for diagnostic purposes.

Disease

- Disease is a change in the individual's normal physical, mental, and social well-being, which disrupts homeostasis.
- Effect of disease is impacted by the organ or tissue affected, and the cause of disease.
  - Disease causes
    - Intrinsic
      - Age, gender, hereditary traits
    - Extrinsic
      - Infectious agents, stressors, behaviors
  - Disease processes
    - Identification
      - Identification of signs and symptoms
    - Occurrence
      - How often symptoms occur
      - When symptoms occur
    - Diagnosis
      - Identification of the specific disease
    - Etiology
      - Causative factors of the disease
    - Prognosis
      - Likelihood of recovery
  - Disease stages
    - Exposure
      - Body is exposed to stimuli that affects cell structure and function.
    - Onset
      - Can be sudden (acute)
        Or
      - Can be insidious (chronic)
    - Acute
      - Short-term illness that develops quickly
      - Distinct signs and symptoms
    - Chronic
      - Develops gradually and can persist for a long time
      - Can cause permanent cell damage

- Latent
  - "Silent" stage
  - No evident signs and symptoms
- Prodromal
  - Early development of disease
  - Individual is aware of a change in the body.
  - Nonspecific signs and symptoms
- Manifestation
  - Clinical signs and symptoms are evident.
- Remission
  - Manifestations of the disease subside.
- Convalescence
  - Recovery period

APPLICATION AND REVIEW

1. Which statement, provided by the nurse to a patient newly diagnosed with type 2 diabetes, demonstrates an understanding of the term pathophysiology?
   1. "It's the study of how your body organs, such as your pancreas, are supposed to work."
   2. "It helps explain how type 2 diabetes will affect the way your body functions."
   3. "Sending your blood to the laboratory to determine your A1C is an example of pathophysiology."
   4. "It's the science that explains how your body is structured."
2. Which assessment data related to a specific client demonstrates the presence of a disease process? **Select all that apply.**
   1. Sleeps 8 hours nightly
   2. Eats a high-fiber, low-fat diet
   3. Reports pain in left knee
   4. Allergic to strawberries and eggs
   5. Reports being depressed since death of partner
3. Which assessment question is focused on identifying an extrinsic cause of a client's migraine headaches? **Select all that apply.**
   1. "At what age did you start experiencing migraine headaches?"
   2. "What kinds of emotional stress are you currently experiencing?"
   3. "Do either of your parents or any of your siblings have a history of migraines?"
   4. "Are there specific foods or activities that trigger your migraines?"
   5. "Do you have any physical indications that you are about to experience a migraine?"
4. What assessment question is focused on identifying the etiology of the client's current cold signs and symptoms?
   1. "What signs and symptoms of a cold are you experiencing?"
   2. "Is your cough worse at night or during the day?"
   3. "Have you been around anyone with a cold within the last 2 weeks?"
   4. "How often do you experience the signs and symptoms of a cold?"

5. Which statement indicates that the disease currently being experienced by a client is acute in nature?
    1. "One minute I was fine and the next I was having trouble breathing."
    2. "I can't really explain it, but I just don't feel well."
    3. "The knee has gotten progressively more swollen over the last 2 years."
    4. "The symptoms will go away for months at a time, but enviably they return."
See Answers on pages 13–16.

Cells

- The cell is the body's basic building block, which, when grouped together, forms tissues, blood, and bone.
- Cells can adapt to changes in the body.
- Cells become specialized and thus carry out different functions.
  - Differentiation (maturation) is the process cells undergo to become specialized.
  - Specialized cellular functions
    - Movement
    - Conductivity
    - Metabolic absorption
    - Secretion
    - Excretion
    - Respiration
    - Reproduction
    - Communication
- When cell structure and function change, disease may develop.
  - Irreversible changes in a cell can cause altered deoxyribonucleic acid (DNA) structure.
- An individual cell is composed of various structures that help maintain cell life and homeostasis (Fig. 1.1).
  - Nucleus
    - Controls the activity of the cell
    - Involved in cellular reproduction
  - Cytoplasm
    - Site where biochemical reactions take place
    - Aqueous solution found between nucleus and plasma membrane
  - Endoplasmic reticulum
    - Helps move materials around the cell
    - Main function is storage and secretion.
    - Responsible for protein folding and recognizing cell stress
  - Mitochondria
    - Generates and transforms energy
    - Assists in generating adenosine triphosphate (ATP)
    - Responsible for cellular respiration
  - Ribosome
    - Aids in protein synthesis
  - Cell membrane
    - Controls the entry and exit of certain substances
    - Composed of lipids and proteins

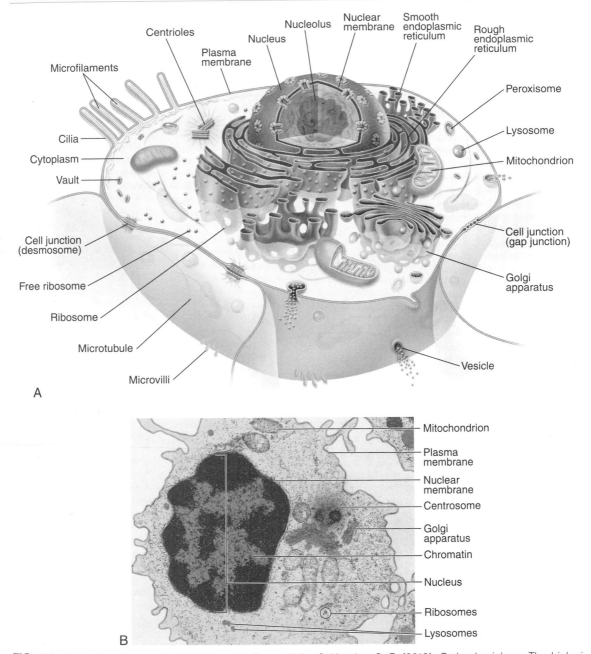

FIG. 1.1 Typical or Composite Cell. (From McCance K. L., & Huether S. E. [2019]. *Pathophysiology: The biologic basis for disease in adults and children* [8th ed.]. St. Louis: Elsevier.)

- Golgi complex
  - Helps move materials within the cell
  - Processes proteins
- Lysosome
  - Breaks down old cell materials
  - Aids in cell recovery

- Peroxisomes
  - Contain catalase and urate oxidase
  - Similar to lysosomes
- Cytosol
  - Found in the cytoplasm
  - Aids in ribosomal protein synthesis
  - Stores fats, carbohydrates, and secretory vesicles
- Cytoskeleton
  - Composed of protein filaments
  - Provides support to the cell
- Plasma membrane
  - Involved in metabolism
  - Protects the cell from the external environment

APPLICATION AND REVIEW

6. Which action is a direct result of a specialized cell function? **Select all that apply**.
   1. Walking up steps
   2. Sweating on a hot day
   3. Healing a broken bone
   4. Digesting a hamburger
   5. Laughing at a joke

7. What is the likely result of a structural change in a cell?
   1. Illness
   2. Skeletal growth
   3. Increase in muscle strength
   4. Death of the cell's ability to reproduce

8. When a cell is incapable of normal reproduction, which cellular structure is malfunctioning?
   1. Nucleus
   2. Endoplasmic reticulum
   3. Cell membrane
   4. Cytoskeleton

See Answers on pages 13–16.

- Cellular functions
  - Movement
    - Enable movement in muscle and bone
  - Conductivity
    - Stimulates the cell into motion
    - Chief function of nerve cells
  - Metabolic absorption
    - Provides energy to the cells
    - Helps cells synthesize proteins and reabsorb fluids
      - As seen in the renal system
  - Secretion
    - Cells absorb substances and also discharge them.
    - New substances are distributed to where they are needed.
      - As seen in mucous secretion
  - Excretion
    - Cells break down nutrients and expel waste products.
      - As seen in urination and defecation
  - Respiration
    - Cells absorb oxygen needed for ATP creation.
      - As seen in the respiratory system

- Reproduction
  - Process of making new cells
  - Needed for bone and tissue growth
- Communication
  - Required to maintain homeostasis of body tissues
- Cell division and reproduction
  - Cells can be eukaryotic (higher animals and plants, fungi, protozoa, most algae) or prokaryotic (blue-green algae, bacteria, rickettsia).
    - Eukaryotic cells have a nucleus and are enclosed in a membrane, whereas prokaryotic cells are unicellular and do not have the characteristics of a typical cell.
  - Mitosis
    - Vegetative division
    - Two daughter cells are identical to the parent cell.
    - Each daughter cell has the same number and kind of chromosomes as the parent cell.
  - Meiosis
    - Sexual reproduction of eukaryotic cells
    - One parent diploid cell reduces to four genetically diverse haploid cells (daughter cells).
    - Produces sex cells (gametes): sperm in males, eggs in females
    - Meiosis I
      - Begins with one diploid parent cell
      - Ends with two haploid daughter cells
      - Has half the number of chromosomes in each cell
    - Meiosis II
      - Begins with two haploid parent cells
      - Ends with four haploid daughter cells
      - Maintains the same number of chromosomes in each cell
    - Meiosis I and meiosis II share the same stages
      - Prophase
        - Chromosomes coil and shorten.
        - Nuclear membrane dissolves.
        - Each chromosome is made up of a pair of strands (chromatids).
        - Chromatids connect to a spindle of fibers called centromeres.
      - Metaphase
        - Centromeres divide.
        - Chromosomes pull apart.
        - Centromeres align in the middle of the spindle.
      - Anaphase
        - Centromeres separate and guide newly created chromosomes to opposite sides of the cell.
        - 46 chromosomes are present on each side of the cell.
      - Telophase
        - New membrane forms around each set of chromosomes.
        - Spindle fibers disappear.
        - Cytoplasm divides.
        - Two identical daughter cells are created.
- Cellular metabolism and energy
  - Anabolism (energy-using)
  - Catabolism (energy-releasing)
  - Proteins, fats, and starches are hydrolyzed in the intestinal tract into amino acids, fatty acids, and glucose.

- Substances are absorbed, circulated, and taken up by the cell where they are used for ATP production and other functions.
  - ATP is energy needed to maintain cell function.
- Oxidative phosphorylation occurs in the mitochondria.
  - It is the manner by which the energy produced from carbohydrates, fats, and proteins is transferred to ATP.
- Catabolism of proteins, lipids, and polysaccharides found in food are divided into three phases.
  - Digestion
    - Secreted enzymes outside the cell break large molecules into smaller units, proteins into amino acids, polysaccharides into simple sugars, and fats into fatty acids and glycerol.
  - Glycolysis
    - The splitting of glucose molecules to create pyruvate and two molecules of ATP
  - Oxidation
    - Loss of electrons during reaction by a molecule
    - Occurs when the oxidation state of a molecule is increased
  - Citric acid cycle (Krebs cycle)
    - Occurs in the mitochondria
    - Creates energy in the form of ATP, nicotinamide adenine dinucleotide, and flavin adenine dinucleotide from the oxidation of pyruvate (end process of glycolysis)
- Cellular transportation
  - Active transport
    - Movement of a substance across a membrane against its concentration gradient
    - Movement of particles from areas of lower concentration to areas of higher concentration
    - Accumulates high concentrations of molecules needed by the cell
    - Helps molecules penetrate the lipid bilayer of the membrane
      - Primary active transport
        - Uses chemical energy (ATP)
      - Secondary active transport
        - Uses electrochemical gradient
  - Passive transport (facilitated diffusion)
    - Spontaneous passive transport
    - Passage of molecules across the membrane via transport proteins
    - Does not require energy input
      - Diffusion
        - Movement from an area of greater concentration to an area of lesser concentration
        - Difference in concentration = concentration gradient
        - Particles move through the permeable membrane to reach equilibrium.
        - Rate of diffusion
          - Differences of electrical potential across the membrane
          - Diffusion coefficient = size of the substance
          - Lipid solubility
            - Smaller molecules that are oil-soluble are hydrophobic and nonpolar.
            - Oil-soluble molecules quickly diffuse across the membrane.
            - Lipophilic substances diffuse rapidly.
          - Water solubility
            - Water-soluble substances diffuse slowly.
            - Water molecules are small and uncharged and diffuse quickly.

- Filtration
  - Movement of water and solutes through a membrane caused by a greater force on one side of the membrane than on the other side
  - Hydrostatic pressure
  - Force of water pushing against cellular membranes
- Osmosis
  - Spontaneous movement of a solvent through a semipermeable membrane to an area of higher solute concentration
  - Osmotic pressure = external pressure needed to prevent movement of a solvent across the membrane
  - Osmotic gradient = difference in concentration between two solutions on either side of a semipermeable membrane
    - Reverse osmosis
      - Pressure is used to force a solvent through a semipermeable membrane against the concentration gradient.
- Vesicle formation transport
  - Endocytosis
    - Section of the plasma membrane that attracts substances from outside the cell, folds inward, and separates from the plasma membrane
    - Forms an endocytic vesicle that moves into the inside of the cell
    - Regulates the plasma membrane owing to changes in the extracellular environment
    - Counterbalances exocytosis
    - Maintains homeostasis
  - Pinocytosis
    - Cell ingests contents of extracellular fluid and small parts of the plasma membrane.
  - Exocytosis
    - Secretion of material from intracellular vesicles at the cell's surface
- Types of cellular adaptation
  - Atrophy
    - Decreased size of cells
  - Hypertrophy
    - Increased size of cells
  - Hyperplasia
    - Increased number of cells that causes large tissue mass
  - Metaplasia
    - One mature cell type is replaced by a different mature cell type.
  - Dysplasia
    - Varying cell size and shape, large nuclei, and increased mitosis
  - Anaplasia
    - Undifferentiated cells with variable cell structures and numerous mitotic figures
  - Neoplasia
    - New growth or tumor
- Cell damage and necrosis (apoptosis) causes
  - Ischemia
    - Decreased oxygenated blood flow to the tissue
  - Physical agents
    - Excessive temperature changes, exposure to radiation, trauma, surgery

- Chemical toxins
  - Chlorine gas, mercury, snake venom
- Mechanical damage
  - Pressure, tearing of tissue
- Microorganisms
  - Bacteria, virus, parasite
- Nutritional deficits
  - Protein, vitamins, minerals
- Fluid and electrolyte imbalance
  - Increased fluid, decreased fluid
  - Cation and anion imbalance
- Cell growth and replication abnormalities
  - Neoplasm
    - Also called a tumor
    - Overgrowth of cells that no longer is able to be controlled by the body
    - Cells continue to reproduce even though there is no physiologic purpose.
    - Usually consists of immature or atypical cells
    - Neoplasms are benign or malignant.
      - A malignant neoplasm is referred to as "cancer."
    - Cell overgrowth causes
      - Nutrition deprivation of normal cells
      - Increased pressure to surrounding tissues
      - Ischemia
      - Reduced blood flow
      - Necrosis
      - Organ death
  - Benign neoplasm
    - Has normal cell qualities
    - Can form anywhere
    - Surrounded by connective tissue
      - Freely moveable on palpation
    - Not able to invade neighboring tissue or metastasize
      - Encapsulated
      - Localized
    - Slower growth rate than a malignant tumor
    - Can be serious if it presses on vital organs and structures
      - Life-threatening only in certain locations
        - Increased pressure on brain
    - Caused by dead cells that remain in the tissue
    - Normal mitosis
      - Rare systemic effects
    - Typically removed by surgery
      - Does not typically return after removal
    - Classified by where it grows
      - Adenoma
        - Forms in a thin layer of tissue that protects organs, glands, and other structures
        - Polyps

- ○ Lipoma
  - ○ Most common type of benign tumor
  - ○ Grows in fat tissue
- ○ Myoma
  - ○ Grows in walls of blood vessels or muscles
  - ○ Can grow in wall of smooth tissue
    - - Uterus
- ▪ Fibroid
  - ○ Grows in fibrous tissue of organs
    - ○ Uterine fibroids
- ▪ Nevi
  - ○ Skin growths
  - ○ Mole
- • Malignant tumor
  - ▪ Composed of dysplastic cells
  - ▪ Typically spreads rapidly to surrounding structures
    - ▪ Secretes growth factors to help tumor grow and spread
  - ▪ Can be in situ
    - ▪ Preinvasive stage that can last for months or years
  - ▪ Has abnormal chromosomes and DNA
    - ▪ Makes nucleus larger and darker
  - ▪ Has a different shape than a benign neoplasm
  - ▪ Can be disrupted or absent
    - ▪ Cell-to-cell communication
    - ▪ Growth inhibition
    - ▪ Organization
    - ▪ Contact controls
  - ▪ Cell membranes and surface antigens are altered.
  - ▪ Secretes enzymes that break down cells and proteins
  - ▪ Causes increased pressure on surrounding structures
    - ▪ Compresses blood vessels
      - ○ Results in necrosis that leads to increased inflammation
      - ○ Results in organ death
  - ▪ Systemic effects
    - ▪ Paraneoplastic syndrome
      - ○ Symptom complexes triggered by cancer
      - ○ Usually caused by substances (e.g., hormones) released from the tumor or tumor-initiated immune response
    - ▪ Other effects
      - ○ Fatigue
      - ○ Weight loss
      - ○ Cachexia
      - ○ Anemia
      - ○ Infection
      - ○ Bleeding
  - ▪ Staging
    - ▪ Detects how far the cancer has spread

- Staging is based on the TNM system.
  - Size of the primary tumor (T)
    - TX: Nonmeasurable
    - T0: No evidence of the tumor
    - Tis: Tumor has not grown into nearby tissue.
    - T1 to T4: Tumor has grown into nearby tissue.
    - Numbers 1 to 4 express how much the tumor has grown.
  - Lymph node involvement (L)
    - NX: Unable to evaluate lymph nodes
    - N0: No cancer found in the lymph nodes.
    - N1 to N3: Cancer has spread to the lymph nodes.
  - Metastasis (M)
    - M0: Cancer has not spread to other parts of the body.
    - M1: Cancer has spread to other parts of the body.
- Grading
  - Describes how the tumor cells look under the microscope
  - The more the cells look like normal cells, the lower the grade and likelihood that the cancer will spread slowly.
  - Grade 3 and 4 tumors do not look like normal cells and tissues; they grow rapidly and spread faster than tumors with lower grades.
  - Grading classification
    - GX: Grade cannot be determined (undetermined).
    - G1: Well-differentiated (low grade)
    - G2: Moderately differentiated (intermediate grade)
    - G3: Poorly differentiated (high grade)
    - G4: Undifferentiated (high grade)

APPLICATION AND REVIEW

9. Which characteristics are associated with sexual reproduction of eukaryotic cells? **Select all that apply.**
   1. Sex cells, including gametes and eggs
   2. Diploid cell reduction
   3. Haploid cell production
   4. Two daughter cells chromosomes identical to those of the parent cell
   5. Four genetically diverse haploid cells
10. Which characteristics are associated with the form of sexual reproduction referred to as Meiosis II? **Select all that apply.**
    1. Begins with one diploid parent cell
    2. Ends with four haploid daughter cells
    3. Has half the number of chromosomes in each cell
    4. Begins with two haploid parent cells
    5. Maintains the same number of chromosomes in each cell
11. Which events take place during the prophase of meiosis? **Select all that apply.**
    1. Chromosomes coil and shorten.
    2. Centromeres align in the middle of the spindle.
    3. The nuclear membrane dissolves.
    4. The chromatids connect to a centromere.
    5. New membrane forms around each set of chromosomes.

12. What substances are required for the cell to produce ATP? **Select all that apply**.
    1. Protein
    2. Fat
    3. Starch
    4. Water
    5. Sodium
13. What role does the mitochondria play in the production of cellular energy?
    1. Protein synthetization
    2. Site of cellular chemical reactions
    3. Protein folding
    4. ATP creation
14. What events occur during the digestion phase of catabolism? **Select all that apply**.
    1. Fats are broken into fatty acids.
    2. Glucose molecules are split to create pyruvate.
    3. Proteins are broken into amino acids.
    4. Polysaccharides are broken into simple sugars.
    5. Fats are broken into glycerol.
15. What is the final product of the Krebs cycle? **Select all that apply**.
    1. Pyruvate
    2. Amino acids
    3. ATP
    4. Simple sugar
    5. Fatty acid
16. What form of cellular transport is dependent on ATP to be effective?
    1. Primary active transport
    2. Filtration
    3. Osmosis
    4. Diffusion
17. What type of cellular adaptation results in a decrease in cell size?
    1. Hypertrophy
    2. Metaplasia
    3. Neoplasia
    4. Atrophy
18. Which agents cause cell damage related to exposure to a physical agent? **Select all that apply**.
    1. Frostbite
    2. Scalding
    3. Radiation exposure
    4. Snake bite
    5. Bacterial infection
19. A client, diagnosed with a Grade 1 tumor, asks for an explanation regarding this grade. What information should the nurse use to formulate a response?
    1. The cells are well differentiated.
    2. The cells' degree of differentiation cannot be determined.
    3. The cells are graded at an intermediate or moderate level.
    4. The cells are highly undifferentiated.

See Answers on pages 13–16.

Tissues

- Tissues are made up of cells.
- How cells are grouped together determine the structure and function of tissues.
- Cover internal and external surfaces of the body
- Can be modified owing to hormonal changes
- Tissue formation
  - Cells communicate to form new cells.
  - Morphogenesis occurs.
    - Cells assemble into tissues.
  - Precursor cells
    - Create specialized cells

- Stem cells
  - Can produce daughter cells
  - Repair and maintain tissues
- Tissue types
  - Epithelial
    - Composed of three cell shapes
      - Squamous
        - Flat, thin
      - Cuboidal
        - Cube or square shaped
      - Columnar
        - Rectangular shape
  - Connective tissue
    - Framework for clusters of epithelial cells to form organs
    - Binds tissues and organs together
    - Provides support to tissues
    - Acts as storage site for nutrients
  - Muscle tissue
    - Composed of contractile myocytes
    - Cardiac, skeletal, smooth
  - Neural tissue
    - Composed of neurons
      - Cell body
      - Single axon
      - Dendrites
    - Receive and transmit electrical impulses across synapses
    - Neurotransmitters help neurons communicate.

APPLICATION AND REVIEW

20. What characteristic is associated with epithelial tissue?
    1. It provides a framework to form organs.
    2. Types include cardiac, skeletal, and smooth.
    3. It is found in the cell body of neurons.
    4. It can present as one of three cell shapes.

See Answers on pages 13–16.

ANSWER KEY: REVIEW QUESTIONS

1. **2 Pathophysiology is the study of how disease processes or injury cause physiologic changes in the body.**
   1 Physiology is the study of the way in which a living organism or bodily part functions normally. **3** Pathology deals with the laboratory examination of samples of body tissue for diagnostic or forensic purposes. **4** Anatomy is the branch of science concerned with the bodily structure of humans, animals, and other living organisms.
   Client Need: Health Promotion and Maintenance; **Cognitive Level:** Analysis; **Nursing Process:** Evaluation

2. **Answers: 3, 4, 5.**
   3 Disease is a change in the individual's normal physical, mental, and social well-being that disrupts homeostasis. Pain would be characteristic of a disease process that, in this case, is affecting the

musculoskeletal system. **4, 5** Disease is a change in the individual's normal physical, mental, and social well-being that disrupts homeostasis. Allergies are manifestations of a disease process that affects the immune system.

1 Sleeping 8 hours a night is an example of a characteristic associated with maintaining normal human homeostasis. **2** Eating a high-fiber, low-fat diet has been proven to support health and so contributes to maintaining normal human homeostasis.

Client Need: Health Promotion and Maintenance; **Cognitive Level:** Analysis; **Nursing Process:** Assessment/Analysis

3. **Answers: 2, 4.**

   2 Disease may be a result of either intrinsic or extrinsic factors. Extrinsic factors occur outside of the body and include infectious agents, stressors, and behaviors. **4** Disease may be a result of either intrinsic or extrinsic factors. Extrinsic factors occur outside of the body and include factors such as eating a specific food or engaging in an activity that triggers a disease process.

   1 This assessment question is not focused on cause, but rather duration of the disease process. **3** Disease may be a result of either intrinsic or extrinsic causes. Intrinsic factors are inherent to the individual and are generally unchangeable, such as hereditary traits. A family history of a disease would be considered an intrinsic cause. **5** This assessment question is not focused on cause, but rather identifying characteristics of the disease process.

   Client Need: Physiological Adaptation; **Cognitive Level:** Analysis; **Nursing Process:** Assessment/Analysis

4. **3 The Etiology is determined by identifying possible causes of the disease.**

   1 Naming the signs and symptoms of a disease is associated with the Identification stage of the assessment process. **2** Concluding when signs and symptoms occur or worsen is associated with the Occurrence stage of the assessment process. **4** Concluding how often signs and symptoms occur is associated with the Occurrence stage of the assessment process.

   Client Need: Physiological Adaptation; **Cognitive Level:** Analysis; **Nursing Process:** Assessment/Analysis

5. **1 Acute illness has a sudden onset with distinct signs and symptoms. Feeling fine one minute and then suddenly having difficulty breathing would be indicative of an acute illness.**

   2 The prodromal stage of disease is characterized by a lack of specific signs and symptoms. **3** Signs and symptoms that develop gradually and persist for a long period of time are considered chronic. **4** Remission is characterized by signs and symptoms of the disease subsiding or going away; these manifestations of the disease will generally reoccur at some time in the future.

   Client Need: Physiological Adaptation; **Cognitive Level:** Analysis; **Nursing Process:** Assessment/Analysis

6. **Answers: 1, 2, 3, 4.**

   1 Cells become specialized and thus carry out different functions. Movement is such a function because some cells, such as muscle and bone tissue, enable movement. **2** Cells become specialized and thus carry out different functions. Excretion is such a function demonstrated by the cells that comprise sweat glands. **3** Cells become specialized and thus carry out different functions. Reproduction is such a function because bone cells reproduce to mend broken bones. **4** Cells become specialized and thus carry out different functions. Metabolic absorption is such a function because some cells synthesize proteins from food we eat.

   5 Laughing is an emotion not directly controlled by a type of cell function.

   Client Need: Physiological Adaptation; **Cognitive Level:** Applying; **Nursing Process:** Assessment/Analysis

7. **1 When cell structure and function change, disease may develop.**

   2 Illness is a result of changes to cell structure or function. Skeletal growth results from effective reproduction of bone cells. **3** Illness is a result of changes to cell structure or function. Muscle strength results from effective reproduction of muscle cells. **4** Illness is a result of changes to cell structure or function. Cellular death is not the direct result of such changes.

   Client Need: Physiological Adaptation; **Cognitive Level:** Understanding; **Nursing Process:** Assessment/Analysis

8. **1 An individual cell is composed of various structures that help maintain cell life and homeostasis. Its nucleus controls the cell's reproduction.**
   2 An individual cell is composed of various structures that help maintain cell life and homeostasis. The main functions of its endoplasmic reticulum are storage and secretion. **3** An individual cell is composed of various structures that help maintain cell life and homeostasis. The cell's membrane controls the entry and exit of certain substances. **4** An individual cell is composed of various structures that help maintain cell life and homeostasis. The cytoskeleton provides structure to the cell.
   Client Need: Physiological Adaptation; **Cognitive Level:** Understanding; **Nursing Process:** Assessment/Analysis

9. **Answers: 1, 2, 3, 5.**
   1 Meiosis is the process of sexual reproduction of eukaryotic cells found in higher animals. This form of reproduction involves gametes and eggs. **2, 3, 5** Meiosis is the process of sexual reproduction of eukaryotic cells found in higher animals. This form of reproduction involves the reduction of a parent diploid cell into four genetically diverse haploid cells.
   4 Mitosis that involves two daughter cells that are identical to the parent cell is not associated with the sexual reproduction of eukaryotic cells.
   Client Need: Physiological Adaptation; **Cognitive Level:** Understanding; **Nursing Process:** Assessment/Analysis

10. **Answers: 2, 4, 5.**
    Meiosis II begins with two haploid parent cells, ends with four haploid daughter cells, and maintains the same number of chromosomes in each cell.
    1, 3 Meiosis I begins with one diploid parent cell, ends with two haploid daughter cells, and has half the number of chromosomes in each cell.
    Client Need: Physiological Adaptation; **Cognitive Level:** Understanding; **Nursing Process:** Assessment/Analysis

11. **Answers: 1, 3, 4.**
    1 The prophase of meiosis is when chromosomes coil and shorten. **3** The prophase of meiosis is when the nuclear membrane dissolves. **4** The prophase of meiosis is when the chromatids connect to a centromere.
    2 The metaphase of meiosis is when the centromeres align in the middle of the spindle. **5** The telophase is when the new membrane forms around each set of chromosomes.
    Client Need: Physiological Adaptation; **Cognitive Level:** Understanding; **Nursing Process:** Assessment/Analysis

12. **Answers: 1, 2, 3.**
    Proteins, fats, and starches are absorbed, circulated, and taken up by the cell where they are used for ATP production.
    4 Water is not an essential component in the cellular production of ATP. **5** Sodium is not an essential component in the cellular production of ATP.
    Client Need: Physiological Adaptation; **Cognitive Level:** Understanding; **Nursing Process:** Assessment/Analysis

13. **4 Oxidative phosphorylation, the process by which energy is transferred to ATP, occurs in the mitochondria.**
    1 Ribosomes aid in protein synthesis. **2** Cytoplasm is where biochemical reactions take place. **3** Endoplasmic reticula are responsible for protein folding
    Client Need: Physiological Adaptation; **Cognitive Level:** Understanding; **Nursing Process:** Assessment/Analysis

14. **Answers: 1, 3, 4, 5.**
    The digestion stage of catabolism is where secreted enzymes outside the cell break proteins into amino acids, polysaccharides into simple sugars, and fats into fatty acids and glycerol.
    2 Glucose molecules are split to create pyruvate and two molecules of ATP during the glycolysis stage of catabolism.
    Client Need: Physiological Adaptation; **Cognitive Level:** Understanding; **Nursing Process:** Assessment/Analysis

15. **3 Citric acid cycle (Krebs cycle) creates energy in the form of ATP.**
    1 Pyruvate is the end process of glycolysis. **2** Protein is broken down into amino acids during the digestion phase of catabolism. **4** Polysaccharides are broken down into simple sugars during the

digestion phase of catabolism. **5** Fat is broken down into fatty acids during the digestion phased of catabolism.

Client Need: Physiological Adaptation; **Cognitive Level:** Understanding; **Nursing Process:** Assessment/Analysis

16. **1 Primary active transport moves particles from areas of lower concentration to areas of higher concentration using chemical energy in the form of ATP.**

    2 Filtration causes the movement of water and solutes through a membrane using hydrostatic pressure. **3** Osmosis causes the spontaneous movement of a solvent through a semipermeable membrane using osmotic pressure to control the process. **4** Diffusion creates movement of an area of greater concentration to one of lesser concentration. This form of transport does not require an input of energy.

    Client Need: Physiological Adaptation; **Cognitive Level:** Understanding; **Nursing Process:** Assessment/Analysis

17. **4 Atrophy is the form of cellular adaptation that produces a decrease in cell size.**

    1 Hypertrophy is the form of cellular adaptation that produces an increase in cell size. **2** Metaplasia is the form of cellular adaptation where a mature cell is replaced by a different type of mature cell. **3** Neoplasia is the form of cellular adaptation that can result in tumor growth.

    Client Need: Physiological Adaptation; **Cognitive Level:** Understanding; **Nursing Process:** Assessment/Analysis

18. **Answers: 1, 2, 3.**

    1 Cell damage caused by physical agents include exposure to excess temperature (heat and cold) and radiation. **2** Cell damage caused by physical agents include exposure to excess temperature (heat and cold) and radiation. **3** Cell damage caused by physical agents include exposure to excess temperature (heat and cold) and radiation.

    4 Cell damage caused by chemical toxins would include a snake bite. **5** Cell damage caused by microorganisms would include a bacterial infection.

    Client Need: Physiological Adaptation; **Cognitive Level:** Understanding; **Nursing Process:** Assessment/Analysis

19. **1 Grade 1 is given when the microscopic examination of the cells shows they are well differentiated (similar to normal cells).**

    2 Grade X is given when the microscopic examination of the cells proves to be indeterminable. **3** Grade 2 is given when the microscopic examination of the cells shows they are moderately differentiated. **4** Grade 4 is given when the microscopic examination of the cells shows indifferentiated cells.

    Client Need: Physiological Adaptation; **Cognitive Level:** Applying; **Nursing Process:** Assessment/Analysis

20. **4 Epithelial tissue is composed of three different cell shapes: squamous, cuboidal, and columnar.**

    1 Connective tissue serves as a framework for clusters of epithelial cells to form organs. **2** Muscle tissue can be either cardiac, skeletal, or smooth. **3** Neural tissue is found in the cell body, single axons, and dendrites of neurons.

    Client Need: Physiological Adaptation; **Cognitive Level:** Understanding; **Nursing Process:** Assessment/Analysis

FLUIDS AND ELECTROLYTES OVERVIEW

- Changes in electrolyte concentrations affect nerve and muscle cell electrical activity.
- Alterations in acid–base balance affect enzyme systems and can cause cell injury and death.
- Disruption in acid–base and electrolyte functions can lead to patient death.

Body Fluid Compartments

- Cells exist in a continuously moving fluid environment.
- Balance between fluid compartments is maintained by the combined action of the renal system, hormones, and the neural system.
- Fluid moves between compartments by osmosis and the action of hydrostatic pressure.
  - Intracellular fluid (ICF) compartment
    - Fluid inside the cell
    - Contains two-thirds of the body's water
    - Movement of water in and out of the intracellular space occurs primarily by osmosis.
    - Potassium, the main electrolyte of the intracellular space, works to maintain balance within the intracellular space.
    - The ICF compartment usually does not experience rapid changes in osmolarity.
  - Extracellular fluid (ECF) compartment
    - Contains one-third of the body's water
    - Primary electrolyte of the ECF is sodium.
    - Two main extracellular compartments
      - Interstitial space
        - Fluid between cells
        - Also known as "third space"
      - Intravascular space
        - Blood plasma
    - ECF also includes lymph and transcellular fluid.
    - Transcellular fluid and lymph fluid do not have an impact on fluid and electrolyte balance.
    - Transcellular fluid includes
      - Synovial (joint fluid)
      - Pericardial (fluid around the heart)
      - Intraocular (eye fluid)
      - Peritoneal (fluid in peritoneal cavity)

Fluid Movement

- Total body water (TBW) is the sum of all fluids in the body.
- TBW changes with age. Infants have 70% to 80% TBW owing to low body fat. With aging, TBW decreases to 60% to 65% of body weight.

- Muscle cells contain more water than do fat cells.
- Males generally have more TBW than females owing to more muscle mass.
- With older age, TBW decreases owing to increased fat and decreased muscle mass.
- Older adults have more difficulty with fluid balance because of less efficient renal function. This becomes a significant factor with stress and illness. Changes in body fluid can be life threatening for this population.
- Water moves between the intracellular and ECF compartments mainly by osmosis.
- Diffusion allows water to move through the lipid bilayer of the cell membrane.
- Potassium provides the osmotic balance of the intracellular space.
- Sodium maintains the osmotic equilibrium of the extracellular space.
- Water, nutrients, and waste products move across the cell membrane as a result of changes in hydrostatic pressure and osmotic forces at the end of capillaries.
- Movement across capillary membranes is a product of net filtration. Hydrostatic pressure and interstitial oncotic pressure favor filtration from the capillary. Interstitial hydrostatic pressure and capillary oncotic pressure oppose movement of fluid from the capillaries.
  - Isotonic fluid movement
    - When fluid is isotonic, it has equal tonicity, and no exchange of fluid occurs at the cell membrane.
    - Isotonic fluid loss causes dehydration and fluid volume deficit.
    - Excessive sweating, wound drainage, and blood loss are examples of isotonic fluid loss.
  - Hypotonic fluid movement
    - Hypotonic fluid contains fewer solutes as compared with other fluids.
    - Hypotonic solutions push fluid from the vascular space into cells.
  - Hypertonic fluid movement
    - Hypertonic fluid contains more solutes than other fluids.
    - Hypertonic fluids pull fluid from the inside of the cell into the vascular space.

Fluid Sources

- Oral intake
  - Ingestion of fluid
    - About 60% of water comes into the body through drinking. This totals about 1400 to 1800 mL in the average adult.
  - Ingestion of solid food, which contains water
    - About 30% of the body water comes from solid food.
    - 700 to 1000 mL of water per day enters the body in the form of solid food.
- Intravenous solutions
  - Fluid can be added to the body through the vascular system using different types of intravenous fluids.
    - Isotonic fluid
      - Has the same solute concentration as blood and body fluids
      - Allows fluid replacement without pushing fluids into or outside of body cells
      - No swelling or shrinking of cells occurs with the introduction of isotonic fluid into the body
        - Examples
          - 0.9% saline (normal saline) (NS)
          - Lactated Ringers (LR) solution

- ○ 5% dextrose in water (D_5W)
  - - D_5W may also be considered a hypotonic solution due to the liver metabolizing the glucose from the solution.
- ▪ Administration of excess isotonic fluid can result in hypervolemia.
- ▪ Hypotonic fluid
- ▪ Contains fewer solutes than blood
- ▪ Causes water to move from the intravascular space into the cell
- ▪ When exposed to hypotonic fluid, cells swell
  - ○ Example
  - ○ 0.45% NS (1/2 NS) (1/2 NS)
- ▪ Hypertonic fluid
- ▪ Contains more solutes than blood
- ▪ Causes water to move from the cell into the intravascular space
- ▪ When exposed to hypertonic fluids, cells shrink
  - ○ Examples
  - ○ 10% dextrose in water ($D_{10}W$)
  - ○ 3% saline

Fluid Loss

- • Two types
  - • Insensible (cannot be measured)
    - ▪ About 10% of body water or 300 to 500 mL is lost through oxidation each day.
      - ▪ Fluid loss through skin via perspiration
      - ○ Exercise and fever increase fluid loss through the skin.
      - ▪ Fluid loss through the respiratory tract via respirations
      - ○ Increased respirations increase the amount of fluid loss via the respiratory system.
  - • Sensible (can be measured)
    - ▪ Fluid **loss**
      - ▪ Urine
      - ○ 60% of daily water is lost through urine. Approximately 1400 to 1800 mL in a healthy adult.
      - ▪ Feces
      - ○ About 100 mL of water is normally excreted in stool each day. This accounts for 2% of the total body water.
      - ▪ Drains
      - ▪ Emesis

Fluid Balance Control

- • Thirst mechanism
  - • Located in the hypothalamus
  - • The level of antidiuretic hormone (ADH) present in the body, along with thirst, work to regulate water balance in the body.
  - • Osmoreceptor cells sense fluid volume and concentration of fluid in the body.
  - • The ability of osmoreceptor cells to sense fluid volume and concentration of fluid in the body diminish with age.
  - • ADH
    - ▪ Regulates the volume of fluid leaving the body through the urine
    - ▪ Stimulates reabsorption of water into the blood from the tubules in the kidneys

- Aldosterone
  - Regulates the reabsorption of water and sodium from the tubules of the kidneys
  - Maintains more fluid when there is a fluid deficit in the body
- Atrial natriuretic peptide
  - Manufactured and released by myocardial cells in the atrium
  - Reduces workload on the heart by controlling fluid, sodium, and potassium levels
  - Works in the kidney to increase the rate of glomerular filtration
  - Decreases sodium reabsorption in the distal convoluted tubules through impeding ADH
  - Reduces renin secretion and impairs the renin angiotensin system
  - Results in ECF loss and lowers blood pressure

Fluid Excess

- Occurs in the extracellular compartment
- Edema
  - Disproportionate collection of fluid in the interstitial space
  - Fluid collection in the interstitial space causes tissue swelling.
  - Can be caused by lymphatic obstruction
  - May be localized (a single area of the body)
    - May be localized edema to an injury site, such as an injured extremity
    - May be localized to a single organ, such as the lungs or brain. Localized edema to organs can be life threatening.
  - May be generalized (all over the body)
  - May be visible or invisible
    - Fluid can build up around internal organs such as the liver or heart.
  - Weight gain can be significant.
  - Usually more severe in dependent areas of the body affected by gravity, such as the legs and feet
    - Dependent edema can be assessed using the fingers to apply pressure over bony prominences and grading the amount of pitting (pitting edema).
    - Important to assess sacrum and buttocks of bedbound patients.
  - Prolonged edema can cause problems.
    - Venous insufficiency
    - Arterial insufficiency
    - Impaired cellular function and tissue death in affected areas
      - Impaired wound healing
      - Increased risk of pressure ulcer formation in bed-bound patients
      - Dehydration can occur from the accumulation of fluid in the interstitial space.
  - Four causes of edema
    - Increased capillary hydrostatic pressure
      - High blood pressure inhibits the return of fluid from the interstitial compartment to the venous ends of the capillaries.
    - Loss of plasma proteins
      - Lack of albumin causes a decrease in plasma osmotic pressure
    - Obstruction of lymphatic circulation
      - Excessive fluid and protein cannot be returned to the circulatory system, which causes localized edema.

- Tumor or infection may damage a lymph node.
      - Increased capillary permeability
        - May result from inflammation or infection
        - Caused by the inflammatory response that increases capillary permeability
  - Isotonic fluid volume excess (hypervolemia)
    - Increased blood volume associated with heart failure, renal failure, excessive isotonic fluid administration, pregnancy
    - Signs and symptoms (Table 2.1)
      - Edema
      - Elevated blood pressure
      - Full and bounding pulse
      - Pulmonary edema
        - Cough
        - Shortness of breath; dyspnea
        - Crackles
      - Distended neck veins
      - Weight gain
    - Associated laboratory values
      - Decreased blood urea nitrogen (BUN)
      - Decreased hematocrit
      - Normal or decreased serum sodium
  - Water intoxication
    - Occurs when a person has excessive intake of water as compared with output
    - Rare
      - Seen occasionally in psychiatric settings with compulsive water drinking.

TABLE 2.1 Comparison of Signs and Symptoms of Fluid Excess (Edema) and Fluid Deficit (Dehydration)

Fluid Excess (Edema)	Fluid Deficit (Dehydration)
Localized swelling (feet, hands, periorbital area, ascites)	Sunken, soft eyes
Pale, gray, or red skin color	Decreased skin turgor, dry mucous membranes
Weight gain	Thirst, weight loss
Slow, bounding pulse; high blood pressure	Rapid, weak, thready pulse, low blood pressure, and orthostatic hypotension
Lethargy, possible seizures	Fatigue, weakness, dizziness, possible stupor
Pulmonary congestion, cough, rales	Increased body temperature

Laboratory values:
  Decreased hematocrit
  Decreased serum sodium
  Urine: low specific gravity, high volume
	Laboratory values:
	  Increased hematocrit
	  Increased electrolytes (or variable)
	  Urine: high specific gravity, low volume

Note: Signs may vary depending on the cause of the imbalance.

From Hubert, R. J., & VanMeter, K. C. (2018). *Gould's pathophysiology for the health professions* (6th ed.). Philadelphia: Saunders.

APPLICATION AND REVIEW

1. What clinical finding does a nurse anticipate when admitting a client with an extracellular fluid volume excess?
   1. Rapid, thready pulse
   2. Distended jugular veins
   3. Elevated hematocrit level
   4. Increased serum sodium level
2. A nurse is caring for a client diagnosed with albuminuria resulting in edema. What pressure change does the nurse determine as the cause of the edema?
   1. Decrease in tissue hydrostatic pressure
   2. Increase in plasma hydrostatic pressure
   3. Increase in tissue colloid osmotic pressure
   4. Decrease in plasma colloid oncotic pressure
3. A nurse is evaluating the effectiveness of treatment for a client with excessive fluid volume. What clinical finding indicates that treatment has been successful?
   1. Clear breath sounds
   2. Presence of pedal pulses
   3. Normal potassium level
   4. Increased urine specific gravity

See Answers on pages 37–39.

Fluid Deficit

- Isotonic fluid volume deficit
  - Deficient fluid volume
  - Caused by poor intake of fluid
    - Elderly population
    - Unconscious clients
    - Lack of access to safe drinking water
  - Caused by excessive loss of fluids
    - Vomiting
    - Diarrhea
    - Excessive sweating
    - Excessive urination
    - Diabetic ketoacidosis
    - Hyperventilation
    - Arid climates
  - Can occur when output of fluid exceeds intake of fluid
  - More serious for newborns and elderly population
  - Signs and symptoms
    - Dry, mucous membranes
    - Decreased skin turgor
    - Lowered blood pressure
    - Weak, rapid pulse
    - Increased thirst
    - Elevated heart rate
    - Pale skin
    - Decreased urine output
    - Increased hematocrit level

Electrolyte Balance

- Sodium
  - Primary electrolyte in the ECF
    - Normal serum sodium level is 135 to 145 mEq/L.
      - Average dietary intake of sodium is around 6 g daily; 500 mg are the minimum required.
    - Important for maintaining ECF volume
    - Necessary for muscle contraction and conduction of nerve impulses
    - Important electrolyte in the maintenance of acid–base balance in the body
    - Transport of sodium controlled by sodium-potassium pump
    - Secreted in body fluids, such as mucus
    - Occurs in the body in the form of sodium bicarbonate and sodium chloride
    - High ratios of sodium-to-potassium in the blood are associated with hypertension, heart disease, and increased morbidity.
    - Taken in the body with food and drink
    - Excreted in urine, feces, and sweat
    - Increased sweating increases the body's need for sodium.
    - Sodium and water equilibrium are closely related. Water imbalance can result in changes in serum sodium levels.
    - Sodium amounts are primarily controlled by aldosterone hormone and renal function.
  - Hypernatremia
    - Serum sodium levels greater than 145 mEq/L (146 mmol/L)
    - Excessive sodium in the intravascular fluid
    - Increased sodium levels result from either an increase in the sodium level or a decrease in the total body water.
    - Sodium is mainly controlled by the kidneys through the action of aldosterone.
    - Causes of hypernatremia
      - Elderly patients are at an increased risk for developing high sodium levels.
      - Patients with impaired mental status are at increased risk.
      - Patients with fever, diarrhea, and vomiting have an increased risk of developing hypernatremia.
      - Excessive sodium intake in foods and beverages
      - Deficient water intake
        - Can result from loss of thirst mechanism and decreased function of osmoreceptors in elderly patients
      - Insufficient ADH as in diabetes insipidus
      - Uncontrolled diabetes mellitus
      - Watery diarrhea
      - Tube feedings
      - Use of diuretic medications
      - Prolonged periods of rapid respirations found in diabetic ketoacidosis, respiratory alkalosis, and improper mechanical ventilator settings
      - Inability of the kidneys to adequately concentrate urine
    - Signs and symptoms of hypernatremia (Table 2.2)
      - Increased thirst
      - Dry mucous membranes
      - Firm subcutaneous tissues
      - Weakness
      - Agitation

TABLE 2.2 Signs of Sodium Imbalance	
Hyponatremia	**Hypernatremia**
Anorexia, nausea, cramps	Thirst; tongue and mucosa are dry and sticky
Fatigue, lethargy, muscle weakness	Weakness, lethargy, agitation
Headache, confusion, seizures	Edema
Decreased blood pressure	Elevated blood pressure

From Hubert, R. J., & VanMeter, K. C. (2018). *Gould's pathophysiology for the health professions* (6th ed.). Philadelphia: Saunders.

- Headache
- Confusion
- Decreased reflexes
- Seizures and coma (severe hypernatremia)
  - Hyponatremia
    - Most frequent electrolyte imbalance found in a hospitalized client
      - Decreased sodium levels in the intravascular fluid of less than 135 (mEq/L or 3.8 to 5 mmol/L
      - Causes water to move from the vascular space into the cell
    - Causes of hyponatremia
      - Inadequate sodium intake is a rare cause.
      - Excessive water intake that dilutes serum sodium concentration
      - Use of diuretic drugs in combination with salt-restricted diets
      - Loss from excessive sweating
      - Vomiting
      - Diarrhea
      - Insufficient aldosterone
      - Adrenal insufficiency
      - Excess ADH secretion in conditions such as syndrome of inappropriate ADH
      - Renal failure
      - Diuretic medication
    - Signs and symptoms of hyponatremia (see Table 2.2)
      - Muscle cramps
      - Fatigue
      - Abdominal cramps
      - Nausea
      - Vomiting
      - Diarrhea
      - Decreased reflexes
      - Headache
      - Disorientation; lethargy
      - Seizures and coma (severe hyponatremia)
  - Chloride
    - Important electrolyte necessary for maintaining acid–base balance
      - Normal serum level 96 to 106 mEq/L (98 to 106 mmol/L)
      - Sodium and chloride are attracted to each other owing to the electrical ion charge.

- Hyperchloremia
  - Serum chloride level of greater than 106 mEq/L (101 mmol/L)
  - Chloride is attracted to sodium. High sodium levels lead to high chloride levels.
  - Causes of hyperchloremia
    - Increased intake of sodium chloride
    - Excessive administration of intravenous sodium chloride
    - Hypernatremia
  - Signs and symptoms of hyperchloremia
    - Increased weight
    - Edema
- Hypochloremia
  - Serum chloride level less than 96 mEq/L (98 mmol/L)
  - Usually occurs in combination with hyponatremia
  - May coincide with high bicarbonate levels in the blood
  - Causes
    - Vomiting
    - Loss of hydrochloric acid from the stomach, such as from gastrointestinal (GI) suctioning
    - Increased loss of fluid through perspiration or fever
    - Restricted sodium diet
    - Diuretic medication
  - Signs and symptoms of hypochloremia
    - Muscle twitching
    - Decreased level of consciousness
    - Feeling fatigued
    - Confusion
    - Nausea
    - Vomiting
    - Diarrhea
- Potassium (K^+)
  - Major intracellular electrolyte
  - Necessary electrolyte for cardiac function, smooth muscle contraction, and skeletal muscle movement
  - Required for proper metabolic functions of the body
  - The ICF contains 150 to 160 mEq/L of potassium.
  - The normal extracellular potassium level is 3.5 to 5.0 mEq/L (3.6 to 5.2 mmol/L).
  - Normal serum potassium levels are imperative in diseases requiring administration of insulin, such as diabetes mellitus.
  - The sodium-potassium pump maintains the balance of potassium between the ECF and ICF by active transport.
  - Insulin stimulates the active transport system and drives potassium into cells with glucose.
  - Low insulin levels can cause potassium to exit the cells and enter the vascular system, increasing the serum potassium level.
  - The recommended daily dietary intake of potassium is 40 to 150 mEq/day.
    - Lower risk of hypertension and stroke have been associated with diets enriched in potassium.
    - Those with impaired renal function must use caution when considering the potassium content of their diet.
  - 5 to 10 mEq of potassium are excreted within the stool each day.

- Most potassium is absorbed by the GI system.
- The renal system is responsible for the excretion of potassium. Patients with renal failure have problems with potassium regulation.
- Disease processes that impair aldosterone can have an impact on potassium excretion.
- Sudden increases in serum potassium levels can be fatal.
- Hyperkalemia
  - Defined as a serum potassium level greater than 5 mEq/L or 2.6 mmol/L
  - Potassium adaptation allows the body to respond slowly to increased potassium intake. Rapid increases in potassium in the intravascular system can lead to severe complications.
  - Causes of hyperkalemia
    - Renal failure
    - Aldosterone deficiency
    - Potassium-sparing diuretic drugs
    - Angiotensin-converting enzyme (ACE) inhibitors and angiotensin receptor blockers used to treat hypertension
    - Burns or crushing injuries, which cause intracellular potassium to escape into the vascular space
    - Acidosis
    - Hypoxia diminishes the active transport system that exchanges potassium and sodium at the cellular level.
    - Excessive intake of foods high in potassium
      - Citrus fruits
      - Bananas
      - Tomatoes
      - Lentils
      - Salt substitutes, which contain potassium
    - Use of stored whole blood
    - Insulin deficiency
    - Excess of potassium replacement
    - Administration of penicillin G by intravenous bolus
    - Digitalis overdose
  - Signs and symptoms of hyperkalemia
    - Cardiac dysrhythmias with associated electrocardiographic (ECG) changes
      - Hallmark sign: tall, tented T waves
      - Decreased QR interval
      - ST segment depression with prolonged PR intervals and a widened QRS complex
      - Bradydysrhythmias
      - Ventricular fibrillation and cardiac arrest
      - Muscle weakness
      - Fatigue
      - Nausea
      - Sense of restlessness
      - Paresthesias
      - Tingling in fingers and lips
      - Intestinal cramping
      - Diarrhea
      - Paralysis

- Hypokalemia
  - Defined as serum potassium level less than 3.5 mEq/L or 2 mmol/L
  - Causes
    - Excessive loss owing to diarrhea
      - 100 to 200 mEq of K^+ can be lost per day with diarrhea.
    - Intestinal drainage from any source, including gastric suction
    - Laxative abuse
    - Diuresis caused by diuretic drugs
      - Patients taking non–potassium-sparing diuretics may need a potassium supplement.
    - Cushing syndrome or other endocrine disorders causing increased aldosterone secretion
    - Deficient dietary intake
      - May appear with alcoholism, starvation, and some eating disorders
      - May occur in elderly patients with poor dietary intake
    - Treatment of diabetic ketoacidosis with insulin
      - Insulin pushes potassium inside cells
      - Recommend a potassium supplement with insulin administration
  - Signs and symptoms of hypokalemia
    - Severity of symptoms of hypokalemia depend on the rate of potassium depletion. Rapid depletion can cause more severe symptoms. Mild losses of potassium usually produce no symptoms in the body.
    - Cardiac dysrhythmias
      - Sinus bradycardia
      - Atrioventricular block
      - Paroxysmal atrial tachycardia
      - Hypokalemia increases the risk of digitalis toxicity.
    - Electrocardiogram changes
      - Flat T waves are a hallmark sign.
      - ST segment depression
      - Appearance of a U wave
      - Severe hypokalemia:peaked P waves and lengthening of the QT interval
    - Fatigue
    - Muscle weakness
      - Usually occurs in large muscles of the body, such as legs and arms
      - Can affect muscles necessary for breathing
    - Leg cramps
    - Paresthesias
    - Decreased appetite, nausea, constipation
    - Decreased GI motility, distention, decreased bowel sounds, ileus
    - Shallow respirations
    - Impaired renal function
    - Concentrated urine
    - Polyuria
- Calcium
  - Normal serum calcium level is 9.0 to 10.5 mg/dL.
  - 50% of the body's calcium is bound to albumin. Low albumin levels can produce false low calcium levels.

- Delivers strength for bone and teeth
- Required electrolyte for nerve conduction
- Necessary component for muscle contractions
- Required for enzyme reactions needed for blood clotting
- Most of the body's calcium is stored in the bones of the body.
- Excreted in urine, feces, and bone
- Taken in the body by nutritional sources, such as milk and dairy products
- Balance controlled by parathyroid hormone (PTH), which pulls calcium from the bone to the vascular system to maintain normal calcium levels in the circulating blood system
- Balance controlled by calcitonin, which pushes calcium into the bone from the vascular system to maintain normal calcium levels in the circulating blood system
- Requires adequate vitamin D (cholecalciferol) levels obtained from supplementation or ultraviolet rays for adequate absorption and use in the body
  - Persons with lack of exposure to sunlight may experience low vitamin D levels.
  - Sunscreen with a sun protection factor greater than 15 may reduce synthesis of vitamin D.
  - Vitamin D is a necessary component for calcium to move from the bone and blood into the intestines.
  - Some cancers and the development of multiple sclerosis have been linked to low vitamin D levels.
- Calcium and phosphate have a reciprocal relationship. When calcium levels are high, phosphate levels are low. When calcium levels are low, phosphate levels are high.
- Precipitate or crystals of calcium phosphate formation occurs in soft tissue if calcium and phosphate levels are high at the same time.
- Hypercalcemia
  - Serum calcium level greater than 10.5 mg/dL
  - Causes
    - Hyperparathyroidism
    - Prolonged immobility causing demineralization of the bone
    - Increased intake of dietary calcium
    - Excessive vitamin D intake
    - Excessive intake of milk and antacids
    - Malignant bone disease or tumors
    - Decreased binding of calcium to albumin can occur with acidosis causing high serum calcium levels.
  - Signs and symptoms of hypercalcemia
    - Polyuria
    - Cardiac dysrhythmias with electrocardiogram changes
      - Shortened QT segment
      - Depressed T waves
      - Heart block
      - Bradycardia
    - Muscle weakness
    - Lethargy
    - Decrease muscle tone
    - Nausea
    - Decreased appetite
    - Constipation

- Behavior changes; possible stupor
- Pathologic bone fractures
- Possible formation of calcium kidney stones in the renal system
- Hypocalcemia
  - Serum calcium level less than 9 mEq/L
  - Causes
    - Calcium must bind to albumin. Decreased albumin in the body results in a decreased calcium level.
    - Deficient intake of calcium in the diet
    - Inability of the body to absorb calcium or vitamin D in the intestine
    - Hypoparathyroidism
    - Blood administration
    - Alkalosis from an increased blood pH
    - Renal failure
  - Signs and symptoms of hypocalcemia
    - Trousseau's sign—when a blood pressure cuff is inflated on the arm: a carpopedal spasm (contraction) occurs in the hand and fingers.
    - Chvostek's sign: tapping of the facial nerve in front of the ear results in a spasm of the lip and face.
    - Hyperactive reflexes
    - Tetany
    - Parethesias
    - Laryngospasm
    - Arrhythmias from weak heart contractions
- Magnesium
  - Normal serum level of 1.5 to 3.0 mg/dL
  - Major intracellular electrolyte, second to potassium
  - Imbalances of magnesium are rare.
  - The kidneys and small intestine are responsible for magnesium metabolism.
  - Half of the body's magnesium is stored in bone.
  - Ingested with dietary intake of green vegetables
  - Necessary electrolyte for DNA synthesis
  - Normal levels required for many enzyme reactions
  - Associated with calcium and potassium levels
  - Magnesium supplementation may be used for the treatment of preeclampsia in pregnancy.
  - Magnesium has also been found to be beneficial in the treatment of depression, migraine headaches, heart disease, and asthmatic respiratory conditions.
  - Hypermagnesemia
    - Total serum magnesium level greater than 3.0 mEq/L
    - Rare
    - Causes
      - Renal failure
      - Excessive use of antacids containing magnesium
    - Signs and symptoms of hypermagnesemia
      - Diminished reflexes
      - Lethargy
      - Cardiac arrhythmias
      - Weakened neuromuscular function

- Hypomagnesemia
  - Total magnesium level less than 1.5 mEq/L
  - Low magnesium levels can cause potassium to move outside of cells.
  - Causes
    - Hyperaldosteronism
    - Diabetic ketoacidosis or metabolic acidosis
    - Use of diuretics
    - Prolonged use of proton pump inhibitors
    - Hyperparathyroidism
    - Alcoholism
    - Diabetes mellitus
    - Widespread inflammation of the body
  - Signs and symptoms of hypomagnesemia
    - Tremors
    - Chorea: repetitive involuntary movements
    - Decreased sleep
    - Behavior changes
    - Tachycardia
    - Cardiac arrhythmias
    - Irritability
- Phosphate
  - Normal level: 2.5 to 4.5 mg/dL (0.85 to 1.45 mmol/L)
  - Circulates in ECF and ICF
  - Important portion of the cell membrane
  - Located mainly in the bone
  - Required for tooth and bone mineralization
  - Has an inverse relationship with calcium
  - Necessary component in cellular processes requiring adenosine phosphate (ATP)
  - Part of the phosphate buffer system necessary for the body to maintain acid–base balance
  - Hyperphosphotemia
    - Serum phosphorous level greater than 4.5 mg/dL
    - Increased levels of phosphate lower serum calcium levels.
    - Causes
      - Chemotherapy
      - Tissue damage
      - Long-term use of laxatives or enemas
      - Hypoparathyroidism
      - Renal failure
    - Signs and symptoms of hyperphosphotemia
      - Because calcium and phosphorous have an inverse relationship, symptoms of hyperphosphotemia are the same as symptoms of hypocalcemia.
      - Trousseau's sign: when a blood pressure is inflated on the arm, a carpopedal spasm (contraction) occurs in the hand and fingers.
      - Chvostek's sign: tapping of the facial nerve in front of the ear results in a spasm of the lip and face.
      - Hyperactive reflexes
      - Tetany
      - Parethesias

- Laryngospasm
- Arrhythmias from weak heart contractions
- High levels of both phosphate and calcium can cause deposits to form in soft tissues and bone.
- Hypophosphatemia
  - Serum phosphate level less than 2.5 mg/dL
  - Symptoms of hyphosphotemia do not become evident until serum levels are severely low.
  - Causes of hypophosphatemia
    - Alcoholism
    - Diarrhea
    - Overuse of antacids containing aluminum or magnesium, which bind to phosphate
    - Refeeding syndrome after starvation
    - Respiratory alkalosis
    - Hyperparathyroidism
    - Intestinal malabsorption
  - Signs and symptoms of hypophosphatemia
    - Decreased appetite
    - Diminished reflexes and muscle weakness that can impair respirations
    - Dysphagia
    - Behavior and level of consciousness changes, which can progress to stupor
    - Hypoxia
    - Bradycardia that may progress to heart block
    - Paresthesias
    - Tremors
    - Decreased cellular function increases risk for bleeding and infection.

APPLICATION AND REVIEW

4. Which notations in the medical histories of various clients increase their risk for developing hypokalemia? **Select all that apply**.
   1. Severely malnourished
   2. Prescribed a non–potassium-sparing diuretic
   3. Diagnosed with Cushing syndrome 5 years ago
   4. Currently being treated for diabetic ketoacidosis with insulin
   5. Currently being treated for malignant bone tumors of the spine
5. What clinical manifestations would support the diagnosis of hyperkalemia? **Select all that apply.**
   1. Muscle spasms
   2. Grand mal seizure
   3. Diarrhea lasting 24 hours
   4. Generalized weakness
   5. Bradycardia
6. A nurse is concerned that a client is at risk for developing hyperkalemia. Which pre-existing diagnosis supports the nurse's concern?
   1. Crohn disease
   2. Cushing disease
   3. End-stage renal disease
   4. Gastroesophageal reflux
7. Which events place clients at risk for the development of hyperkalemia? **Select all that apply.**
   1. Extensive burns
   2. Metabolic alkalosis
   3. Respiratory alkalosis
   4. Potassium-sparing diuretic drugs
   5. Crushing injury of the right femur

8. A client is admitted to the hospital with a diagnosis of chronic kidney failure. Which electrolyte imbalance would the nurse expect?
   1. Hypokalemia
   2. Hypocalcemia
   3. Hypernatremia
   4. Hyperglycemia
9. A client diagnosed with hypokalemia is placed on a cardiac monitor to evaluate cardiac activity during intravenous (IV) potassium replacement. Before starting the potassium infusion, what cardiac change is the nurse most likely to identify when observing the monitor?
   1. Flattening of the T wave
   2. Elevation of the ST segment
   3. Shortening of the QRS complex
   4. Increased deflection of the Q wave
10. What clinical finding indicates to a nurse that a client may be experiencing hypokalemia?
    1. Edema
    2. Muscle spasms
    3. Kussmaul breathing
    4. Abdominal distention

See Answers on pages 37–39.

Acid–Base Balance

- pH is a measure of hydrogen ions in the body. The more hydrogen ions in the body, the lower, or more acidic, the pH of the blood becomes.
- The fewer hydrogen ions in the body, the higher the pH becomes, and the blood becomes more basic or alkaline.
- Arterial blood gases are obtained to determine the pH level of the blood. Laboratory results can also be evaluated for a base excess or deficit and anion gap to determine acid–base status.
- Normal arterial blood pH is 7.35 to 7.45.
- Normal pH is required for cellular function. There is a narrow pH range; when hydrogen ions exceed this concentrated range, death may occur.
- A pH of less than 7.35 indicates acidosis.
- A pH of greater than 7.45 is indicative of alkalosis.
- To determine the presence of an acid–base imbalance pH, partial pressure of carbon dioxide in arterial blood ($PaCO_2$), and sodium bicarbonate are assessed.
- $PaCO_2$ is an indicator of respiratory function. Normal $PaCO_2$ is 38 to 42 mm HG.
- HCO_3 levels are indicative of metabolic involvement. Normal HCO_3 levels 22 to 28 mEq/L.
- To determine if an acid–base imbalance is present, the following approach is recommended.
  - First, assess pH.
  - Second, assess $PaCO_2$ to determine if the cause of the disorder is respiratory.
    - The respiratory system is most likely the cause of the imbalance if the $PaCO_2$ value indicates the same acid–base imbalance as the pH. (Example: pH 7.30; $PaCO_2$ 50 mm Hg) In this case, both values indicate acidosis, thus the acid–base imbalance is respiratory acidosis.
    - If the $PaCO_2$ value is normal, the metabolic system should be considered the source of the imbalance. (Example: pH 7.30; $PaCO_2$ 40 mm Hg; HCO_3 20 mEq/L); in this case, the pH indicates acidosis, the $PaCO_2$ is normal, and the HCO_3 indicates acidosis; thus the imbalance is metabolic acidosis.
  - Next, assess the $PaCO_2$ and HCO_3 levels to determine if compensation is occurring. Laboratory values will indicate a normal pH level, but alterations in either the $PaCO_2$ or the HCO_3. Compensation is the process by which one system has adjusted to normalize the blood pH.

- Owing to the body's production of carbon dioxide (CO_2), carbonic acid (H_2CO_3), and lactic acid, the body has a tendency toward acidosis.
- 50 to 100 mEq/day of acid are formed as end products of cellular metabolism.
- The body controls pH levels by blood buffers, respirations, and renal function.
- The lungs can alter the rate of respiration to change the pH level of the body.
- The kidneys can alter the acidity or alkalinity of the urine to affect the pH of the blood.

APPLICATION AND REVIEW

11. A client is in a state of uncompensated acidosis. What arterial blood pH would support this diagnosis?
    1. 7.20
    2. 7.35
    3. 7.45
    4. 7.48

See Answers on pages 37–39.

Buffer System

- Weak acids and alkaline salts combine to make buffers in the vascular system that work to balance pH levels.
- Located in both intracellular and ECF compartments
- Buffers react with acids and alkali in the blood to maintain a pH of 7.35 to 7.45.
- Buffer systems act immediately when a change in pH is recognized by the body, but are the weakest of the body's pH control systems.
- Four major buffer pairs
  - Sodium bicarbonate–carbonic acid system
    - Major buffer of the ECF compartment
    - Main buffer system used to clinically diagnose a client's acid–base imbalance
    - Ratio of bicarbonate ion to carbonic acid (carbon dioxide) must be 20:1 to maintain pH balance.
    - More bicarbonate (alkaline base) is necessary to neutralize acid.
    - Changes in bicarbonate ion and carbonic acid must be equal to maintain pH balance.
    - Works in both lungs and kidneys
  - Phosphate system
    - Attaches protein and phosphate
    - Intracellular buffer
    - Acts to defend the body first against acid–base imbalance.
    - Ammonia and phosphate attach to hydrogen ions and act as buffers in the renal system.
  - Hemoglobin system
    - Intracellular blood buffer
    - Able to bind with hydrogen ions and carbon dioxide
    - Hemoglobin weakens acid.
  - Protein system
    - Negative charged proteins in both ICF and ECF work as hydrogen ion buffers.
  - Respiratory system
    - The respiratory system controls the rate of respirations in order to maintain pH balance of the blood.

- Chemoreceptors recognize changes in pH and $PaCO_2$.
- Respirations increase when serum carbon dioxide levels increase in an attempt to rid the body of more acid in the form of carbon dioxide.
- Respirations decrease when alkalosis develops in an attempt to retain acid in the form of carbon dioxide and normalize the acid–base balance in the body.
- Responds to changes in pH balance within minutes or hours
  - Renal system
    - Kidneys provide the bicarbonate ion necessary to form buffer pairs.
    - The renal system can reduce body acid by exchanging hydrogen ions for sodium and extracting acid through urination.
    - Changes the pH of urine as needed to regulate blood pH.
    - Most powerful body system to correct acid–base imbalance, but may take hours or days to work
    - The renal buffer ammonia does not carry an electrical charge allowing it to cross the cell membranes in the kidneys, bind with hydrogen, and then be eliminated from the body with urination.
    - Kidneys are able to reabsorb bicarbonate in order to neutralize acid in the blood.
    - Normal urine pH is 4.5 to 8.

Acid–Base Imbalances

- Four types of acid–base imbalance
  - Respiratory acidosis
  - Respiratory alkalosis
  - Metabolic acidosis
  - Metabolic alkalosis
- Respiratory acidosis
  - Results from an increase in carbon dioxide levels from a respiratory origin.
  - Laboratory values
    - Decreased pH
    - Increased $PaCO_2$
  - Causes
    - Airway obstruction
    - Chest injuries
    - Sedation
    - Pneumonia
    - Any condition that depresses the respiratory system
      - Patients with chronic obstructive pulmonary disease may experience chronic respiratory acidosis.
  - Signs and symptoms of respiratory acidosis
    - Lethargy
    - Blurred vision
    - Headache
    - Tremors
    - Convulsions
    - Coma is possible

- Hypotension
- Cardiac conduction changes are possible.
- Metabolic acidosis
  - Results from a renal or metabolic problem that causes a decreased level of bicarbonate in the body.
  - Laboratory values
    - Increased pH
    - Decreased HCO_3
    - The anion gap can be assessed to determine if metabolic acidosis is caused by retention of chloride or loss of bicarbonate.
      - Anion Gap = Sodium − (Chloride + Bicarbonate)
      - An anion gap of less than 11 mEq/L is considered normal
      - An increased anion gap usually is caused by an increase in unmeasured anions, and that most commonly occurs when there is an increase in unmeasured organic acids, that is, an acidosis.
      - A low anion gap is relatively rare but may occur from the presence of abnormal positively charged proteins, as in multiple myeloma.
  - Causes
    - Diarrhea
    - Lactic acid accumulation
    - Ketoacidosis in diabetes
    - Hypoxemia
    - Starvation
    - Renal failure
  - Signs and symptoms of metabolic acidosis
    - Weakness
    - Lethargy
    - Confusion
    - Headache
    - Kussmaul respirations
    - Can progress to coma and death
- Respiratory alkalosis
  - Develops from a decrease in carbon dioxide levels from a respiratory origin.
  - Laboratory values
    - Increased pH
    - Decreased $PaCO_2$
  - Causes of respiratory alkalosis
    - Hyperventilation
    - High fever
      Anxiety
    - Aspirin overdose
    - Tumors or head injuries, which impact the respiratory control center in the brain
  - Signs and symptoms of respiratory alkalosis
    - Dizziness
    - Tachypnea
    - Carpopedal spasm
    - Confusion

- ■ Tingling of the extremities
- ■ Convulsions
- ■ Coma
- Metabolic alkalosis
  - Occurs from a loss of hydrogen ions through the kidneys or the GI system
  - Laboratory values
    - ■ Increased pH
    - ■ Increased HCO_3
  - Causes
    - ■ Vomiting
    - ■ GI suctioning
    - ■ Extreme ingestion of acids
    - ■ Hypokalemia
  - Signs and symptoms
    - ■ Muscle twitching
    - ■ Tingling and numbness of fingers
    - ■ Tingling around the mouth
    - ■ Restlessness
    - ■ Hyperactive reflexes
    - ■ Decreased respiratory rate
    - ■ Seizures
    - ■ Tetany
    - ■ Coma
- Mixed acid–base disorders
  - Two or more acid–base disorders co-occurring
  - Common in critically ill patients
  - Requires evaluation of clinical history and medications
  - Evaluation of laboratory values, such as anion gap, electrolytes, urine osmolality, and plasma osmolality, may provide a basis for treatment.
- Correction
  - An acid–base imbalance has been corrected by the body when the pH has returned to normal and the $PaCO_2$ and HCO_3 levels are also normal.
- Compensation
  - The body attempts to normalize the pH of the blood by increased activity by the opposite system. For example, if acidosis is caused by the respiratory system, the renal system will work to retain more bicarbonate ions in order to balance the ratio of bicarbonate to carbonic acid.
  - Compensation has been achieved if the body system is able to return the pH to a normal level despite the presence of underlying disease.
  - Laboratory values in compensated cases of acid–base imbalance will indicate a pH level of 7.35 to 7.45 and will also indicate an altered $PaCO_2$ and/or HCO_3 level.
- Decompensation
  - A patient experiencing an acid–base imbalance who is in a compensated state (normal pH level owing to compensation) must be monitored closely.
  - Often the body system providing compensation will fail from overuse and stress to the system and produce a more complicated acid–base imbalance and system failure. An example would be a patient who experiences renal failure after a period of respiratory acidosis.

APPLICATION AND REVIEW

12. A client is admitted with metabolic acidosis. What body systems should the nurse assess for compensatory changes?
    1. Skeletal and nervous
    2. Circulatory and urinary
    3. Respiratory and urinary
    4. Muscular and endocrine
13. The nurse is caring for a client who has gastric lavage. Which result from arterial blood gases will the nurse expect?
    1. Decreased pH
    2. Increased oxygen level
    3. Increased bicarbonate level
    4. Decreased carbon dioxide level
14. An arterial blood gas report indicates the client's pH is 7.25, $PaCO_2$ is 35 mm Hg, and HCO_3 is 20 mEq/L. Which acid–base disturbance should the nurse identify based on these results?
    1. Metabolic acidosis
    2. Metabolic alkalosis
    3. Respiratory acidosis
    4. Respiratory alkalosis
15. A client's arterial blood gas report indicates the pH is 7.52, $PaCO_2$ is 32 mm Hg, and HCO_3 is 24 mEq/L. The nurse should identify what as a possible cause of these results?
    1. Airway obstruction
    2. Inadequate nutrition
    3. Prolonged gastric suction
    4. Increased respiratory rate and depth

See Answers on pages 37–39.

ANSWER KEY: REVIEW QUESTIONS

1. **2 Because of fluid overload in the intravascular space, the neck veins become visibly distended.**

   1 Rapid, thready pulse occurs with a fluid deficit. **3** Elevated hematocrit level occurs with a fluid deficit. **4** If sodium causes fluid retention, its concentration is unchanged; if fluid is retained independently of sodium, its concentration is decreased.

   Client Need: Physiological Adaptation; **Cognitive Level:** Applying; **Nursing Process:** Assessment/Analysis

2. **4 Because the plasma colloidal oncotic pressure (COP) is the major force drawing fluid from the interstitial spaces back into the capillaries, a drop in COP caused by albuminuria results in edema.**

   1 Hydrostatic tissue pressure is unaffected by an alteration of protein levels; colloidal pressure is affected. **2** Hydrostatic pressure is influenced by the volume of fluid and the diameter of the blood vessel, not directly by the presence of albumin. **3** The osmotic pressure of tissues is unchanged.

   Client Need: Physiological Adaptation; **Cognitive Level:** Understanding; **Nursing Process:** Assessment/Analysis

3. **1 Excess fluid can move into the lungs, causing crackles and shortness of breath; clear breath sounds indicate that treatment was effective.**

   2 Although it may make palpation more difficult, excess fluid will not diminish pedal pulses. **3** A normal potassium level can be maintained independently of fluid excess correction. **4** As the client excretes excess fluid, the urine-specific gravity will decrease, not increase.

   Client Need: Physiological Adaptation; **Cognitive Level:** Analysis; **Nursing Process:** Evaluation/Outcomes

4. **Answers: 1, 2, 3, 4.**

   1 Deficient dietary intake can cause hypokalemia because of insufficient intake. **2** The effects of a non–potassium-sparing diuretic can cause hypokalemia owing to the excretion of potassium. **3** Cushing syndrome causing increased aldosterone secretion results in decreased serum potassium. **4** Treatment of diabetic ketoacidosis with insulin pushes potassium inside cells.

   5 Malignant bone disease or tumors can cause hypercalcemia.

   Client Need: Physiological Adaptation; **Cognitive Level:** Analysis; **Nursing Process:** Assessment/Analysis

5. **Answers: 3, 4, 5.**

    3 Because of potassium's role in the sodium-potassium pump, hyperkalemia will cause diarrhea. **4** Because of potassium's role in the sodium-potassium pump, hyperkalemia will cause weakness. **5** Because of potassium's role in the sodium-potassium pump, hyperkalemia can cause cardiac dysrhythmias.

    1 Tetany (spasms) is caused by hypocalcemia. **2** Seizures caused by electrolyte imbalances are associated with low calcium or sodium levels.

    Client Need: Physiological Adaptation; **Cognitive Level:** Analysis; **Nursing Process:** Assessment/Analysis

6. **3 One of the kidneys' functions is to eliminate potassium from the body; diseases of the kidneys often interfere with this function and hyperkalemia may develop, necessitating dialysis.**

    1 Clients with Crohn disease have diarrhea, resulting in potassium loss. **2** Clients with Cushing disease will retain sodium and excrete potassium. **4** Clients with gastroesophageal reflux disease are susceptible to vomiting that may lead to sodium and chloride loss with minimal loss of potassium.

    Client Need: Physiological Adaptation; **Cognitive Level:** Analysis; **Nursing Process:** Assessment/Analysis

7. **Answers: 1, 4, 5.**

    1 Burns cause intracellular potassium to escape into the vascular space. **4** Potassium-sparing diuretic drug therapy can result in an accumulation of potassium. **5** Crushing injuries cause intracellular potassium to escape into the vascular space.

    2 Hyperkalemia results in an acidotic state. **3** Hyperkalemia results in an acidotic state.

    Client Need: Physiological Adaptation; **Cognitive Level:** Analysis; **Nursing Process:** Assessment/Analysis

8. **2 Hypocalcemia, decreased calcium in the blood, occurs because of the reciprocal relationship with phosphorus, which is increased by the decreased glomerular filtration rate commonly noted in chronic kidney failure.**

    1 Hyperkalemia, not hypokalemia, is more likely to occur because of decreased kidney function. **3** Hypernatremia, an increase in serum sodium, generally will not be present because fluid is retained in the same proportion as sodium. **4** Hyperglycemia, an increased serum glucose level, is not a clinical manifestation of chronic kidney failure.

    Client Need: Physiological Adaptation; **Cognitive Level:** Analysis; **Nursing Process:** Assessment/Analysis

9. **1 Hypokalemia causes a flattening of the T wave on an electrocardiogram, because of its effect on muscle function.**

    2 Hypokalemia causes a depression of the ST segment. **3** Hypokalemia causes a lengthening of the QT interval. **4** Hypokalemia does not cause a deflection of the Q wave.

    Client Need: Physiological Adaptation; **Cognitive Level:** Analysis; **Nursing Process:** Assessment/Analysis

10. **4 Hypokalemia diminishes the magnitude of the neuronal and muscle cell resting potentials. Abdominal distention results from flaccidity of intestinal and abdominal musculature.**

    1 Edema is a sign of sodium excess. **2** Muscle spasms are a sign of hypocalcemia. **3** Kussmaul breathing is a sign of metabolic acidosis.

    Client Need: Physiological Adaptation; **Cognitive Level:** Applying; **Nursing Process:** Assessment/Analysis

11. **1 The pH of blood is maintained within the narrow range of 7.35 to 7.45. When hydrogen ions increase, the respiratory, buffer, and renal systems attempt to compensate to maintain the pH. If compensation is not successful, acidosis results and is reflected in a lower pH.**

    2 This is within the acceptable range for pH. **3** This is within the acceptable range for pH. **4** This is a slightly alkaline pH.

    Client Need: Physiological Adaptation; **Cognitive Level:** Analysis; **Nursing Process:** Assessment/Analysis

12. **3 Increased respirations blow off carbon dioxide (CO_2), which decreases the hydrogen ion concentration and the pH increases (less acidity). Decreased respirations result in CO_2 buildup, which increases hydrogen ion concentration and the pH falls (more acidity). The kidneys either conserve or excrete bicarbonate and hydrogen ions, which helps to adjust the body's pH. The buffering capacity of the**

renal system is greater than that of the pulmonary system, but the pulmonary system is quicker to respond.

1 Neither the skeletal nor the nervous systems are involved in maintaining pH. **2** Although the circulatory system carries fluids and electrolytes to the kidneys, it does not interact with the urinary system to regulate plasma pH. **4** Neither the muscular nor the endocrine systems are involved in maintaining pH.

Client Need: Physiological Adaptation; **Cognitive Level:** Understanding; **Nursing Process:** Assessment/Analysis

13. **3 Gastric lavage causes an excessive loss of gastric fluid, resulting in excessive loss of hydrochloric acid (HCL) that can lead to alkalosis; the HCL is not available to neutralize the sodium bicarbonate ($NaHCO_3$) secreted into the duodenum by the pancreas. The intestinal tract absorbs the excess bicarbonate, and alkalosis results.**

    1 Gastric lavage will lead to alkalosis, which is associated with increased pH. **2** Gastric lavage will not affect oxygen levels. **4** Gastric lavage may lead to metabolic alkalosis; the $PaCO_2$ will either be normal or increased (if compensation occurs).

    Client Need: Physiological Adaptation; **Cognitive Level:** Analysis; **Nursing Process:** Assessment/Analysis

14. **1 A low pH and low bicarbonate levels are consistent with metabolic acidosis.**

    2 pH indicates acidosis. **3** The $PaCO_2$ concentration is within normal limits, which is inconsistent with respiratory acidosis; it is elevated with respiratory acidosis. **4** The pH indicates acidosis.

    Client Need: Physiological Adaptation; **Cognitive Level:** Analysis; **Nursing Process:** Assessment/Analysis

15. **4 The high pH and low carbon dioxide levels are consistent with respiratory alkalosis, which can be caused by hyperventilation.**

    1, 2, 3 These levels are not consistent with airway obstruction, inadequate nutrition, or prolonged gastric suction.

    Client Need: Physiological Adaptation; **Cognitive Level:** Analysis; **Nursing Process:** Assessment/Analysis

3 Genetic Disorders

PATHOPHYSIOLOGY

Genes and Chromosomes

- All genetic diseases involve defects at the cell level.
- Errors occur during replication of genetic material or during translation of genes into proteins.
  - Single-gene disorders
- Errors during cell division may lead to disorders involving entire chromosomes.
- Genes are composed of deoxyribonucleic acid (DNA).
  - Deoxyribonucleic acid
  - Genetic blueprint for proteins
  - Influence all aspects of the body structure and function
- Each cell contains chromosomes that contain genetic information.
  - Twenty-three pairs of chromosomes in each cell
    - Twenty-two pairs are autosomes
      - Arranged by size and shape
    - Twenty-third pair is the pair of sex chromosomes
      - Males XY
        - Males receive X chromosome from mother and Y chromosome from father.
      - Females XX
        - Females receive X chromosome from each parent.
- Meiosis
  - Each sperm and ovum receives 23 chromosomes.
    - One chromosome from each pair
    - Zygote then has 46 chromosomes (23 pairs).
  - Unlikely that any two persons (aside from identical twins) would have the same genes and DNA sequence.
    - Many combinations of genes possible
- DNA
  - Three basic components
    - Pentose sugar
    - Deoxyribose
      - Phosphate group
    - Four nitrogenous bases
      - Cytosine (C) and thymine (T)
        - Single carbon-nitrogen rings
        - Called pyrimidines
      - Adenine (A) and guanine (G)
        - Double carbon-nitrogen rings
        - Called purines
  - Gene mutation
    - Change in DNA sequence
  - Located in the cell nucleus

- A unique, identifying characteristic for an individual
- Molecule
- Carries genetic directions for growth, development, functioning, and reproduction
- Nucleotides
  - Chemical units
  - Four types
    - Adenine
    - Thymine
    - Cytosine
    - Guanine
  - Form chain-like molecules called polynucleotides
- Gene
  - Basic physical and functional unit of heredity
  - Sequence of DNA that codes function for each cell
  - An allele is a form of a gene.
  - Contained in chromosomes
  - Humans have approximately 20,000 to 25,000 genes.
    - An error in one gene may lead to a recognizable genetic disease.
  - Composed of DNA strands
  - Controls all physical characteristics and all metabolic processes
  - Alterations lead to genetic disorders.
  - Microscopic
- Mendelian laws
  - Patterns of inheritance
  - Include recessive and dominant patterns
  - Can be predicted using algebra or Punnett square
    - Punnett square
      - Predictive tool
      - Requires knowledge of the genetic composition of each parent
      - Created by Reginald Punnett
        - Geneticist
      - Looks at all potential combinations of genotypes
      - Graphical representation of discovering potential combinations of genotypes that can occur
- Ribonucleic acid (RNA)
  - RNA
    - Communication link
    - Aids in maintaining control of cell activity
  - Polymeric molecule
  - Essential in several biological roles
    - Coding
    - Decoding
    - Regulation
    - Expression of genes
  - Comparing DNA and RNA
    - Nearly identical
      - Same bonding patterns
      - Both bind to form nuclei acid in the same way.

- Three differences
  - RNA has ribose sugar.
    - DNA has deoxyribose sugar.
  - RNA is a single-stranded nuclei acid (tertiary structure).
    - DNA is a double helix (double-stranded).
  - RNA nucleotides contain uracil base.
    - DNA contains thymine.
- Mitosis
  - Somatic cell division
  - Occurs during embryonic and fetal development
  - Replication of chromosomes
    - Each daughter cell receives an identical parent cell DNA copy.
  - Changes can occur owing to an error during this process.
    - Mutation
      - Alteration in genetic material
      - Spontaneous or results from exposure to harmful substances
        - Teratogenic agents
          - Radiation
          - Chemicals
          - Drugs

APPLICATION AND REVIEW

1. When considering genetic diseases, who is likely to share genes and DNA sequencing?
   1. Father and son
   2. Mother and daughter
   3. Identical twin sisters
   4. Grandfather and grandson

2. What information would be included in a discussion of the form and function of genes? **Select all that apply**.
   1. The slightest error can result in disease.
   2. Heredity is based on this structure.
   3. It is made up of DNA strands.
   4. It is found in chromosomes.
   5. It is macroscopic in size.

3. When discussing genetics with a client, what is the best explanation of the use of a Punnett square?
   1. It is a tool used to predict the genetic characteristic of an offspring of two specific parents.
   2. It explains the process of meiosis in the production of offspring.
   3. It is the concept that explains patterns of genetic inheritance.
   4. It is a tool used to predict genetic mutations in a human.

4. Which statement by a client indicates an understanding of the process of genetic mutations?
   1. "Mutations can occur without an apparent trigger."
   2. "Mutations are a result of changes in RNA sequence."
   3. "Mutations are not common among mitosis-based division."
   4. "Radiation exposure is the primary cause of gene mutations."

See Answers on pages 58–61.

BOX 3.1 Examples of Genetic Disorders and Their Inheritance

Single-Gene Disorders
Autosomal-Dominant Disorders
Adult polycystic kidney disease
Huntington chorea
Familial hypercholesterolemia
Marfan syndrome
Autosomal-Recessive Disorders
Cystic fibrosis
Phenylketonuria
Sickle cell anemia
Tay-Sachs disease
X-Linked Dominant Disorders
Fragile X syndrome
X-Linked Recessive Disorders
Color blindness
Duchenne muscular dystrophy
Hemophilia A

Multifactorial Disorders
Anencephaly
Cleft lip and palate
Clubfoot
Congenital heart disease
Myelomeningocele
Schizophrenia
Chromosomal Disorders
Down syndrome
Monosomy X (Turner syndrome)
Polysomy X (Klinefelter syndrome)
Trisomy 18 (Edwards syndrome)

From Hubert, R. J., & VanMeter, K. C. (2018). *Gould's pathophysiology for the health professions* (6th ed.). Philadelphia: Saunders.

Congenital Abnormalities

- Present at birth
- Cognitive disorders
  - Genetic
    - Changes in genes
  - Inherited
    - Gene mutation passed on from parent
  - Developmental disorders
- Can be a single-gene trait or from a chromosomal defect, or be multifactorial (Box 3.1)
- Clinical signs may not appear at birth; they may occur months or years later.
  - Clinical signs of Huntington disease do not appear until adulthood.
- Disorders often have social and psychological implications.
- Other disorders may result from premature birth, complicated labor and delivery, or the fetus being exposed to a damaging agent during development.
  - Teratogenic agents
    - Cause damage during fetal development
    - Difficult to define the causative agent

APPLICATION AND REVIEW

5. What is an example of a genetic disorder that does not manifest until the individual reaches adulthood?
   1. Huntington disease
   2. Neurofibromatosis
   3. Marfan syndrome
   4. Tay-Sachs disease

See Answer on pages 58–61.

Mendelian Inheritance

- Mendelian conditions
  - Homozygous
    - When the two alleles that form the pair for a trait are identical
  - Heterozygous
    - When the two alleles are different
- Mandel's law of inheritance
  - Law of segregation
    - For each trait, the alleles split and one gene passes from each parent to the offspring.
  - Law of independent assortment
    - Different pairs of alleles are passed onto offspring independently.
    - Inherited genes at one location do not influence inherited genes at another location.

Single-Gene Defects

- Caused by a change in one gene within reproductive cells
- More than 6000 abnormalities are known.
  - 1:200 live births
    - Signs may not be present at birth; therefore, may not be diagnosed immediately.
  - Serious defects usually cause spontaneous miscarriage.
- Single, mutated gene is transmitted to subsequent generations following a specific pattern for that gene.
- Body cell mutations (other than the reproductive cells) may cause dysfunction; however, they are not transmitted to offspring.
- Examples of single-gene disorders
  - Cystic fibrosis (CF)
  - Sickle cell disease
  - Hemophilia
- Autosomal-dominant
  - Recognizing autosomal-dominant inheritance
    - Affected offspring has one affected parent; unless gene was result of a new mutation.
    - Unaffected individuals do not transmit the trait to offspring.
    - Males and females equally likely to transmit trait to both sons and daughters.
    - Trait is expected in every future generation.
    - Affected parent has 50% probability of passing on to offspring.
    - Presence of two mutant alleles presents with more severe phenotype.
    - Detrimental dominant traits rarely seen in homozygous state.
  - Presence of the defect in only one of the alleles produces clinical signs.
  - Recurrence risk
    - If one parent is affected by an autosomal-dominant disease (heterozygote) and the other is normal, the recurrence risk for each child is 50%.
    - Recurrence risk for future children remains 50%.
      - Law of independence
  - Examples of autosomal-dominant disorders
    - Huntington disease
      - Affects about 1 in 20,000 individuals of European descent
      - Less common among Japanese and Africans

- Manifests between 30 and 50 years of age
- Progressive loss of motor control, dementia, and psychiatric disorders
- Although all parts of the brain are affected, most notably damaged is the corpus striatum.
- In some cases, can lead to a 25% brain weight loss.
- Marfan syndrome
  - Transmitted by dominant gene
  - Fibrillin-1 protein
    - Defect in the gene that controls production of this protein
  - Connective tissue
    - Found throughout the body
    - Commonly affects heart, blood vessels, bones, joints, and eyes
    - 50% chance of passing along to offspring (both male and female)
    - No cognitive deficits
- Neurofibromatosis type I (NF1) and II (NF2)
  - NF1
    - Mutation in the neurofibromin gene
    - Characterized by patches of light brown skin spots and neurofibromas (fleshy growths) on/under the skin
      - Multisystem
      - Growths can be benign or malignant; commonly they are benign.
    - Symptoms
      - Several café au lait spots (6 or more)
        - Brown skin spots
      - Freckles in armpit and/or groin area(s)
      - Lisch nodules
        - Tiny growths in the iris
        - Usually do not affect eyesight
      - Neurofibromas
        - Growths that develop under skin; sometimes deeper in the body
        - Tumors along optic nerve may cause eyesight problems.
      - Nerve pain
      - Bone deformities
        - Scoliosis
        - Bowed legs
  - NF2
    - Mutation or deletion of the *NF2* gene
    - Less common than NF1
    - Multiple tumors on cranial and spinal nerves
    - Adult onset
      - Symptoms typically appear between 18 and 24 years of age.
    - Symptoms
      - Hearing loss
      - Weakness to facilitate muscles
      - Poor balance
        - Uncoordinated walking
      - Dizziness

- ○ Cataracts
  - Develop at unusually early age
- Autosomal-recessive
  - Recognizing autosomal-recessive inheritance
    - Most commonly, affected individuals are children of phenotypically normal parents.
    - Often more than one offspring affected.
      - Characterized by a clustering of the disease among siblings
      - One-fourth of the offspring will be homozygous for the gene and affected.
    - Both males and females equally likely to be affected.
    - Affected individuals who have children with normal persons tend to have phenotypically normal children.
    - When trait is very rare, most likely the responsible allele is recessive if there is an undue proportion of relations between close relatives.
      - Consanguineous unions
  - Both parents must pass on the defective gene.
    - Homozygous
    - Affected child
    - One normal gene and one disease gene present in pair.
      - Heterozygous
        - ○ Child is carrier, does not show clinical signs.
    - Examples of autosomal-recessive disorders
      - Phenylketonuria (PKU)
        - ○ Amino acid metabolism disorder
        - ○ A deficiency of the enzyme phenylalanine hydroxylase
          - ○ Required to convert phenylalanine into tyrosine
            - Results in toxic levels of phenylalanine
          - ○ Toxic levels of phenylalanine may cause
            - Intellectual disability
            - Seizures
            - Behavioral problems
            - Mental disorders
        - ○ Blood test is used to confirm diagnosis.
          - Will test for presence of the enzyme
      - Tay-Sachs disease
        - ○ Destroys nerve cells in the spinal cord and brain
          - ○ Progressive neurologic disorder
        - ○ Caused by absence of the enzyme hexosaminidase
          - ○ Needed by the body to break down a fatty waste substance found within brain cells
    - Signs and symptoms usually appear around 3 to 6 months of age.
    - Always fatal
      - ○ Typically, life expectancy is 4 to 5 years of age.
    - Signs and symptoms
      - ○ Deafness
      - ○ Decreased muscle strength
      - ○ Progressive blindness
      - ○ Seizures

- ○ Spasticity
  - ○ Muscle stiffness
- ○ Social and mental developmental delays
- ○ Slow, delayed growth
- ○ Muscle paralysis
- CF
  - Exocrine glands affected
    - ○ Mucous
    - ○ Sweat
    - ○ Salivary
    - ○ Mammary
    - ○ Ceruminous
    - ○ Lacrimal
    - ○ Sebaceous
  - Normally, secreted fluids are thin and slippery.
    - ○ Secretions work as a lubricant.
  - Defective gene causes the secretions to become thick and sticky.
    - ○ Secretions plug up tubes, ducts, and other important passageways.
  - Primarily affects lungs and digestive system
    - ○ Can also affect other organs of the body
  - Life-threatening
    - ○ Individuals with CF may live into mid- to late 30s and even into 40s and 50s in some cases.
  - Occurs in all races, but more common in individuals of Northern European ancestors.
  - Signs and symptoms
    - ○ High level of salt in sweat
      - ○ Parents may report tasting salt when kissing child.
    - ○ Recurrent bouts of pancreatitis
      - ○ Inflamed pancreas
    - ○ Infertility
    - ○ Respiratory problems
      - ○ Recurrent lung infections
        - - Pneumonia
        - - Bronchiectasis
      - ○ Pneumothorax
        - - More common in older individuals
      - ○ Persistent cough that produces thick mucus
        - - Wheezing
        - - Exercise intolerance
        - - Stuffy nose
          - • Inflamed nasal passages
    - ○ Digestive problems
      - ○ Poor growth and poor weight gain
      - ○ Intestinal blockage
        - - Common in newborns
          - • Meconium ileus

- Constipation that can be severe
  - Straining may cause rectum and large intestine to protrude outside the anus (rectal prolapse)
- Greasy, foul smelling stools
- Reproductive system problems
- Most men are infertile.
  - Vas deferens (tube that connects testes and prostate gland) becomes blocked.
- Females may be less fertile.
  - Pregnancy may be possible.
  - Pregnancy can worsen the signs and symptoms of CF.
  - Complications of CF
- Osteoporosis
  - Thinning of bones
- Electrolyte imbalances and dehydration
  - Imbalances result in increased heart rate, fatigue, weakness, and low blood pressure
- Sickle cell disease
  - Defective hemoglobin
  - Transmitted as a recessive trait
  - May also be incomplete dominant inheritance
    - Heterozygotes may display clinical signs and symptoms.
      - Sickle cell trait
    - Homozygotes show full range of expression.
      - Sickle cell anemia
- Comparing autosomal-dominant and autosomal-recessive inheritance patterns
  - Usual recurrence risk
    - Autosomal-dominant
      - 50%
    - Autosomal-recessive
      - 25%
  - Transmitting pattern
    - Autosomal-dominant
      - Vertical
      - Seen in generation after generation
    - Autosomal-recessive
      - Seen in many siblings
      - Not typically seen in earlier generations
  - Sex ratio
    - Autosomal-dominant
      - Usually an equal number of females and males affected
    - Autosomal-recessive
      - Usually an equal number of females and males affected
  - Other
    - Autosomal-dominant
      - Father-to-son transition of gene is possible.
    - Autosomal-recessive
      - In rare recessive cases consanguinity is sometimes seen.

APPLICATION AND REVIEW

6. A woman with a history of a sickle cell disease has just given birth to a baby with no signs or symptoms of the disorder. What response should the nurse provide when the woman states, "I'm so relieved the disease has not affected my baby"?
   1. "I'm so thrilled for you and your family."
   2. "This disease isn't always diagnosable at birth."
   3. "Sickle cell disease is seldom passed from parent to child."
   4. "A fetus with sickle cell disease is usually spontaneously aborted."
7. On what assessment foci should the nurse concentrate to best monitor the status of a client diagnosed with Huntington disease? **Select all that apply**.
   1. Development of depression-related behaviors
   2. Periods of either tachycardia or bradycardia
   3. Presence of involuntary muscular jerking
   4. Dementia-related memory lapses
   5. Difficulty swallowing
8. What is the chance that a client diagnosed with Marfan syndrome will pass the disorder on to offspring?
   1. 25%
   2. 50%
   3. 75%
   4. 100%
9. What safety precaution should the nurse implement when admitting a child for surgery who experienced toxic levels of phenylketonuria at birth?
   1. Falls
   2. Seizure
   3. Suicide
   4. Neutropenic

- X-linked dominant
  - Disorders resulting from X-linked dominant inheritance are much less common than other forms of inheritance.
  - There are no carriers.
    - Occurs in both females and males
    - Only one mutant allele needed
  - An inheritance of a gene mutation on the X chromosome
    - Males have one X chromosome and one Y chromosome.
    - Females have two X chromosomes and no Y chromosomes.
      - Even though women have two X chromosomes, one is used for gene production and the other is switched off.
        - X-inactivation
  - Examples of X-linked dominant disorders
    - Rett syndrome
      - Genetic brain disorder
      - Becomes apparent after 6 months of age
      - Primarily affects females
      - Signs and symptoms
        - Coordination problems
          - Walking difficulties
          - Repetitive movements
        - Language problems

- Slow, delayed growth
- Seizures
- Scoliosis
- Sleeping problems
- Fragile X syndrome
  - Also called FXS, Martin-Bell syndrome
  - Most common cause of intellectual disability, cognitive deficit, and learning disorders
    - Intellectual disability
      - Neurodevelopmental disorder
      - Significantly impaired intellectual and adaptive functioning
    - Cognitive deficit
      - Mental process impairment
      - Decline in cognitive abilities
    - Learning disorders
      - Disability that distrusts learning
      - About one-third have autism
  - Onset
    - Noticeable by age 2
    - Physical characteristics may not be noticeable until puberty.
  - Duration
    - Lifelong
    - No cure
    - Early intervention aids in providing developmental opportunity in building skills.
  - Cause
    - Carried on X chromosome
      - Fragile X mental retardation 1 (*FMR1*) gene
  - Gender role
    - One in 4000 boys
      - More common in males
      - Males are more severely affected
    - One in 8000 girls
      - Displays a penetrance of about 50%
        - Result of having a second, normal X chromosome
      - Symptoms range from mild to severe.
  - X chromosome appears constricted or broken.
  - Physical features
    - Long and narrow face
    - Large ears
    - Flexible fingers
    - Large testicles in males
    - Hypotonia
      - Low muscle tone
  - Behavioral characteristics
    - Stereotypical movements
      - Hand-flapping
    - Atypical social development
      - Limited eye contact

- ○ Shyness
- ○ Difficulty with face encoding
- ○ Memory problems
- X-linked recessive
  - Sex-linked recessive disorders are commonly carried by X chromosome.
  - Genes are recessive.
    - Manifested in heterozygous males who lack matching normal gene on the Y chromosome
      - Males will pass the defect to all female offspring.
        - ○ Carriers
      - Male offspring will not be affected nor be carriers.
        - ○ Male passes only the Y chromosome to sons.
    - Heterozygous females are carriers.
      - No clinical signs or symptoms
      - Have 50% chance of producing affected male
      - Have 50% chance of producing carrier female
  - Examples of X-linked recessive disorders
    - Hemophilia A
      - Deficiency of functional plasma clotting factor VIII
    - Duchenne muscular dystrophy (DMD)
      - Progressive muscular degeneration and weakness
        - ○ Voluntary muscles progressively weaken
      - Most common form of muscular dystrophy in children
        - ○ Appears between ages 2 and 6 years
      - Cause
        - ○ Absence of dystrophin
          - ○ Protein that aids in keeping muscle cells intact
      - Passed on by mother
        - ○ Carrier
      - Gender role
        - ○ Commonly in males
        - ○ In rare cases may affect females
      - In some forms of the disease the heart and other organs may become affected.
      - Signs and symptoms
        - ○ First affects muscles in hip, pelvic, thigh, and shoulder areas
        - ○ Later affects voluntary (skeletal) muscles of arms, legs, and trunk
        - ○ By puberty, heart and respiratory muscles are affected.
      - Other types of X-linked recessive muscular dystrophy
        - ○ Becker
          - ○ Similar to Duchenne
            - - Much milder
            - - Symptoms appear later
            - - Progresses slower
        - ○ Onset usually between 2 and 16 years of age; can appear as late as 25 years of age
    - Red and green color blindness
      - X chromosome
      - Most common form of color blindness

- Normal vision sees seven different hue colors.
- Found primarily in male population
  - Found in about 6% of the male population
- Difficulty distinguishing between reds, greens, browns, and oranges
  - Red and green are the main problem colors.
- Typically inherited
- Subtypes
  - Deuteranopia
    - Green-blind
    - Can only distinguish two to three different hues
  - Deuteranomaly
    - Green-weak
    - Green sensitive cones are present
    - Peak of sensitivity is toward the red sensitive cones

APPLICATION AND REVIEW

11. What information should be included in a discussion concerning color blindness? **Select all that apply**.
    1. Red-green is the most common form of color-blindness.
    2. Color-blindness is associated with the X chromosome.
    3. Color-blindness is usually passed on from parent to child.
    4. About 16% of the male population experiences color-blindness.
    5. Males are primarily affected by color-blindness.
12. Considering the progressive nature of Duchenne muscular dystrophy, what interventions will be required to meet the needs of a post-pubescent client?
    1. Active and passive range-of-motion exercises
    2. Airway clearance management
    3. Lower limb braces
    4. Speech therapy
13. What X-linked recessive gene disorder is associated with a deficiency in clotting factor VIII
    1. Hemophilia A   3. Sickle cell disease
    2. Fragile X syndrome   4. Neurofibromatosis type I

See Answers on pages 58–61.

Chromosomal Disorders

- A change in the number or structure of chromosomes
  - Entire chromosomes or large segments missing, duplicated, or altered
- Each chromosome has a characteristic structure.
- Chromosomes can be looked at and studied under a microscope.
  - Karyotype
    - Any deviation from normal karyotype is considered a chromosome abnormality.
- Some chromosome abnormalities are harmless, others cause disorders.
- Severe chromosome disorders result in spontaneous abortions.
- Major abnormalities that survive to term
  - Down syndrome
    - Abnormality
      - Trisomy 21

- Incidence
  - 15 in 10,000
- Edwards syndrome
  - Abnormality
    - Trisomy 18
  - Incidence
    - 3 in 10,000
- Patau syndrome
  - Abnormality
    - Trisomy 13
  - Incidence
    - 2 in 10,000
- Turner syndrome
  - Abnormality
    - Monosomy X
  - Incidence
    - 2 in 10,000 (very rare)
    - Female births
- Klinefelter syndrome
  - Abnormality
    - XXY
  - Incidence
    - 10 in 10,000
    - Male births
- XXX Syndrome
  - Abnormality
    - XXX
  - Incidence
    - 10 in 10,000
    - Female births
- XYY Syndrome
  - Abnormality
    - XYY
  - Incidence
    - 10 in 10,000
    - Male births
- Trisomy 21
  - Most common form of Down syndrome
  - Born with three copies of chromosome 21
    - Individuals have a total of 47 chromosomes.
  - Most common genetic condition in the United States
    - Occurs in 1 of every 800 newborns
    - As many as 6000 cases a year
  - Parent involvement
    - In 90% of cases the extra chromosome comes from the mother parent (egg).
  - Characteristics
    - Distinct facial appearance
    - Intellectual disability

- Developmental delays
- Possible association with thyroid and heart disease
- Health supervision
  - Atrioventricular canal abnormalities are a common heart defect seen in newborns with Down syndrome.
    - If detected early (before age 1) surgical intervention may be appropriate.
    - If detected later (past age 1) surgery may not be successful because of pulmonary hypertension being present for too long.
  - Strabismus
    - Deviation of the eye from its normal visual axis
  - Hypothyroidism
    - Commonly seen during adolescent years
  - Sensorineural and conductive hearing loss
  - Vertebrae instability
    - First and second vertebrae
    - May lead to spinal cord injuries
      - Commonly seen in older individuals
- Turner syndrome (Fig. 3.1)
  - Affects females
  - Most common feature is short stature
    - Evident by about age 5
  - Early loss of ovarian function is common
    - Ovarian hypofunction or premature ovarian failure
  - Most females will not undergo puberty without hormone therapy.
  - Characteristics
    - Extra folds of skin on the neck
      - Webbed neck
    - Low hairline at the back of the neck
    - Lymphedema
      - Puffiness or swelling to hands and feet
    - Skeletal abnormalities
    - Kidney problems
    - Nearly one-third to one-half of individuals are born with a heart defect.
      - Coarctation of the aorta
        - Narrowing of the large artery
      - Aortic valve abnormalities
      - Complications associated with heart defects may be life-threatening.
- Klinefelter syndrome
  - Affects males
  - Physical and cognitive development
  - Low production of testosterone, small testes
    - Testosterone directs male sexual development before birth and during puberty.
    - Shortage of testosterone
      - Delayed or incomplete puberty
      - Gynecomastia
        - Breast enlargement
      - Reduced facial and body hair
      - Infertility

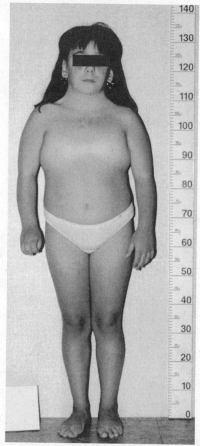

FIG. 3.1 A 14-year-old female with Turner syndrome showing the characteristic short stature and webbed neck. (From Moore, K., Persaud, T. V. N., & Torchia, M. G. [2016]. *Developing human: Clinically oriented embryology* [10th ed.]. Philadelphia: Elsevier.)

- Genital differences
  - Cryptorchidism
    - Undescended testes
  - Hypospadias
    - Opening of urethra on underside of penis
  - Micropenis
    - Unusually small penis
- Older children and adults tend to be taller than peers.
- Adults are at increased risk of developing breast cancer and chronic inflammatory disease.
  - Systemic lupus erythematosus
- Children with Klinefelter syndrome
  - Learning disabilities
  - Delayed speech and language development
  - Tend to be quiet, sensitive, and unassertive (although this may vary)
  - May not affect voice quality during childhood; however, around puberty voice may remain feminine in pitch.

APPLICATION AND REVIEW

14. A nurse is conducting an interview with the parents of a child diagnosed with Klinefelter syndrome. Which statements made by the parents support the presence of the characteristic signs and symptoms of this genetic disorder? **Select all that apply**.
    1. "He attends a special class to help with his reading and math skills."
    2. "He is 3 years old and still has a very limited vocabulary."
    3. "He is shorter and less muscular than his peers."
    4. "His voice is low pitched and gravelly."
    5. "His feelings are very easily hurt."
15. Which assessment finding would tend to support the diagnosis of Klinefelter syndrome in a 25-year-old male?
    1. Prolific body hair
    2. Enlarged breasts
    3. Enlarged penis
    4. Facial acne
16. What specialized information should the nurse provide the family of a pre-teen female diagnosed with Turner syndrome concerning medication therapy?
    1. Asthma medication therapy will include both rescue and prevention inhalers.
    2. Puberty will be triggered and managed with hormone medication therapy.
    3. The characteristic depression will require an antidepressant medication.
    4. Juvenile arthritis will be treated with nonsteroidal antiinflammatory drug therapy.
17. What chromosomal abnormality is associated with Down syndrome?
    1. Trisomy 21
    2. Monosomy X
    3. XXY
    4. XYY

See Answers on pages 58–61.

Multifactorial Inheritance

- Multifactorial disorders represent a relatively small number of diseases.
  - Affects approximately 10% of the population
- May be polygenic or result of a family tendency
  - Polygenic
    - Caused by multiple genes
  - Family tendency
    - Family members are at increased risk of developing the disorder.
    - Not every family member will deveop the disorder.
- Caused by alterations in the small cytoplasmic mitochondrial chromosome
- Unique characteristics of multifactorial inheritance
  - The greater the number of predisposing risk genes possessed by the parent, the greater the probability offspring will be affected.
  - Recurrence is higher when more than one family member is affected.
  - Risk increases with severe malformations.
- More complex
- May be either
  - Polygenic
    - Caused by multiple genes, or
  - Results from an inherited tendency toward a disorder expressed after exposure to environmental factors.

- Typically, factors include a familial tendency.
  - Atherosclerosis
    - Heart and vascular disease
  - Certain cancers
    - Breast cancer
  - Schizophrenia
    - Psychiatric disorder
- Cleft lip/palate
  - Orofacial cleft
    - Opening in the lip and/or roof of the mouth (palate)
  - A common craniofacial anomaly
  - Multiple gene mutations in combination with lifestyle and environmental factors
  - Three categories
    - Cleft lip by itself
      - Common in boys
    - Cleft palate by itself
      - Common in girls
    - Cleft lip and cleft palate together
      - Common in boys
    - Unilateral clefting
      - On one side of the mouth
    - Bilateral clefting
      - On both sides of the mouth
- Diabetes mellitus
  - Caused by oligo- and polygenetic factors in addition to nongenetic factors
    - Nongenetic factors
      - Lacking balance between intake and output
      - Other lifestyle factors
- Hypertension
  - Both male and females affected
  - Higher prevalence in older age groups
  - Genetic and environmental factors
  - Environmental factors
    - Chronic stress
    - Obesity
    - Alcohol intake
    - Salt intake
    - Physical inactivity
- Cancer
  - Chromosome rearrangements can take place in somatic cells, which are responsible for a number of cancers.
  - Leukemias
    - Chronic myelogenous leukemia
      - Abnormality identified as a reciprocal translocation between chromosomes 9 and 22
    - Acute myeloblastic leukemia
    - Acute promyelocytic leukemia
    - Acute myeloid leukemia
    - Acute lymphocytic leukemia

- Solid tumors
  - Burkitt lymphoma
    - Childhood jaw tumor
    - Translocation involving chromosomes 8 and 14
  - Ewing sarcoma
  - Meningioma
  - Retinoblastoma
  - Wilm's tumor
  - Neuroblastoma
  - Breast cancer

APPLICATION AND REVIEW

18. Which disease processes typically tend to present within families? **Select all that apply.**
    1. Atherosclerosis
    2. Breast cancer
    3. Cystic fibrosis
    4. Down syndrome
    5. Schizophrenia
19. Which assessment questions are directed at the identification of environmental factors that contribute to the development of hypertension? **Select all that apply.**
    1. "How do you manage everyday stress?"
    2. "What kinds of problems does your weight cause you?"
    3. "What allergies do you have, including medications?"
    4. "How much alcohol do you consume over a 7-day period?"
    5. "What kinds of physical exercise do you engage in on a weekly basis?"
20. When considering genetic craniofacial clefting, what anomaly is most commonly seen in males?
    1. Tongue
    2. Chin
    3. Palate
    4. Lip and palate combination

See Answers on pages 58–61.

ANSWER KEY: REVIEW QUESTIONS

1. **3 It is unlikely that any two persons, aside from identical twins, would have the same genes and sequence of DNA.**
   1 It is unlikely that any two persons, aside from identical twins, would have the same genes and sequence of DNA. 2 It is unlikely that any two persons, aside from identical twins, would have the same genes and sequence of DNA. 4 It is unlikely that any two persons, aside from identical twins, would have the same genes and sequence of DNA.
   Client Need: Physiological Adaptation; **Cognitive Level:** Understanding; **Integrated Process:** Teaching and Learning

2. **Answers: 1, 2, 3, 4.**
   1 An error in the composition of even one gene can result in the development of a chronic disease. 2 A gene is the basic physical and functional unit of heredity. 3 A gene is composed of DNA strands. 4 Genes are contained in chromosomes.
   5 A gene is microscopic in size.
   Client Need: Physiological Adaptation; **Cognitive Level:** Understanding; **Integrated Process:** Teaching and Learning

3. **1 A Punnett square is a predictive tool used to look at the potential combinations of genotypes in a specific offspring.**

   2 The Punnett square does not propose an explanation for the process of meiosis. **3** The Punnett square is not a concept, but rather a predictive tool. **4** The Punnett square is not used to predict mutations, but rather general combinations of genotypes.

   Client Need: Physiological Adaptation; **Cognitive Level:** Understanding; **Integrated Process:** Teaching and Learning

4. **1 Mutations occur either spontaneously or from exposure to a harmful substance.**

   2 Mutations are a result of changes in the gene's DNA sequence. **3** Mitosis-based division can often result in mutations. **4** Radiation exposure is only one of several different triggers for genetic mutations.

   Client Need: Physiological Adaptation; **Cognitive Level:** Understanding; **Integrated Process:** Teaching and Learning

5. **1 Clinical signs of genetic disorders may not be apparent until adulthood; they may not show up at birth, they may occur months or years later, such as in the case of Huntington disease.**

   2 The manifestations of neurofibromatosis occur before adulthood. **3** The manifestations of Marfan syndrome occur before adulthood. **4** The manifestations of Tay-Sachs disease can occur in infancy.

   Client Need: Physiological Adaptation; **Cognitive Level:** Understanding; **Integrated** Process: Teaching and Learning

6. **2 Signs of sickle cell disease may not be present at birth; therefore, may not be diagnosed immediately.**

   1 It is premature to give such assurance since sickle cell disease may not be present at birth; therefore, may not be diagnosed immediately. **3** Sickle cell disease is a disorder passed genetically from parent to child. **4** Serious genetic defects can cause a spontaneous miscarriage, but that is not typical in the case of sickle cell disease.

   Client Need: Physiological Adaptation; **Cognitive Level:** Applying; **Nursing Process:** Implementation

7. **Answers: 1, 3, 4, 5.**

   1 Huntington disease presents with the progression of psychiatric disorders such as depression. **3** Progressive loss of motor control, such as involuntary jerking is noted with Huntington disease. **4** Progressing dementia is characteristic of Huntington disease. **5** Progressive loss of motor control, such as dysphagia, is noted with Huntington disease.

   2 Cardiac symptoms are not generally associated with Huntington disease.

   Client Need: Physiological Adaptation; **Cognitive Level:** Applying; **Nursing Process:** Assessment

8. **2 There is a 50% chance that an affected client will pass the disease to offspring.**

   1, 3, 4 The other percentages do not reflect the chance that an affected client will pass the disease to offspring.

   Client Need: Physiological Adaptation; **Cognitive Level:** Understanding; **Integrated Process:** Teaching and Learning

9. **2 Toxic levels of phenylalanine may cause risk for seizures.**

   1 Exposure to toxic levels of PKU is not associated with motor dysfunction that could result in falls. **3** Exposure to toxic levels of PKU may be associated with psychiatric disorders, but suicide precautions are generally not required. **4** Exposure to toxic levels of PKU is not associated with suppression of the immune system.

   Client Need: Physiological Adaptation; **Cognitive Level:** Applying; **Nursing Process:** Implementation

10. **2 Tay-Sachs disease is always fatal; life expectancy is 4 to 5 years.**

    1 Tay-Sachs disease does not require a low-fat diet. **3** Intravenous feeds may or may not be required. **4** Although physical growth is slowed or even delayed, the child will experience much greater disabilities.

    Client Need: Physiological Adaptation; **Cognitive Level:** Applying; **Nursing Process:** Planning

11. **Answers: 1, 2, 3, 5.**

    1 Red-green color-blindness is the most common form of color blindness. **2** Color blindness is associated with the X chromosome. **3** Color blindness is typically inherited. **5** Color-blindness is found primarily in the male population.

4 Color blindness is found in about 6% of the male population. **5** Color blindness is found primarily in the male population.

Client Need: Physiological Adaptation; **Cognitive Level:** Understanding; **Integrated Process:** Teaching and Learning

12. **2 By puberty the child diagnosed with Duchenne multiple dystrophy will begin to experience respiratory muscle weakness. This progression of weakness will require frequent clearing of the airway to minimize the increasing risk of respiratory infections.**

     1 Range-of-motion exercises are added early into the plan of care because muscle weakness and the risk of contractures, exist prior to puberty. **3** Muscle weakness is an early characteristic; bracing to provide improved mobility generally occurs early in the disease's progression. **4** The characteristic muscle weakness may impair speech, but this is not always noted and would likely be experienced before puberty.

     Client Need: Physiological Adaptation; **Cognitive Level:** Applying; **Nursing Process:** Planning

13. **1 Hemophilia A causes a deficiency of functional plasma clotting factor VIII, which causes increased bleeding.**

     2 Fragile X syndrome is an X-linked dominant gene disorder that causes intellectual disability, behavioral and learning challenges, and various physical characteristics. **3** Sickle cell disease is an autosomal-recessive disorder that is caused by the production of defective hemoglobin that results in impaired oxygenation and obstructed blood flow. **4** Neurofibromatosis type I is an autosomal-dominant disorder that is caused by a mutation of the neurofibromin gene resulting in both benign and malignant growth on or under the skin.

     Client Need: Physiological Adaptation; **Cognitive Level:** Understanding; **Integrated Process:** Teaching and Learning

14. **Answers: 1, 2, 5.**

     1 Characteristics of Klinefelter syndrome include learning disabilities. **2** Characteristics of Klinefelter syndrome include delayed speech and language development. **5** Characteristics of Klinefelter syndrome include the tendency to be quiet and sensitive.

     3 Older children and adults diagnosed with Klinefelter syndrome tend to be taller than their peers. **4** Klinefelter syndrome does not affect the voice quality of a child; however, around puberty, the voice may remain feminine in pitch.

     Client Need: Physiological Adaptation; **Cognitive Level:** Analysis; **Nursing Process:** Analysis

15. **2 Gynecomastia (breast enlargement) is a sign of Klinefelter syndrome resulting in the low production of testosterone.**

     1 Body hair would be expected to be sparse. **3** A small penis is expected in a client with this disorder. **4** Facia acne is not an expected clinical manifestation of this disorder.

     Client Need: Physiological Adaptation; **Cognitive Level:** Applying; **Nursing Process:** Assessment

16. **2 Turner syndrome, which affects females, requires hormone therapy to stimulate typical puberty.**

     1 Asthma is not a characteristic comorbid condition associated with Turner syndrome. **3** Depression is not a characteristic comorbid condition associated with Turner syndrome. **4** Arthritis is not a characteristic comorbid condition associated with Turner syndrome.

     Client Need: Physiological Adaptation; **Cognitive Level:** Applying; **Nursing Process:** Planning

17. **1 Down syndrome, also known as trisomy 21, is a genetic disorder caused by the presence of all or part of a third copy of chromosome 21.**

     2 Turner syndrome, also known as Monosomy X, is a genetic condition caused by an abnormality on one of the sex chromosomes. **3** Individuals with Klinefelter syndrome inherit one or more extra X chromosomes; the genotype is XXY or more rarely XXXY or XY/XXY mosaic. **4** XYY syndrome (Jacob syndrome) is a rare chromosomal disorder that affects males. It is caused by the presence of an extra Y chromosome.

     Client Need: Physiological Adaptation; **Cognitive Level:** Understanding; **Integrated Process:** Teaching and Learning

18. **Answers: 1, 2, 5.**

    1, 2, 5 Genetic conditions with strong familial tendencies include atherosclerosis, breast cancer, and schizophrenia.

    3, 4 Although genetic in nature, neither cystic fibrosis nor Down syndrome has a strong familial relationship.

    Client Need: Physiological Adaptation; **Cognitive Level:** Understanding; **Integrated Process:** Teaching and Learning

19. **Answers: 1, 2, 4, 5.**

    1, 2, 4, 5 Environmental factors that affect the development of hypertension include chronic stress, obesity, alcohol intake, and physical activity.

    3 Allergies are not considered to be a factor in developing hypertension.

    Client Need: Physiological Adaptation; **Cognitive Level:** Analysis; **Nursing Process:** Planning

20. **4 The combination of lip and palate clefting is most common in males.**

    1, 2 Research has not determined a tendency for this anomaly to occur in one gender over another. **3** Cleft palates are more common in females.

    Client Need: Physiological Adaptation; **Cognitive Level:** Understanding; **Integrated Process**: Teaching and Learning

4 Environmental Disorders

OVERVIEW

- Environmental agents can cause harm to the cell and organs of the human body.
  - As agent(s) collect in the body, the damage can occur slowly over time.
  - Researchers gather and analyze data to identify the cause years after signs and symptoms have occurred.
  - Childhood cancer, hypersensitivities, asthma, and anaphylaxis have increased at a rate that has raised concern for environmental factors.
- Hypersensitivities
  - There has been a substantial increase in responses to the recent chemical substances that have been produced.
  - An increasing array of chemicals is being utilized in the production of food, cosmetics, toiletries, and synthetic building and furnishing materials.
  - Throughout the globe, food and water safety from contamination caused by microbes and chemicals is a major concern.
  - Because many chemicals cannot be metabolized and excreted from the human body, a greater risk exists of increasing the toxin levels within cells.
  - In addition to chemicals, physical factors can be an integral part of environmental disease.
    - For example, exposure to the sun
- Workplace
  - In the workplace, extra safety policies have been instituted to protect people.
  - Regulations exist for a multitude of different work environments.
    - Industrial
    - Health care facilities
  - The Occupational Safety and Health Administration (OSHA) is responsible for ensuring safe work environments for employees in the United States.
  - In Canada, workers are required to take mandatory training regarding the handling, use, and storage of potentially hazardous materials (Workplace Hazardous Materials Information System).
  - Examples of workplace safety initiatives and regulations include
    - Infection control
    - Protective equipment
  - Workers are empowered to question and seek information regarding potentially risky elements in the workplace setting.
    - Resources include toxicology texts or reference material regarding environmental factors.
  - Examples of workplace safety initiatives include
    - Improved ventilation systems for industrial settings
    - Soil testing prior to construction of a dwelling
  - Other workplace initiatives to assure and promote safety include
    - Safety-monitoring committees
    - Employee participation in training regarding supply safety information
    - Standard symbol for hazardous material and handling precautions

- Chemicals
  - Exposure to chemicals can occur at home, in the workplace, at school, and while traveling.
  - Undesirable exposure to chemicals can result from
    - Inhalation in the lungs
    - Swallowing contaminated liquid or food
    - Absorption through the skin
  - Industrial by-products can contaminate the local water and food.
    - Example: Freshwater fish absorb mercury in the lakes and streams.
    - For example, Farmed salmon contain toxic chemicals from the feed.
  - Water processing plants screen for over 300 chemicals in the water, including polychlorinated biphenyls (PCBs) dioxin, lead, and mercury.
    - Often toxic chemicals that drain into the water supply can remain in their original form.
    - Toxic chemical wastes can transform into harmless products or transform into a more toxic product(s).
- Ecosystems
  - Community of organisms
  - Balance in these systems can be disrupted by pesticides.
    - Some microorganisms can become pathogenic or cause disease.
    - Organic fruits and vegetables are a source of food that reduces consumer's exposure to ingesting chemicals.
    - Damage to tissues can result from a single exposure with a large dose or ongoing exposure to smaller doses of an unwanted material.
    - Chemical damage can occur at the entrance site or by circulating through the blood to other areas of the body.
    - The process of chemical exposure can be insidious and happen without the individual being aware of the situation.
    - Often there are no signs of symptoms that the exposure has occurred or the foreign chemicals are accumulating.
  - Detoxification to substances usually occurs by the liver. Foreign chemicals are inactivated or removed from the body.
    - Chemicals that bypass the liver can be stored elsewhere in the body's tissues.
    - Chemicals can accumulate with repeated exposure to dangerous levels over the years.
    - Often accompanied by no visible signs
    - For example, hexachlorophene was once widely used in health care and in homes as an antiseptic in lotions, soaps, and powders.
      - Later it was discovered hexachlorophene was absorbed through the skin, especially open skin. Excessive use causes brain damage.
    - Currently, antibacterial soaps and lotions are being used by the public.
      - It may take years to determine if there are any health-related impacts.
  - Exposure to plastics in the environment is a major concern.
    - Soft plastic contain phthalates to prevent breakage.
      - However, toys, baby bottles, and pacifiers that were manufactured with phthalates have been removed from the market in the United States and Canada.
      - Items made overseas may still be made with this chemical.
    - Hard plastic contains bisphenol A that is used in water bottles and plastic baby bottles.
      - Bisphenol A is classified as a toxin in Canada.
    - Plastics mimic hormones such as estrogen and act within tissues as endocrine disrupters.
      - These can lead to infertility and promote the growth of endocrine-sensitive cancers.

- Surveys have linked solvents in the environment to
    - Alterations in menstrual cycles
    - Spontaneous abortions
    - Stillbirths
- Chemicals can affect the body in several ways.
    - Injuring cells directly by impairing the cell membrane, resulting in swelling and rupture of the cell.
    - Cell damage results in inflammation and tissue necrosis.
    - Alterations in metabolic pathways in the cell can result in degenerative changes.
    - Chemicals can be carcinogenic and result in the cell mutations that result in the onset of cancers, such as leukemia.

APPLICATION AND REVIEW

1. What is the most critical factor contributing to the dangers posed by chemical poisoning to humans?
    1. The lack of public education about the dangers associated with environmental chemicals
    2. The inability of the body to metabolize and excrete environmental chemicals
    3. The rise in individuals developing environmentally triggered chemical sensitivities
    4. The increasing amount of chemicals being introduced into water, soil, and air
2. What is the role of the Occupational Safety and Health Administration (OSHA) concerning safety in the American workplace? **Select all that apply.**
    1. Assisting employers in providing safe work environments
    2. Unionizing employees to promote safe work places
    3. Evaluating the safety of the work environments
    4. Enforcing established safety requirements
    5. Formulating national safety policies
3. Which individual is demonstrating the empowerment afforded employees by the OSHA?
    1. A staff member receiving prompt treatment for an infection resulting from a work-related accident
    2. A nurse attending a seminar on the use of a new form of protective equipment during working hours
    3. A pregnant woman assigned to housekeeping asks the manager about risks related to chemical exposure
    4. A nurse receiving training on the appropriate way to manage the disposal of hospital-generated hazardous waste
4. Which medical diagnosis would place a client at an increased risk for toxicity-related health issues?
    1. Cirrhosis of the liver
    2. Kidney failure
    3. Cardiomegaly
    4. Lung cancer
5. Parents should be educated to inspect plastic toys, bottles, and pacifiers made outside of North America for the presence of what potentially hazardous chemical?
    1. Lead
    2. Phthalate
    3. Asbestos
    4. Hexachlorophene
6. The medical diagnosis of which reproductive system has been linked to the exposure to plastic solvents? **Select all that apply.**
    1. Irregular menstrual cycle
    2. Spontaneous abortion
    3. Uterine fibroids
    4. Uterine cancer
    5. Stillbirth

7. What processes are associated with the chemical effects on the human body? **Select all that apply**.
   1. Alterations causing metabolic degeneration
   2. Damage to cell membranes
   3. Inflammation of tissue
   4. Cell mutation
   5. Cell shrinkage

See Answers on pages 81–84.

Heavy Metals

- Heavy metals such as lead and mercury can collect in tissues with long-term exposure.
- Lead is stored in the bone and is ingested in food and water, or is inhaled.
  - Lead, which is utilized by the manufacturing industry, is found in batteries and pipes.
  - Lead-based paint is used on furniture, walls, and woodwork or toys.
    - Children ingest lead by chewing on items painted with lead-based paint or eating paint flakes from walls or woodwork.
    - Toys and other items manufactured abroad have been recalled because of lead-based paints.
    - Lead vaporizes over time from unregulated (imported) vinyl window blinds.
    - Pica is a craving for food or nonfood material (e.g, clay), and ingestion can result in high levels of lead.
  - Toxic side effects of lead
    - Hemolytic anemia
      - Low hemoglobin levels owing to the destruction of erythrocytes
    - Lead colic
      - Inflammation and ulceration of the digestive tract
  - Impairment of the nervous system
    - Neuritis: inflammation and demyelination of peripheral nerves
    - Encephalopathy: swelling and degrading of neurons in the brain
    - In children, lead toxicity is characterized by
      - Seizures
      - Developmental delays
      - Intellectual impairment
  - Irreversible brain damage (even on exposure to low levels of lead)
  - Lead poisoning can be identified by bone defects (known as lead lines) on the bone and gums (gingiva) near the teeth.
- Arsenic
  - Associated with other minerals; it is a metalloid
  - Arsenic occurs naturally in groundwater and is toxic in its inorganic form.
  - Water contaminated with arsenic (either drinking water or food grown with contaminated water) can be carcinogenic.

APPLICATION AND REVIEW

8. Which mineral, if present in drinking water, should raise concerns for public consumption?
   1. Fluoride
   2. Iodine
   3. Lead
   4. Chloride

9. The nurse is assessing a 2-year-old child. Which findings would indicate possible lead poisoning? **Select all that apply**.
1. Has tantrums when frustrated
2. Is unable to balance on one foot
3. Is unable to put together a three-piece puzzle
4. Has a vocabulary of approximately 250 words
5. History of two previous seizures of unknown cause

See Answers on pages 81–84.

Acids and Bases

- Chemical burns can occur when acids or bases damage living tissue.
  - Classification of chemical burns follows the same standard as a thermal burn.
  - Products containing acids and bases can be found in
    - Household products in the home
    - Other products in laboratories, hospitals, and industries
  - Other products that can cause a chemical burn include
    - Acids and bases
    - Potent oxidizers
    - Reducing agents
    - Other solvents

Inhalants

- Can be classified as particulates or solvents
  - Particulates
    - Asbestos
    - Silica
    - Gaseous (sulfur dioxide and ozone)
  - Solvents
    - Tetrachloride
- Signs and symptoms
  - Local irritation to eyes or nose is obvious initially.
  - Later, inflammation of the respiratory tract occurs.
    - Effects on the central nervous system become apparent.
  - Inhaled or aspirated solvents (e.g., carbon tetrachloride) spread through the blood stream, causing
    - Inflammation of the liver cells
    - Irreversible hepatic damage
    - Pneumonitis
    - Other inhalants directly affect lung tissue.
- Other sources of toxic inhalants
  - Factories
  - Laboratories
  - Mines
  - Insecticides
  - Aerosols
- Sources of toxic inhalants in the home
  - Paints

- Glues
- Furniture
- Floor coverings
- Smog
  - Visible air pollution
  - Contains both toxic gases (hydrogen sulfide), and particles of dust and smoke
  - Areas that are closed in without a supply of fresh air, such as apartment buildings or airplanes, have raised concerns about inhaled substances, infectious disease, and lower oxygen levels.
  - Inhaled particles of iron oxide and silica often cause lung damage in coal mine or in factory workers of industries that use these chemicals. These chemicals can cause
    - Episodes of acute inflammation
    - Low-grade chronic inflammation
    - Fibrosis in the lung
    - Chronic cough and frequent lung infections owing to irritation and inflammation of respiratory mucosa
    - Increase in chronic lung disease in areas with heavy air pollution
    - Particles in the air can be carcinogenic and increase the risk of lung disease.
- Other gases that can result in lung inflammation are
  - Sulfur dioxide
  - Carbon monoxide
    - Produced from incomplete combustion from automobile exhaust
    - Carbon monoxide displaces oxygen from hemoglobin for a significant time period.
    - Prolonged exposure to carbon monoxide can be a serious situation for individuals with respiratory or cardiovascular disease.
    - Carbon monoxide monitors are available to alert individuals to the presence of the colorless and tasteless gas.
- Cigarette smoke
  - Predisposes individuals to a variety of lung and other diseases.
    - Emphysema
    - Bronchitis
    - Lung cancer
    - Bladder cancer
    - Peptic ulcers
    - Cardiovascular disease
  - Other health conditions related to smoking tobacco are
    - Impaired fertility
    - Impaired fetal development (stillbirth, low-birth-weight infant, increase in fetal complications)
  - Secondhand smoke
    - Health concerns related to exposure to secondhand cigarette smoke have resulted in smoking restrictions in the workplace or any indoor dwelling.
    - Many facilities and cities have laws banning smoking in public places.
- Asbestos
  - Originally used for insulation and is still found in old buildings
  - Exposure to asbestos can lead to
    - Severe acute inflammation
    - Scarring of the lung
    - Chronic problems, such as mesothelioma

> ▪ Malignant mesothelioma: rare lung cancer that develops in the mesothelium; it is caused by exposure to asbestos.
- Chronic asbestos-related diseases take a long time to occur so this can delay diagnosis and prognosis for recovery.

APPLICATION AND REVIEW

10. A client who has inhaled tetrachloride should be monitored frequently for signs/symptoms of irreversible damage to what organ?
    1. Brain
    2. Eyes
    3. Liver
    4. Kidney
11. What environmentally triggered public health concerns are increased for people living in large apartment complexes? **Select all that apply**.
    1. Exacerbation of existing emphysema
    2. Developing tuberculosis
    3. Developing skin cancer
    4. Impaired concentration
    5. Spread of measles
12. A client has been a coal miner for 40 years. What assessment data support the client's exposure to environmental iron oxide? **Select all that apply**.
    1. Currently being treated for lung cancer
    2. Diagnosed with lung fibrosis 3 years ago
    3. Reports a chronic cough that worsens at night
    4. Treated for bronchitis four times in the last 2 years
    5. Is screened regularly for increased serum levels of carbon monoxide
13. Which client is at greatest risk if exposed to carbon monoxide?
    1. A teenager diagnosed with migraines
    2. A child diagnosed with Down syndrome
    3. A middle-aged adult being treated for asthma
    4. An older adult recovering from a fractured hip
14. Which health problems have a strong link with tobacco smoking? **Select all that apply**.
    1. Peptic ulcer
    2. Emphysema
    3. Bladder cancer
    4. Mesothelioma
    5. Low birthweight newborns

See Answers on pages 81–84.

Pesticides

- A group of diseases and complications can be caused by some type of exposure to pesticides.
  - Depending on the type of pesticide and length of exposure, resulting health effects can be acute or chronic.
  - Health problems can occur as a result of pesticides draining into creeks, rivers, and other bodies of water.
  - Infants and children are particularly sensitive to health risks resulting from exposure to pesticides.
  - The organs and bodies of infants and children are still in the process of developing.
- Signs and symptoms
  - Acute exposure
    - ▪ Diarrhea
    - ▪ Nausea and vomiting

- Pinpoint pupils
- Rashes
- Headaches
- Irritation of the eyes, skin, and throat
- Chronic exposure
  - Exasperate asthma or other lung issues
  - Damage to the immune system
  - Increased risk for certain cancers
  - Increased risk for birth defects

Thermal Injury

- Hyperthermia: a significant elevation in body temperature
  - Can occur when the temperature in the environment is excessively elevated
  - Prevents effective cooling of the body
  - Inadequate replacement of salt and fluid lost in perspiration can lead to hyperthermia.
  - Individual is most at risk of overheating owing to effective physiologic compensation mechanism.
    - Eldery
    - Infants
    - Individuals with cardiac disorders
  - Syndromes associated with hyperthermia
    - Heat cramps associated with skeletal muscle spasms owing to a loss of electrolytes
    - Heat exhaustion owing to a loss of water and sodium and subsequent hypovolemia
      - Signs and symptoms include
        - Headache
        - Sweating
        - Nausea
        - Syncope (fainting)
    - Heat stroke, the most serious complication, is associated with an extremely high core body temperature.
      - Commonly occurs in infants, elderly, or debilitated individuals
      - Early signs and symptoms include
        - Red, dry skin
        - Headache
        - Dizziness
        - Rapid, weak pulse
      - Heat stroke symptoms are manifested by
        - General vasodilation
        - Significant decrease in circulating blood volume
        - Damage to the heart
- Hypothermia
  - Exposure to cold tempcratures
  - Can have localized or systemic effects
  - Increased cases of hypothermia in cold climates owing to homelessness
  - Children are vulnerable because they are unaware of the risk.
  - Syndromes associated with hypothermia
    - Localized frostbite: affects exposed parts of face, fingers, toes, and ears
      - Wet clothing increases the danger of frostbite.

- Vascular occlusion occurs and can lead to necrosis and gangrene.
- Sensation is lost initially, and the individual is not aware of the danger.
- Observe exposed body areas for color changes, such as white or bluish spots.
- Systemic exposure to cold temperatures can occur with submersion in cold water, inadequate clothing in cold weather, or wet clothing on a particularly windy day.
- Low temperatures can affect body tissues.
- Shivering occurs initially as the body tries to generate heat.
- Body becomes numb; lethargy and confusion become pronounced.
- Pulse and respiratory rates decrease.
- The individual becomes unresponsive.
- Reflex vasoconstriction and increased blood viscosity lead to ischemia and reduced metabolism.
- Core body temperature drops, and capillaries and cell membranes are injured.
- Abnormal shifts in fluid and sodium occur leading to hypovolemic shock (low blood pressure).
- Results in cell necrosis

APPLICATION AND REVIEW

15. Which client should be assessed for possible acute pesticide exposure?
    1. A 3-year-old presenting with diarrhea and skin irritation around the mouth
    2. A 15-year-old reporting joint pain and vomiting
    3. A 25-year-old who is confused and delusional
    4. A 40-year-old experiencing chest pain and syncope
16. Which signs and symptoms are associated with heat exhaustion? **Select all that apply**.
    1. Nausea
    2. Headache
    3. Diaphoresis
    4. Red, dry skin
    5. Rapid, weak pulse
17. Which situation places an individual at the greatest risk for developing frostbite?
    1. Going hatless and gloveless when conditions are windy and cold
    2. Being outside in temperatures below 20° F for 20 minutes
    3. Spending 3 hours in a car trapped in a snowbank
    4. Wearing wet socks and boots on a hike in the snow

See Answers on pages 81–84.

Injury Caused by Radiation

- Ionizing radiation: derived from natural sources; for example, the sun and radioactive materials in the soil
  - Concerns about ionizing radiation are increasing due to changes in the protective ozone layer of the earth's atmosphere, and the resulting risk of additional radiation.
  - Additional sources of radiation
    - Homes; radon gas (a by-product of the natural decay of uranium in the soil) can flow in through water or soil.
    - Industry and defense systems

- Electrical production by nuclear generators
- Medication for use with diagnostic procedures (x-rays and tracer studies) and treatments
  - This also presents a potential exposure risk for health care workers and patients.
- Health care employees with a risk of exposure are given a lead shield and wear monitoring devices to measure and track individual exposure.
  - Radiation absorbed by the body is measured in 'rads' or radiation-absorbed doses.
  - Radiation affects cells that are experiencing rapid mitosis, for example
    - Epithelial tissue
    - Bone marrow
    - Gonads (ovaries and testes)
- With exposure to small doses of radiation, the cells can repair the impacted DNA strands.
- With exposure to larger doses of radiation, the DNA is altered and frequently cross-linkages form.
  - This results in mutations to the cells, which can lead to the development of cancer, and the original cells are destroyed.
  - Radiation sickness results from exposure to large amounts of radiation, and this results in harm to the
    - Bone marrow
    - Digestive tract
    - Central nervous system
  - Damage from radiation can occur from a single (often accidental) or small, repeated exposures to small doses.
  - Effects of repeated small-dose exposure to radiation has not been extensively studied versus the aftermath of an expansive exposure such as the atomic bombs used in Japan in 1945 and the nuclear meltdown of Chernobyl nuclear reactor in Ukraine in 1986.
- Light energy
- Damage to skin and eyes can result from exposure to visible light and ultraviolet (UV) rays.
- Repeated exposure to the sun and subsequently the UV rays can result in the development of skin cancer.
  - Skin cancer is usually seen in older individuals.
  - The UV exposure can harm the nucleotides in the cell's DNA.
  - To reduce the risk of skin cancer it is recommended to
    - Reduce exposure
    - Use skin lotions that block harmful UV rays (UVA and UVB).
  - Depending on the specific wavelength, exposure to intense UV radiation can permanently damage an individual's eyes.
    - Shorter wavelengths can damage the corneal cell.
    - UVA and UVB rays can damage the lens of the eye.
    - Longer wavelength exposure has been linked to
      - Development of macular degeneration
      - Retinal tissue damage
- Visible laser light can seriously harm the eyes.
  - A laser light can cause two types of eye damage
    - Thermal burns to the tissues, such as the cornea
    - Photochemical damage to the retina
  - Thermal harm to unprotected skin can occur with exposure to powerful lasers.

APPLICATION AND REVIEW

18. Which human cells are most at risk from radiation exposure? **Select all that apply.**
    1. Epithelial
    2. Bone marrow
    3. Ovarian
    4. Testicular
    5. Brain
19. Which activity most increases an individual's risk for developing an environmentally triggered chemical-related disease?
    1. Drinking well water
    2. Sunbathing without use of sunscreen
    3. Living in an urban area
    4. Allergy to an airborne allergen

See Answers on pages 81–84.

Noise Hazards

- Extreme noise can result in hearing impairment. A lone loud noise, such as a gunshot, or a variety of intense noise can result in additive hearing damage.
  - A quick, intense noise can rupture a tympanic membrane (eardrum) or damage nerve cells in the inner ear.
  - Aggregate noise can come from many sources.
    - Workplace
    - Urban areas
    - Recreation (loud music)
  - Noisy work environments require ear protection (ear plugs) to be worn.
  - Hearing loss involves initially soft or high-pitched sounds, so the effects of trauma are slow and go unnoticed until hearing loss has progressed.
  - Tinnitus or ringing of the ears is often the initial warning sign of hearing loss.

Food and Waterborne Hazards

- Food and waterborne illnesses
  - Can be caused by the contamination of food or water
  - Some bacteria secrete two substances: toxins and enzymes.
    - Toxins: two types (exotoxins and endotoxins)
      - Exotoxins: produced by gram-positive bacteria
        - Diffuse through the body fluids
        - Interfere with nerve conduction
        - Enterotoxins stimulate the vomiting center and cause gastrointestinal distress.
      - Endotoxins occur in the cell wall of gram-negative organisms.
        - Endotoxins are released when the bacterium dies.
        - This release can cause fever, malaise, or even severe circulatory system effects by
          - Increasing capillary permeability
          - Loss of vascular fluid
          - Ultimately endotoxic shock
  - Signs and symptoms include
    - Vomiting

- ▪ Diarrhea
- ▪ Gastroenteritis
- Because of a lack in personal hygiene or community health standards, organisms are transmitted from the fecal-oral route.
  - ▪ *Escherichia coli* is part of the normal intestinal flora that can be transmitted through contaminated food or water.
  - ▪ An example of this type of infection is traveler's diarrhea.
  - ▪ Swimming in water areas can be a source of contamination owing to improper sewage treatment or water runoff from cattle or other pastures.
  - ▪ Water in deep wells is filtered underground and is deemed safe for drinking.
  - ▪ Heavily contaminated water, which can flow into wells and water tables, can serve as a source of contamination and cause widespread illness.
- Organisms such as *E. coli* have been responsible for serious outbreaks of food and water contamination in North America.
  - ▪ Toxic strains of *E. coli* have resulted in deaths from kidney damage.
  - ▪ Virulent strains of *E. coli* invade the bloodstream and then damage the renal tubules.
  - ▪ Other sources of contamination are ground or processed meats that have not been thoroughly cooked to temperatures recommended to eradicate the bacteria.
- Salmonella is another opportunistic infection associated with tainted poultry products or through food handlers that are carriers (an individual who is asymptomatic but is a reservoir for infection and can spread disease).
  - ▪ Infection has been spread in nurseries and daycare centers owing to lack of effective handwashing and other infection control measures.
  - ▪ Stool cultures can identify the infectious organism.
  - ▪ Often infection can run its course without treatment.
  - ▪ Greatest risk is for the elderly, infants, and children who can easily become dehydrated.
- Other foodborne outbreaks have been linked to the organisms such as listeria and shigella.
  - ▪ Listeria occurs often in processed sausage or ham and is commonly present in the environment.
  - ▪ Shigella is a bacterium transmitted through contaminated hands and only a small dose is need to cause a serious outbreak.
- Melamine is a plastic which, in some areas of the world, is added to food and milk, to increase product volume and profit margins.
  - ▪ Melamine reacts similar to a protein and can go unnoticed unless additional testing occurs.
  - ▪ Ingestion of melamine can result in acute renal failure and potentially death.

Biologic Agents—Bites and Stings

- Injections of animal toxins into the human body
  - Sources of toxins involve the neurotoxins that affect the nervous system are produced by poisonous
    - ▪ Snakes
    - ▪ Spiders
      - ▪ Result in paralysis, respiratory failure, or seizures
      - ▪ Insect or animal vectors transmit infectious agents to human host.
    - ▪ Rabies (or hydrophobia), which is caused by the RNA virus, is transmitted through
      - ▪ A bite from wild animals (e.g., raccoons, skunks, foxes)
      - ▪ Occasionally a domestic animal (dog or cat) that has previously been bitten by an infected wild animal

- Following a bite, the animal is quarantined and monitored for signs of infection.
  - Rabies can result in nerve paralysis and death if immediate treatment is not given.
- Ticks and mosquitoes are another potential source of disease transmission.
  - Rocky Mountain spotted fever and Lyme disease are caused by the organism spirochete, which is transmitted by ticks.
- Allergic reactions
  - Can occur owing to sensitivity to an insect's secretions
  - Bee or wasp stings can result in a life-threatening, anaphylactic reaction in certain individuals.
    - Hypersensitivity or circulatory allergic reactions
    - Anaphylaxis is identified by respiratory impediment in an individual who has just been bitten.

Alcohol Effects

- Alcohol (ethyl alcohol, ethanol) in moderation can have some medicinal benefits, such as reduced risk for dementia and cardiovascular disorders.
- Alcohol, when consumed in excess, can have profound negative effects on the psychological and physiologic well-being of an individual.
- Alcohol metabolism and oxidation
  - Alcohol is metabolized both in the stomach and liver, but the primary site is the liver.
  - Alcohol is converted to acetaldehyde, and this reaction is catalyzed by alcohol dehydrogenase.
    - Reaction is slow and restricts the rate of alcohol inactivation.
    - Once acetaldehyde is formed, it quickly converts to acetic acid.
    - Acetic acid is then synthesized to cholesterol, fatty acids, and other compounds.
    - As the blood content of alcohol increases, no change in the rate of alcohol conversion occurs.
      - The kinetics of alcohol metabolism is opposite of most drugs; when plasma levels rise, the rate of drug metabolism also increases.
      - Alcohol is metabolized at a constant rate regardless of how much is present in the blood stream.
      - Because alcohol is metabolized at a constant rate, there is a limit how much can be consumed without accumulation.
      - For most individuals, one drink per hour prevents alcohol buildup.
    - The transformation of alcohol to acetaldehyde is short-lived and quickly converts to acetic acid.
      - Acetaldehyde is a toxic by-product; it can damage cells and can produce acetaldehyde toxicity.
  - Another by-product of alcohol metabolism is reactive oxygen species (ROS).
    - Alcohol metabolism by the enzyme CYP2E1 produces ROS, and these can damage DNA or combine with other materials to form carcinogenic compounds.

Adverse Drug Reactions

- The World Health Organization (WHO) defines adverse drug reactions (ADR) and any unintended, harmful, and undesired effect that occurs at normal drug dosages.
  - Definition excludes undesired drug effects that result from improper dosing owing to accidental poisoning, drug abuse, and medication errors.
  - Reactions can range from mild to life threatening.
  - With proper drug usage, many ADR can be avoided or reduced.

- In the United States, more than 700,000 emergency department visits a year are owing to ADR.
- Among hospitalized patients annually
  - 770,000 patients will experience an ADR
  - 110,000 patients will die from an ADR.
- ADRs most commonly occur in children and older adults.
  - The potential for an ADR increases with age.
    - Older adult patients are more likely to have multiple health problems.
    - With advanced age, the liver cannot metabolize drugs as efficiently as younger patients.
    - Older patients are twice as likely to suffer from an ADR than younger patients.
    - With age, the percent of fat tissues compared with water increases.
      - Drugs that are water-soluble obtain higher concentrations.
      - Drugs that dissolve in fat are readily stored owing to the higher amount of fat tissue.
    - In the older adult, the kidneys are less efficient at excreting drugs in the urine.
    - In the older adult, the liver is less efficient at metabolizing many drugs.
    - Because of these age-related processes, many drugs will remain in the body of an older individual (relative to a younger individual).
      - Extending the length of a drug's effect results in an increase in the likelihood of a side effect.
  - Infants and young children have an increased risk of ADR because their capacity to metabolize the drug has not been fully researched.
    - Neonates under the age of 8 weeks have immature renal tubular function, and, therefore, administration of certain drugs (digoxin, nonsteroidal anti-inflammatories) should be avoided.
    - Neonates have low body fat, which can affect fat-soluble drugs.
    - At less than 8 weeks of age, the immature blood brain–barrier can increase the anesthetic effects of certain drugs.
    - Neonates myocardium has less contractile force than adults and therefore predisposes the neonate to hypotension, exacerbated by an ADR.
- Other factors impacting the chance of an ADR are
  - Gender
    - Biological differences between males and females can affect the action of drug(s).
    - Variations that exist between male and females include
      - Body weight and composition
      - Liver metabolism rates
      - Gastrointestinal factors
      - Renal function
    - The differences between females (compared with males) that can increase a female's risk of an ADR owing to pharmacokinetics and pharmacodynamics of drugs are
      - Drug absorption
      - Drug distribution
      - Drug metabolism
      - Drug elimination
    - Drug metabolism in females can be altered owing to a hepatic enzyme; CYP3A4 is more active in females than males.
    - Isoenzymes CYT P450 activity is higher in females than in males and can lead to differences is pharmacodynamic responses.
    - Pregnancy exposes the fetus and the mother to the drug.

- The fetus is exposed to drugs and chemicals in the maternal blood supply.
  - The small size of the fetus makes it vulnerable to drug effects.
  - Owing to fetal size, it has few plasma proteins to bind with drug molecules.
  - Reduces capacity to metabolize and excrete drugs
  - When drugs reach the fetus, teratogenicity, anatomic malformations, or other ADR can result.
  - ADR are most likely to occur in the fetus during the first trimester.
- Alcohol ingestion and ADR
  - Alcohol alters the metabolism of drugs and can result in the development of an ADR.
  - Alcohol drug interaction
    - Alcohol can change the intensity of an ADR development.
    - Alcohol can increase the toxicity of an ADR.
    - Alcohol can be harmful owing to pharmacokinetic or pharmacodynamics influences.
      - Acetaminophen is contraindicated when consuming alcohol because it can be metabolized into a toxic product and cause liver damage.
    - Alcohol combined with certain drugs can result in ADRs, such as
      - Nausea and vomiting
      - Headaches
      - Drowsiness
      - Fainting
      - Loss of coordination
      - Hypotension
- Individuals with peptic ulcer disease can have severe internal bleeding because of the consumption of alcohol while taking nonsteroidal anti-inflammatory drugs and aspirin.
- Chronic alcohol ingestion can damage the liver and other organs by activating enzymes that can transform some drugs into toxic chemicals.
- Alcohol potentiates the inhibitory effects of sedatives and narcotics at specific sites of the brain.
- Liver function can be altered with chronic alcohol consumption, resulting in damage (liver cirrhosis and liver hepatitis).
  - The ability of the liver to metabolize drugs is impaired, especially drugs with first-pass metabolism.
  - Beta blocker toxicity increases with liver damage.
- Negative impact of alcohol and the potential for ADR are increased if additional risk factors are present, such as age and other comorbidities.
- Race and ethnicity
  - Drug activity can vary greatly among individuals.
  - Genetic factors are controlled by ethnic background.
  - Interindividual differences are owing to
    - Polymorphisms in genes encoding drug metabolism enzymes
    - Drug transporters
    - Drug receptors
  - Smoking
  - Smoking is a risk factor for diseases, such as cardiovascular conditions, cancer, and peptic ulcers.
  - Smoking influences liver enzymes by altering the metabolic process and is a potent inducer of hepatic cytochrome P-450 and various isoenzymes.

- There can be a significant decrease in pharmacologic effects of some medications because of smoking.
- Polypharmacy (receiving multiple drugs) increases the likelihood of individuals experiencing an ADR than individuals taking only one drug.
- Polypharmacy is an increase in the number of medications or the use of more medications than are medically necessary.
- The more medication that is prescribed, the greater the risk of polypharmacy; however, this does not necessarily dictate that the patient should not take medications.
  - Individuals can have multiple chronic diseases requiring a variety of medications.
  - Individuals can have more than one prescriber at the same time for acute and chronic diseases.
- ADR can occur owing to drug interactions, duplication of medications, additive effect, synergism, skipping medications, lowering dosages to save money, and physiologic antagonism.
- Severe or chronic illness increases the risk of ADR.
- The presence of multiple diseases can make an individual more susceptible to encountering an ADR.
  - Owing to the presence of one or more diseases
  - Owing to the use of multiple drugs to treat disease(s)
  - Drugs that can treat one disease can be harmful for another disease.
    - For example, an individual with hypertension may take a beta-blocker, but a beta-blocker can exacerbate asthma.
- A side effect of medication is an almost unavoidable secondary effect of a drug that may occur at therapeutic levels. Listed below are examples of side effects.
- Drowsiness with the use of antihistamines
- Gastric irritation with the use of aspirin therapy

Drug Abuse

- Substance abuse is a broadly used term to describe the nonmedical use of pharmaceuticals or chemicals to impair an individual's function to some degree and induce a state of euphoria.
  - Substance abuse can lead to serious social, occupational, and medical impairment resulting from a destructive pattern of using drugs.
  - Abuse of drugs does not require the dependence on the drug or tolerance to its effects.
    - Tolerance describes a reduction in effect with repeated use of a medication and, therefore, higher doses are required to provide the same effect.
      - Drug tolerance does not occur for all effects of a drug. For example, a chronic heroin abuser many increase dosage and die from respiratory depression.
    - Dependence is a physiologic or behavioral change that occurs after the discontinuation of drug use.
      - Psychological dependence is distinguished by compulsive drug-seeking behavior.
      - Physical dependence is distinguished by withdrawal symptoms when the drug is not used.
    - Cocaine
      - Naturally occurring opiate, 3-methoxymorphine
      - Derived from the South American coca bush
      - Cocaine (and other stimulants) has the ability to activate the mesolimbic dopamine reward pathway in the brain.

- Administered intravenously (IV), the effects are noted in seconds; Inhaled cocaine takes 5 to 10 minutes to take effect; and both routes last for about 30 minutes. Oral doses of cocaine take longer to absorb, and the intensity of the effect is lessened.
    - Absorbed into the bloodstream, metabolized in the liver, and excreted in the urine; urine metabolites can be present for a week.
  - Heroin
    - Synthetic or natural compound 3, 6-diacetylmorphine
    - Most commonly abused opioid (compounds isolated from the opium poppy that interface with opioid receptors)
    - Three times as potent as morphine, but with different effects
    - Heroine is transformed to 6-acetylmorphine and morphine in order to employ its effects.
    - Poor oral bioavailable owing to first-pass metabolism in the liver
    - Heroine routes of administration: IV, inhalation, or intranasal
      - Rapid euphoria in 7 to 8 seconds if administered IV
      - Delay of 10 to 15 minutes if inhaled or used intranasally
      - Duration of 4 to 6 hours
      - Rapid euphoria contributes to addictive properties.
  - Marijuana (cannabis)
    - Dried leaf material (buds and flowering tops) of the hemp plant cannabis sativa
    - Most commonly abused illegal drug in the United States
    - Active chemical is 9-tetrahydrocannabinol (9-THC) and related modules
    - Usually smoked in cigarettes or in pipes, but can be taken orally
    - Oral administration has lowered blood levels owing to first-pass metabolism and high lipid solubility.
    - Oral administration has effect in 1 to 4 hours. Because of its high lipophilicity, the cannabinoids remain in the body for weeks.

Physical Agents Causing Injury

- An important health issue in the United States involves unintentional and intentional injuries.
  - Significant numbers of people have to manage the mental, physical, and financial challenges that can last a lifetime.
  - Injuries resulted in 2.5 million people being hospitalized in 2014 and 26.9 million people treated for injuries in emergency departments.
- Basis of healing: cell injury and death
  - Can be a result of exposure to toxic chemicals, infections, and physical trauma
  - Injured cells may recover and have reversible injury.
  - Injured cells may die and have irreversible injury.
  - The degree of cell injury depends on several factors
    - Type of injury (e.g., chemical, electrical, physical)
    - State of injury (level of cell differentiation)
    - Adaptive properties of the cell
    - Severity and duration of injury stimulus
  - Other associated factors are nutritional status and age of the individual (elderly and young are more vulnerable).
  - Common biochemical process for cell injury/death regardless of the injury type (Table 4.1)
    - Adenosine triphosphate (ATP) depletion
    - Mitochondrial damage

TABLE 4.1 Common Mechanisms in Cell Injury and Cell Death

Theme	Comments
ATP depletion	Loss of mitochondrial ATP and decreased ATP synthesis; results include cellular swelling, decreased protein synthesis, decreased membrane transport, and lipogenesis, all changes that contribute to loss of integrity of plasma membrane (see text)
Oxygen and oxygen-derived free radicals	Lack of oxygen is key in progression of cell injury in ischemia (reduced blood supply); activated oxygen species (free radicals, H_2O_2, $O_2^{\bullet-}$, NO) cause destruction of cell membranes and cell structure
Intracellular calcium and loss of calcium steady state	Normally intracellular cytosolic calcium concentrations are very low; ischemia and certain chemicals cause an increase in cytosolic Ca^{2+} concentrations; sustained levels of Ca^{2+} continue to increase with damage to plasma membrane; Ca^{2+} causes intracellular damage by activating a number of enzymes (see text)
Defects in membrane permeability	Early loss of selective membrane permeability found in all forms of cell injury (see text)

ATP, Adenosine triphosphate.
From McCance, K. L., & Huether, S. E. (2019). *Pathophysiology: The biologic basis for disease in adults and children* (8th ed.). St. Louis: Elsevier.

- Reserve of oxygen and oxygen-derived free radicals
- Membrane damage (owing to depletion of ATP)
- Protein folding defects
- DNA damage defects
- Calcium level alterations
- Normal cellular communication and function, and diseases are impacted by the ROS from aerobic metabolism.
  - ROS signaling modulates intracellular pathways.
  - ROS are involved in the signaling of transduction pathways and cell rates.
  - ROS can affect protein function.
- An important part of the cell is the free radicals; they disturb the balance between the production of ROS and antioxidant defenses (oxidative stress).
- Oxidative stress can initiate several intracellular pathways, because ROS can regulate enzymes and transcription factors, a process called redox signaling.
- Redox systems are critical for cell defense, such as inflammation.
- ROS generation is reported to result in vascular endothelial damage and ultimately atherosclerosis.
- Systemic characteristics of cellular trauma and resulting injury include
  - Fatigue
  - Malaise
  - Loss of well-being
  - Alterations in appetite
  - Fever (biochemical produced in inflammatory response)
  - Cell death
    - Described as necrosis or apoptosis
    - Necrosis is marked by a rapid loss of the plasma membrane, organelle swelling, and mitochondrial dysfunction. Occurs after severe and unexpected injury.
    - Apoptosis is a type of cell death, an active process of cellular self-destruction; it is distinguished by the dropping of cellular fragments called apoptotic bodies.

- Mechanical injury
  - Injuries to the body resulting in tearing, shearing, or crushing caused by a blow or impact
    - Most frequent injury encountered in health care
      - Usually caused by a fall or motor vehicle accident
  - Types of injuries
    - Contusion (bruise)
      - Bleeding occurs into the skin in underlying tissue.
      - Discoloration begins as red-purple, progresses to black-blue, and transitions to yellow-brown or green.
      - Duration of the discoloration depends on the location, severity, and degree of vascularization.
      - Hematoma is described as a gathering of blood in the soft tissue.
      - Subdural hematoma is a collection of blood between the dura mater and the surface of the brain.
        - Can result from a fall or blow to the head or rapid acceleration/deceleration such as in shaken baby syndrome
      - Epidural hematoma results from blood between the inner surface of the skull and dura.
    - Lacerations
      - When the tensile strength of skin or other tissue is surpassed, a rip or tear occurs.
      - Internal organs can be injured or lacerated owing to a blunt force trauma, such as an automobile accident. Examples include laceration of the liver or kidneys.
    - Fracture
      - Impact or blunt force blow that results in a breaking or shattering of a bone
    - Cutting and piercing wounds
      - Incised wound is longer rather than deeper, and can have jagged edges or straight edges. It has distinct edges without abrasion (no deeper than the dermis). An example is a sharp force injury suicide.
      - A stab wound is deeper rather than longer. The depth of the wound may be clean but abraded, if the penetrating object has a wider portion.
      - External bleeding is decreased after initial blood loss. A puncture wound is made with an object or instrument with a sharp point but not sharp edges.
        - Can be deep and susceptible to infection
        - Classic example is stepping on a nail or some other sharp foreign object
      - A chopping wound by a heavy, sharp-edged instrument (ax, hatchet, propeller blades) results in blunt and sharp force laceration.
- Electrical Injury
  - Direct contact with high-voltage or low-voltage electrical lines can result in severe burns (Fig. 4.1).
  - Usually a result of risk-taking behavior by children or young adults
  - Trauma occurs at the site where there was contact with the electrical energy source.
    - Additional injury occurs to organs, muscles, nerves, and vascular pathways where the electricity flowed.
    - Lightning strikes can also result in electrical burns.
    - Electrical burns may appear to have resulted in minimal damage, but this can be deceiving. There may be substantial injury to internal structures.
    - Young children are a risk for electrical injury from chewing on electrical cords or inserting an object into an outlet.

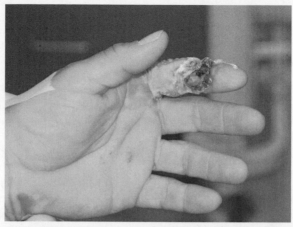

FIG. 4.1 Severe full-thickness electrical burn to anterior left index finger. (From Trinquero, P., & Levine, M. R. [2017]. High voltage electrical injury. *Visual Journal of Emergency Medicine*, 6, 35–36.)

ANSWER KEY: REVIEW QUESTIONS

1. **2 Because many chemicals cannot be metabolized by and excreted from the human body there is a greater risk of increasing toxin levels within cells.**
   1 Education of the public on this topic would certainly affect the degree of dangers chemicals pose, but it does not have as great an impact as the body's inability to effectively metabolize and excrete them. 3 Whereas the sensitivity to chemicals plays a role in this issue, it does not have as much impact as the body's inability to effectively metabolize and excrete them. 4 Although the amount of existing environment chemicals is a factor in chemical poisoning, it does not have as great an impact as the body's inability to effectively metabolize and excrete them.
   Client Need: Physiological Adaptation; **Cognitive Level:** Understanding; **Nursing Process:** Teaching and Learning

2. **Answers: 1, 3, 4, 5.**
   1 OSHA's mission is to assure safe and healthful working conditions for working men and women by working with employers to keep the work environment safe. 3 OSHA's mission is to assure safe and healthful working conditions for working men and women by monitoring workplaces for compliance with standards of safety. 4 OSHA's mission is to assure safe and healthful working conditions for working men and women by setting safety standards. 5 OSHA's mission is to assure safe and healthful working conditions for working men and women by setting safety standards.
   2 Unionization is not a function of OSHA.
   Client Need: Physiological Adaptation; **Cognitive Level:** Understanding; **Nursing Process:** Teaching and Learning

3. **3 Empowerment infers the ability to be proactive; the woman is demonstrating this by initiating a discussion about chemical risks.**
   1 Treatment for a work-related infection is an expected employee right the employer must provide. 2 In-services on new equipment is an expected employee right the employer must provide. 4 In-services on safety practices is an expected employee right the employer must provide.
   Client Need: Physiological Adaptation; **Cognitive Level:** Analysis; **Nursing**

4. **1 Detoxification to substances usually occurs by the liver causing foreign chemicals to be inactivated or removed from the body. Failure results in the accumulation of these chemical in body tissues.**
   2 It is the liver not the kidney that is primarily responsible for detoxification. 3 It is the liver not the heart that is primarily responsible for detoxification. 4 It is the liver not the lungs that is primarily responsible for detoxification.
   Client Need: Physiological Adaptation; **Cognitive Level:** Appling; **Nursing Process:** Assessment

5. **2 Phthalate is used to strengthen plastics; has been removed from the market in the United States and Canada. Items made overseas may still be made with this chemical.**

   1 Lead is a toxic substance found in water and in certain paint products. **3** Asbestos was used commonly in house insulation products. **4** Hexachlorophene was once widely used in health care and in homes as an antiseptic in lotions, soaps, and powders.

   Client Need: Physiological Adaptation; **Cognitive Level:** Understanding; **Nursing Process:** Teaching and Learning

6. **Answers: 1, 2, 5.**

   1, 2, 5 Surveys have linked solvents in the environment to alterations in women's menstrual cycles, spontaneous abortions, and stillbirths.

   3, 4 No such relationship has been found between uterine fibroids and cancers with exposure to plastic-based solvents.

   Client Need: Physiological Adaptation; **Cognitive Level:** Understanding; **Nursing Process:** Teaching and Learning

7. **Answers: 1, 2, 3, 4.**

   1 Chemical effects on the human body include causing changes to metabolic pathways resulting in some degenerative changes. **2** Chemical effects on the human body include causing damage to cell membranes. **3** Chemical effects on the human body include causing inflammation of the body tissues. **4** Chemical effects on the human body include causing cell mutation that can result in the formation of cancers.

   5 Chemical effects on the human body include causing membrane damage that result in swelling and rupturing of the cell rather than shrinkage.

   Client Need: Physiological Adaptation; **Cognitive Level:** Understanding; **Nursing Process:** Teaching and Learning

8. **3 Lead is a toxic mineral and should be monitored closely.**

   1 Fluoride is added to water supplies to facilitate dental health. **2** Iodine is a mineral that has been shown to have health benefits, especially for thyroid health. **4** Chlorine in the water supply actually helps prevent water contamination.

   Client Need: Physiological Adaptation; **Cognitive Level:** Understanding; **Nursing Process:** Teaching and Learning

9. **Answers: 2, 3, 5.**

   2 In children, lead poisoning is characterized by developmental delays; a 2-year-old should be able to stand on one foot. **3** In children, lead poisoning is characterized by intellectual impairment; a 2-year-old should be able to put together a puzzle consisting of three to four pieces. **5** In children, lead poisoning is characterized by a history of seizures.

   1 Tantrums in response to frustration is typical of a 2-year-old. **4** The vocabulary of a 1-year-old should consist of 200 or more words.

   Client Need: Physiological Adaptation; **Cognitive Level:** Analysis; **Nursing Process:** Analysis

10. **3 Inhaled or aspirated carbon tetrachloride spreads through the blood stream, causing the possibility of irreversible hepatic damage.**

   1 The brain is not as likely to be affected as is the liver. **2** The eyes are not as likely to be affected as is the liver. **4** The kidneys are not as likely to be affected as is the liver.

   Client Need: Physiological Adaptation; **Cognitive Level:** Understanding; **Nursing Process:** Teaching and Learning

11. **Answers: 1, 2, 4, 5.**

   1 Areas that are enclosed and lack sufficient circulating air, such as apartment complexes, raise concerns for lower oxygen levels that can worsen chronic lung diseases such as emphysema. **2** Areas that are enclosed and lack sufficient circulating air, such as apartment complexes, raise concerns related to the spread of infectious diseases such as tuberculosis. **4** Areas that are enclosed and lack sufficient circulating air, such as apartment complexes, raise concerns for lower oxygen levels that can result in poor brain oxygenation and resulting impaired concentration. **5** Areas that are enclosed and lack sufficient circulating air, such as apartment complexes, raise concerns related to the spread of infectious diseases such as measles.

3 Although skin cancer can be a result of environmental triggers related to sun exposure, this is not associated with the closed environment of an apartment complex.
Client Need: Physiological Adaptation; **Cognitive Level:** Analysis; **Nursing Process:** Teaching and Learning

12. **Answers: 1, 2, 3, 4.**

    1 Inhaled particles of iron oxide often cause lung damage such as lung cancer in coal miners. **2** Inhaled particles of iron oxide often cause lung damage in the form of fibrosis in coal miners. **3** Inhaled particles of iron oxide can cause lung damage resulting in chronic coughing in coal miners. **4** Inhaled particles of iron oxide often cause lung damage in the form of lung infections such as bronchitis in coal miners.

    5 Carbon monoxide poisoning is not associated with iron oxide inhalation.
    Client Need: Physiological Adaptation; **Cognitive Level:** Analysis; **Nursing Process:** Analysis

13. **3 Prolonged exposure to carbon monoxide can be a serious situation for individuals with a respiratory disease such as asthma.**

    1 A teen with no respiratory or cardiac complications is at minimal risk when exposed to carbon monoxide. **2** A child with no respiratory or cardiac complications is at minimal risk when exposed to carbon monoxide. **4** An older adult with no respiratory or cardiac complications is at minimal risk when exposed to carbon monoxide.
    Client Need: Physiological Adaptation; **Cognitive Level:** Analysis; **Nursing Process:** Analysis

14. **Answers: 1, 2, 3, 5.**

    1 Tobacco smoke predisposes the smoker to the increased risk of developing a peptic ulcer. **2** Tobacco smoke predisposes the smoker to the increased risk of developing emphysema. **3** Tobacco smoke predisposes the smoker to the increased risk of developing bladder cancer. **5** Tobacco smoke predisposes the smoker to the increased risk of delivering a low-birth-weight newborn.

    4 Mesothelioma, a rare lung cancer that develops in the mesothelium layer of the lung, is caused by exposure to asbestos not tobacco smoke.
    Client Need: Physiological Adaptation; **Cognitive Level:** Understanding; **Nursing Process:** Teaching and Learning

15. **1 Infants and children are particularly sensitive to health risks resulting from exposure to pesticides. A 3-year-old presenting with diarrhea and oral skin irritation should be assessed for pesticide exposure.**

    2 This client is neither in the critical age group nor demonstrates signs/symptoms associated with pesticide poisoning. **3** This client is neither in the critical age group nor demonstrates signs/symptoms associated with pesticide poisoning. **4** This client is neither in the critical age group nor demonstrates signs/symptoms associated with pesticide poisoning.
    Client Need: Physiological Adaptation; **Cognitive Level:** Analysis; **Nursing Process:** Analysis

16. **Answers: 1, 2, 3.**

    1, 2, 3 Heat exhaustion owing to a loss of water and sodium and results in nausea, headache, and sweating.
    4, 5 Heat stroke is a serious complication associated with extremely high core body temperate and will present with red, dry skin, and a rapid, weak pulse.
    Client Need: Physiological Adaptation; **Cognitive Level:** Understanding; **Nursing Process:** Teaching and Learning

17. **4 Wet clothing increases the danger of frostbite.**

    1 Although unadvisable, going hatless and gloveless is less of a risk for frostbite than by wearing wet clothes. **2** Although unadvisable, being outside in temperatures described is less of a risk for frostbite than by wearing wet clothes. **3** Although unadvisable, spending hours in a car trapped in the snow is less of a risk for frostbite than by wearing wet clothes.
    Client Need: Physiological Adaptation; **Cognitive Level:** Analysis; **Nursing Process:** Analysis

18. **Answers: 1, 2, 3, 4.**

    1, 2, 3, 4 Radiation affects cells that experience rapid mitosis (reproduction), including epithelial, bone marrow, gonads (ovaries and testes).

5 Brain cells do not experience rapid mitosis and so are not at as great a risk from radiation exposure.
Client Need: Physiological Adaptation; **Cognitive Level:** Understanding; **Nursing Process:** Teaching and Learning

19. **2 Unprotected exposure to the sun is a known risk for the development of skin cancers.**

   1 Well water may or may not be contaminated with ground chemicals, making the risk less than regular sun exposure. **3** Living in an urban area may or may not increase the risk of airborne allergies and diseases, making the risk less than regular sun exposure. **4** Airborne allergies are triggered by a variety of substances, not all being chemical in nature.
   Client Need: Physiological Adaptation; **Cognitive Level:** Applying; **Nursing Process:** Assessment

PATHOPHYSIOLOGY

Nutrients

- Nutrients are the chemical substances found in foods.
- The utilization of foods by living organisms is essential for normal growth, reproduction, and health maintenance.
- Humans require more than a dozen different minerals in their diets.
  - Minerals vary depending on concentration of the mineral in the soil or the water in which it grows.
- Two groups of nutrients
  - Organic (carbon-containing)
    - Make up the majority of the human diet
    - Synthesized by living cells from simpler compounds
    - Green plants and photoplankton form the base of the organic nutrient chain.
      - Able to make organic compounds from inorganic compounds
    - Organic nutrients
      - Proteins
      - Carbohydrates
        - Sugars and starches
      - Fats
        - Essential fatty acids
      - Vitamins
        - 13 essential vitamins
    - Organic compounds are primarily made up of six elements
      - Hydrogen
      - Carbon
      - Nitrogen
      - Oxygen
      - Sulfur
      - Phosphorus
  - Inorganic
    - Minerals and water
      - Do not need to come from living sources (plants or animals)
  - Other nutrients
  - Macronutrients
    - Nutrients the body needs in large amounts
    - Provide the body with energy
    - The three basic components of every diet
      - Carbohydrates
        - Major energy source
        - Fruits, vegetables, legumes, and cereal grains

- ○ Carbohydrate classification
  - ○ Available
    - - Those that are absorbed in the small intestine and enter the path of carbohydrate metabolism
  - ○ Unavailable
    - - Not hydrolyzed by digestive enzymes; however, may be partially fermented by large intestine bacteria. This forms short-chain fatty acids that can be absorbed and which assist in meeting the body's energy needs.
- ■ Proteins (polypeptides)
  - ○ Composed of amino acid residues linked by peptide bonds
  - ○ Promote wide diversity of functions in the human body
  - ○ Functions
    - ○ Enzymes
    - ○ Transcription factors
    - ○ Binding proteins
    - ○ Transmembrane transporters/channels
    - ○ Hormones
    - ○ Immunoglobulins
    - ○ Motor proteins
    - ○ Receptors
    - ○ Structural proteins
    - ○ Signaling proteins
  - ○ Examples of proteins: Egg whites, wheat gluten, plasma albumin, and fibrin
- ■ Lipids
  - ○ Small molecules that are unified by their solubility in nonpolar solvents
  - ○ Functions
    - ○ Structural components of cell membranes
    - ○ Form of energy storage
    - ○ Body surface lubrication
    - ○ Signaling molecules
    - ○ Receptors
    - ○ Antigens
    - ○ Sensors
    - ○ Electrical insulators
    - ○ Membrane anchors for proteins
  - ○ Examples of lipids: Lard, tallow, butterfat, soybeans, canola, cottonseed, peanuts, sunflower, corn, and olive oils
  - ○ Chemical classification
    - ○ Nonesterified fatty acids
      - - Saturated fatty acids
      - - Unsaturated fatty acids
      - - Trans fatty acids
      - - Conjugated fatty acids
    - ○ Glycerolipids
      - - Monoacylglycerols
      - - Diacylglycerols
      - - Triacylglycerols

- ○ Glycerophospholipids
  - Common phospholipids
  - Including sulfate
- ○ Phosphatidylglycerol
  - Lysophospholipids
  - Diphosphatidylglycerols
  - Ether phospholipids
- ○ Sphingolipids
  - Sphingosine
  - Ceramics
  - Sphingomyelin
  - Neutral glycosphingolipids
  - Acidic glycosphingolipids
- ○ Isoprenoids
  - Carotenoids
  - Retinoids
  - Prenols
- ○ Steroids
  - Sterols
  - Steroid hormones
  - Bile acids
- ○ Biological waxes
  - Long-chain ester waxes
  - Related compounds
- ○ Eicosanoids
  - Cyclooxygenase products
  - Lipoxygenase products
  - Cytochromes P450 products
- ○ Other lipids
  - Acyl-coenzyme A (acyl-CoA)
  - Acylcarnitine
  - Anandamide
  - Lipopolysaccharides
- Micronutrients
  - Nutrients the body needs in small amounts
  - Enable the body to produce essential substances for proper development and growth
    - Enzymes
    - Hormones
  - Absence of these has a negative impact on human health.
    - Pregnant women and children particularly
  - Consists of
    - Iron
    - Copper
    - Zinc
    - Fluoride
    - Iodine

APPLICATION AND REVIEW

1. What is a direct outcome for the human body when there is an ineffective use of dietary nutrients? **Select all that apply.**
   1. Infertility
   2. Stunned growth
   3. Immunosuppression
   4. Ineffective oxygenation
   5. Increased formation of tumors
2. What information should be included when planning a discussion regarding macronutrients and human nutrition? **Select all that apply.**
   1. They are especially vital to child growth.
   2. They are required in large amounts.
   3. Their focus is energy production.
   4. They are found in egg whites.
   5. They include iron and copper.

See Answers on pages 103–105.

Dietary Reference Intakes

- Reference for recommended intakes and safe upper levels of intake nutrients
- Introduced in 1994
  - Superseded the recommended dietary allowance (RDA)
    - The RDA had been the standard since 1941.
- Nutrient-based reference values
  - Estimated average requirement
    - The predicted dietary energy intake average needed to maintain energy balance in a healthy adult within a certain age, gender, weight, height, and physical activity level
  - RDA
    - The average daily dietary nutrient intake level that would adequately meet the nutrient requirements for most healthy individuals within a particular life stage and gender group
      - Meets requirements for 97% to 98% of healthy individuals
  - Adequate intake
    - A set, recommended average daily nutrient intake level
  - Tolerable upper intake level
    - Highest nutrient intake level that is likely to pose no significant health risks for most healthy individuals
  - For macronutrients
    - Acceptable macronutrient distribution range
      - Intake range associated with reduced risk of chronic disease while allowing adequate intake of essential nutrients
        - Carbohydrates
          - 45% to 65%
        - Lipids
          - 20% to 35%
        - Protein
          - 10% to 35%

- Estimated energy requirement
  - Average energy intake needed to maintain energy balance in healthy, normal-weight individuals

APPLICATION AND REVIEW

3. What human characteristics are considered when the estimated average requirements for energy are calculated? **Select all that apply**.
1. Age
2. Gender
3. Weight
4. Activity
5. Allergies

4. A client is found to have a diet that is composed of 50% carbohydrates, 40% protein, and 10% fats. What nutritional counseling should the nurse provide to this client? **Select all that apply**.
1. "We need to work on making more healthy choices in all the food categories."
2. "Your carbohydrate consumption is within the acceptable, healthy range."
3. "You're not getting enough fat so let's discuss sources of healthy fats."
4. "Let's discuss ways to increase your daily protein intake."
5. "On a daily basis, your diet is very well balanced."

See Answers on pages 103–105.

Digestion, Absorption, Transportation, and Excretion of Nutrients

- Gastrointestinal (GI) tract
  - Essential in nutritional process
  - One of the largest organs in the body
    - About 9 meters long (mouth to anus)
  - Functions
    - Digests macronutrients from ingested foods
    - Absorbs fluids, micronutrients, and trace elements
    - Provides a physical and immunologic barrier
      - Pathogens
      - Foreign material
      - Potential antigens
    - Provides regulatory and biochemical signals to the nervous system
      - Gut–brain axis
        - Pathway
  - Common GI nutrition diagnoses
    - Imbalance of nutrient uptake
    - Altered GI function
    - Altered nutrient utilization
    - Altered nutrient biomarkers
    - Food–drug interaction
    - Inadequate or excessive fluid intake

Nutritional Disorders

- Malnutrition
  - Deficiencies
    - Lack of important vitamins and minerals
    - Underweight, wasting
  - Excesses
    - Excess of micronutrients
    - Obesity
  - Imbalances
    - Consuming too much or too little
    - Unbalanced diet

Severe Acute Malnutrition

- Marasmus (Fig. 5.1)
  - Severe undernourishment of protein energy in the diet
    - Wasting
      - "Skin and bones"
  - Most commonly occurs in young children
  - Four causes leading to marasmus
    - Improper feeding
    - Infection
      - Syphilis
      - Tuberculosis
    - Congenital weakness of disease
      - Congenital heart disease
    - Poor sanitary and hygienic conditions that spread disease
  - Signs and symptoms
    - Thin
      - Face
      - Ribs and shoulders visible through skin
    - Very loose skin which may hang in folds on the upper arms, thighs, and buttocks
    - Persistent dizziness
    - Diarrhea

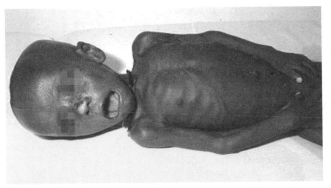

FIG. 5.1 Child with marasmus. (From Kramer, C. V., & Allen, S. [2015]. Malnutrition in developing countries. *Paediatrics and Child Health, 25*[9], 422–427.)

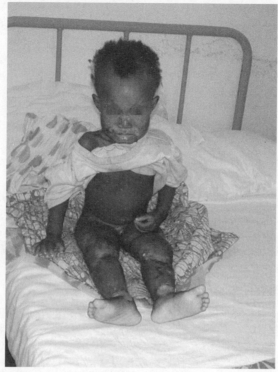

FIG. 5.2 Child with kwashiorkor. (From Kramer, C. V., & Allen, S. [2015]. Malnutrition in developing countries. *Paediatrics and Child Health, 25*[9], 422–427.)

- ▪ Sunken eyes
- ▪ Behavioral issues
  - ▪ Irritable
  - ▪ Active
  - ▪ Alert
  - ▪ Anxious
- ▪ Dehydration
- ▪ Frequent infections
- Kwashiorkor (Fig. 5.2)
  - Severe protein-energy malnutrition
  - Causes individual to retain large amounts of fluid in places such as the lower legs, feet, arms, hands, and face
  - Signs and symptoms
    - ▪ Edema
    - ▪ Loss of appetite
    - ▪ Lack of energy
    - ▪ Behavioral issues
      - ▪ Irritability
      - ▪ Anxiety
    - ▪ Hair color changes
      - ▪ May change to yellow or orange

- Dermatosis
  - Large patches of skin become abnormally light or dark, the skin sheds, skin ulcers develop, and lesions may leak or bleed.
- Prompt, timely diagnosis is critical.
  - More life-threatening than marasmus
  - May result in quick death
- Marasmic-Kwashiorkor
  - Third form of protein-energy malnutrition
  - Individuals experience a combination of marasmus and kwashiorkor.
  - Signs and symptoms
    - Extremely thin
      - Wasting away
    - Edema
    - Severely dehydrated
  - Prompt, timely diagnosis is critical.
    - As condition worsens, individual is at increased risk of death.

APPLICATION AND REVIEW

5. Which nutritional condition is a probable outcome for a client diagnosed with tuberculosis (TB)?
   1. Bulimia
   2. Rickets
   3. Marasmus
   4. Anorexia nervosa
6. Which assessments should the nurse preform to assist in the diagnosis of a protein-energy deficiency in a client diagnosed with Kwashiorkor? **Select all that apply.**
   1. Check the skin for ulcers.
   2. Assess the skin for light patches.
   3. Inspect the hair for orange-yellow tint.
   4. Look at the tongue for deep furrows.
   5. Determine if there is a halo around the pupil of the eyes.

See Answers on pages 103–105.

Anorexia Nervosa and Bulimia

- Eating disorder is a psychiatric disease characterized by a constant disturbance of eating habits and/or weight control negatives that result in significantly impaired physical health and psychosocial functioning.
- Body image distortion
  - Causes individuals to feel overweight despite their often cachectic state
- Diagnostic criteria
  - Diagnostic and Statistical Manual of Mental Disorders V (DSM-V)
  - American Psychiatric Association website: http://www.dsm5.org
  - Anorexia nervosa
    - Voluntary self-starvation leading to emaciation
    - Prevalence
      - Females
        - 0.3% to 3.7%

- Males
  - 0.3%
- Westernized, postindustrialized societies at greater risk
- Physical and clinical signs and symptoms of anorexia nervosa
  - Dizziness
  - Confusion
  - Dry, brittle hair
  - Lanugo-type hair
  - Low blood pressure, pulse, electrocardiogram voltage
  - Orthostasis
  - Cachexia
  - Biochemical changes
    - Decreased white blood cell count
    - Decreased glucose
    - Increased cholesterol
    - Increased carotene
  - Stool retention
  - Acrocyanosis
  - Loss of menses
  - Muscle wasting
  - Diminishing deep tendon reflexes
  - Osteoporosis
  - Dry skin
  - Edema
  - Growth retardation
  - Hypothermia
- Psychological features associated with anorexia nervosa
  - Compulsivity
  - Inflexible thinking
  - Perfectionism
  - Harm avoidance
  - Feelings of ineffectiveness
  - Overly restrained emotional expression
  - Limited social spontaneity
- Psychiatric conditions associated with anorexia nervosa
  - Depression
    - Reported in 50% to 75% of patients
  - Anxiety disorders
  - Personality disorders
  - Obsessive-compulsive disorder (OCD)
    - Reported in 40% of patients
  - Substance abuse
- Mortality
  - Mortality rate of 0% to 8%
- American Psychiatric Association (DSM-V) criteria
  - Refusal to maintain body weight at/above minimally normal weight for age/height.
  - Fear of weight gain

- Disturbance in one's body weight/shape is experienced, undue influence of body weight/shape on self-evaluation, denial of the current low weight.
- Amenorrhea in postmenarcheal females
- Bulimia nervosa
  - Disorder characterized by recurrent episodes of binge eating followed by one or more compensatory behaviors (vomiting, laxative use, diuretic use, compulsive exercise, and/or fasting).
  - Binge refers to the consumption of an unusually large amount of food (1000 to 2000 calories) within a discrete period (usually within 2 hours).
  - Prevalence
    - Females
      - 1% to 3%
    - Males
      - Approximately one-tenth that in women
  - Physical and clinical signs and symptoms of bulimia nervosa
    - Salivary gland enlargement
    - Enamel erosion
    - Esophagitis
    - Arrhythmias
    - Normal weight, underweight, or overweight
    - Callus
    - Biochemical changes
      - Decreased potassium
      - Increased CO_2
      - Increased amylase
    - Diarrhea
    - Edema
  - Psychological features associated with bulimia nervosa
    - Frustration
    - Labile mood
    - Anxiety
    - Impulsivity
  - Psychiatric conditions associated with bulimia nervosa
    - Depression
    - Anxiety disorders
    - Personality disorders
    - Substance abuse
    - Self-injurious behaviors
  - Mortality
    - Mortality rates are lower than those for anorexia nervosa.
    - Mortality rate of 0.4%
  - American Psychiatric Association (DSM-V) criteria
    - Recurrent binge eating
      - Eating an amount of food that is definitely larger than most people would eat within a discrete period (e.g., within a 2-hour period)
      - Inability to gain control of eating during episode
    - Inappropriate compensatory actions to prevent weight gain
      - Self-induced vomiting
      - Misuse of laxatives, diuretics, enemas, and/or other medications

- Binge eating and inappropriate compensatory actions occurring at least twice a week for 3 months
- Self-evaluation unduly influenced by shape/weight of body
- Disturbances not exclusively occurring during anorexia nervosia episode
  - Purging type
    - During episode of bulimia nervosa, regularly engaging in self-induced vomiting and/or misusing laxatives, diuretics, and/or enemas
  - No purging type
    - During episode of bulimia nervosa, use of other inappropriate compensatory behaviors such as excessive exercise or fasting; however, not regularly engaging in self-induced vomiting or the misuses of laxatives, diuretics, and/or enemas
- Eating disorder not otherwise specified
  - Under DSM-V, approximately 50% of individuals with eating disorders fall into this diagnostic group.
  - Individuals in this group meet most, not all, of the criteria for anorexia nervosa or bulimia nervosa.
    - Examples
      - A female may meet diagnostic criteria for anorexia nervosa except amenorrhea.
      - A previously obese individual, despite extreme weight loss, pathological eating behavior, and amenorrhea fails to meet anorexia nervosa diagnostic criteria of body weight less than 85% of expected.
      - An individual who binges and purges; however, with less frequency/shorter duration than specified for bulimia nervosa diagnosis
      - Individual who does not binge eat, however does commit after eating a normal-sized meal

APPLICATION AND REVIEW

7. A nurse is caring for a newly admitted client diagnosed with anorexia nervosa. What is the priority treatment for the client?
   1. Medication therapy to reduce anxiety triggers
   2. Family psychotherapy counseling to minimize dysfunction
   3. Psychotherapy focused on client self-image to minimize risk of low self-esteem
   4. Correction of existing biochemical imbalances to stabilize current physical condition
8. A nurse is caring for an underweight adolescent female who is diagnosed with anorexia nervosa. Which client statement demonstrates a common psychological characteristic of this eating disorder?
   1. "I can only eat breakfast between 8:15 and 8:30 am."
   2. "I wear whatever clothing is soft and comfortable."
   3. "I'm pleased with the Bs and Cs I earn in school."
   4. "I'm always so cold even when it is warm outside."
9. A nurse demonstrates an understanding of the common comorbid conditions associated with anorexia nervosa when asking which assessment questions? **Select all that apply**.
   1. "What is likely to make you feel really anxious?"
   2. "What do the voices you hear say when you are alone?"
   3. "What substances have you used to help cope with stress?"
   4. "What is happening with your life that could cause you to be depressed?"
   5. "Give me an example of something that makes you feel your family is against you."

10. Which client behaviors support the medical diagnosis of bulimia nervosa? **Select all that apply**.
    1. Engages in compulsive exercise
    2. Layers clothing to stay warm
    3. Frequently induces vomiting
    4. Regularly uses laxatives
    5. Restricts food intake
11. Which behavior is associated with a psychiatric condition associated with bulimia nervosa?
    1. Pulling out clumps of hair
    2. Hoarding paper and plastic bags
    3. Compulsively lying about achievements
    4. Acting on the irresistible urge to steal inexpensive items
12. Which client has the greater risk for a diagnosis of anorexia nervosa?
    1. A female living in New York City
    2. A male living in rural Mississippi
    3. A male Army private stationed in Afghanistan
    4. A female born in a refugee camp in southern Africa
13. Which findings would support a diagnosis of bulimia nervosa? **Select all that apply.**
    1. Numerous oral cavities
    2. Irregular heart beat
    3. Callused knuckles
    4. Brittle, dry hair
    5. Amenorrhea

See Answers on pages 103–105.

Vitamin Deficiencies

- Vitamin A
  - Essential during embryonic development
  - Estimated average requirement
    - Adult
      - Males
        - 600 mcg/day
      - Females
        - 500 mcg//day
      - During pregnancy
        - 800 mcg/day
      - During lactation
        - 850 mcg/day
    - Children
      - Birth to 6 months of age
        - 375 mcg/day
      - 7 months to 3 years of age
        - 400 mcg/day
      - Children 4 to 6 years of age
        - 450 mcg/day
      - Children 7 to 10 years of age
        - 500 mcg/day

- Adolescents
  - 600 mcg/day
- Retinol is the alcoholic form of vitamin A.
  - Retinoids have three distinct structural domains.
    - β-Ionone ring
    - Spacer of a polyunsaturated chain
    - Polar end-group
- Functions in a wide spectrum of biological functions
  - Vision
  - Immune function
  - Reproduction
  - Regulation of metabolism
  - Cell proliferation, differentiation, and apoptosis
- Deficiencies
  - Ocular problems
    - Initial symptoms include night blindness and, if left untreated, can lead to irreversible damage to the cornea and blindness.
  - Depressed immune function
  - Lower resistance to infection
- Vitamin A toxicity
  - Three types of toxicity
    - Acute toxicity
      - Occurs after consumption of foods very high in vitamin A in a short time
      - Rare
      - Easily reversible
    - Chronic toxicity
      - Routine intake of smaller, yet still large doses of vitamin A over time
      - Rare
      - Easily reversible
    - Pregnancy toxicity
      - Teratogenic effects which may lead to fetal abnormalities
- Vitamin D
  - Synthesized by humans through the action of sunlight on direct skin
  - Estimated average requirement
    - Adult
      - Males
        - 19 to 70 years of age
          - 600 IU/day
        - >70 years of age
          - 800 IU/day
      - Females
        - 19 to 70 years of age
          - 600 IU/day
        - >70 years of age
          - 800 IU/day
        - During pregnancy
          - 600 IU/day

- During lactation
  - 600 IU/day
- Children
  - Birth to 12 months of age
    - 400 IU/day
  - 1 to 13 years of age
    - 600 IU/day
  - 14 to 18 years of age
    - 600 IU/day
- There are two forms of vitamin D with nutritional relevance.
  - D2 (ergocalciferol)
    - Not synthesized by animals or plants
    - Generated from the precursor ergosterol by phytoplankton, yeast, fungi, and invertebrates in response to ultraviolet (UV) irradiation
    - Can be commercially synthesized
    - May have lower toxicity risk compared with D3
  - D3 (cholecalciferol)
    - Generated in the skin when exposed to UV irradiation
    - Metabolized to 250HD3 in the liver, then to $1a,25(OH)2D3$ in the kidney
      - $1a,25(OH)2D3$ plays critical role in endocrine system
      - Incidence of lifestyle-related diseases (e.g., diabetes and osteoporosis) is significantly associated with 250HD3, but not with $1a,25(OH)2D3$.
    - Can be commercially synthesized
    - May have higher toxicity risk compared with D2
- Vitamin D is fat soluble.
  - Absorbed in the intestine
- Fraction of vitamin D may be absorbed by fat cells.
  - Obese individuals may need higher intake of the vitamin.
- Metabolism
  - Liver metabolism
    - Plays an important role in vitamin D metabolism and vitamin D functions
    - Critical role in hydroxylation pathway and formation of biologically active metabolites
    - Liver is the major productive organ for 250HD3 and sole productive organ for DBH, which aids in delivering 250HD3 to tissues and stores it in the blood circulation.
  - Kidney metabolism
    - Kidneys are abundant in vitamin D receptors and play a major role in turning vitamin D into its active form.
    - A critical step of the endocrine regulatory process is the metabolism of 250HD to 1,25[OH]2D, and this is essential for maintaining homeostatic regulation of plasma calcium and phosphorus concentrations.
      - Promotes bone health
    - Calciferol is hydroxylated by the kidneys; this forms calcitiol (1,25-dihydroxychole-calciferol).
      - Biologically active form of vitamin D

- Functions of vitamin D
  - Intestinal absorption of calcium
    - Vitamin D, along with calcium, promotes bone building and keeps bones strong and healthy.
  - Blocks the release of parathyroid hormone
    - This hormone reabsorbs bone tissue, causing bones to become thin and brittle.
  - Bone mineralization.
- Deficiencies
  - Severely low levels of vitamin D
    - Soft, brittle bones
    - Bone pain
    - Muscle pain and weakness
- Clinical vitamin D deficiency is referred to as rickets in children and osteomalacia in adults.
  - Rickets in children
    - Skeletal condition caused by lack of vitamin D, calcium, or phosphate
    - Failure of cartilage to mature and mineralize normally
    - Signs and symptoms
      - Soft, weak bones
      - Stunted growth
      - Skeletal deformities (severe cases, rare)
    - Diagnosis
      - Blood test to measure calcium, phosphorus, and vitamin D levels
      - X-ray
  - Osteomalacia in adults
    - Softening of the bone owing to a severe deficiency of vitamin D
    - Inadequate bone mineralization
      - Low levels of vitamin D lead to the body not being able to process calcium for bone formation.
    - Signs and symptoms
      - Bones fracture easily
      - Muscle weakness and pain
      - Bone pain
        - Especially common in hips
    - Diagnosis
      - Blood test to measure calcium, phosphorus, and vitamin D levels
      - X-ray
      - Bone biopsy
    - Complete healing of the bones takes approximately 6 months.
    - Certain conditions can interfere with vitamin D absorption.
      - Celiac disease
        - Can damage intestinal lining and prevent absorption
      - Certain cancers
        - Interfere with vitamin D processing
      - Kidney and liver disorders
        - Affect the metabolism of vitamin D

- Certain medications
  - Phenytoin and phenobarbital (medications used to treat seizure disorders) can interfere with absorption of vitamin D.
- Vitamin D toxicity
  - Difficult to achieve
    - Typically from a combination of endogenous production and the consumption of typical supplements and fortified food sources
  - Typically causes hypercalcemia
    - Acute hypercalcemia signs and symptoms
      - Loss of appetite
      - Nausea
      - Vomiting
      - Dehydration
      - Renal impairment
      - Mental status change
      - Coma
        - If it is left untreated, it may be lethal.
    - Chronic hypercalcemia symptoms
      - Ectopic tissue calcification
      - End-organ dysfunction
- Vitamin C
  - Essential micronutrient
    - Humans must ingest vitamin C to survive.
  - Water soluble
  - Estimated average requirement
    - Adult
      - Males
        - 90 mg/day
      - Females
        - 75 mg/day
      - During pregnancy
        - 85 mg/day
      - During lactation
        - 120 mg/day
    - Children
      - Birth to 6 months of age
        - 40 mg/day
      - 7 to 12 months of age
        - 50 mg/day
      - Children 1 to 3 years of age
        - 15 mg/day
      - Children 4 to 8 years of age
        - 25 mg/day
      - Children 9 to 13 years of age
        - 45 mg/day
      - Adolescents
        - Males 14 to 18 years of age
          - 75 mg/day

- ○ Females 14 to 18 years of age
- ○ 65 mg/day
- Ascorbic acid
  - ▪ Reduced form of vitamin C
    - ▪ Six-carbon lactose is synthesized from glucose by many animals.
      - ○ Not synthesized by humans
        - ○ Humans lack gulonolactone oxidase, the terminal enzyme in the biosynthetic pathway of aerobic acid.
- Functions
  - ▪ Hydroxylation of procollagen
    - ▪ Helps the body form and maintain connective tissue, bones, blood vessels, and skin
  - ▪ Powerful antioxidant properties
- Deficiency signs and symptoms
  - ▪ Fatigue
  - ▪ Joint and muscle weakness and pain
  - ▪ Bleeding gums
  - ▪ Leg rash
  - ▪ Scurvy
    - ▪ Prolonged deficiency
    - ▪ Rare
    - ▪ Severe illness
- Sources of vitamin C
  - ▪ Synthesized in all green plants
  - ▪ Found in many fruits and vegetables
    - ▪ Fruits
      - ○ Cantaloupe
      - ○ Kiwi
      - ○ Strawberries
      - ○ Lemons
      - ○ Oranges
    - ▪ Vegetables
      - ○ Broccoli
      - ○ Red pepper
      - ○ Cauliflower
      - ○ Spinach
      - ○ Tomatoes
      - ○ Brussel sprouts
      - ○ Asparagus
    - ▪ Juices
      - ○ Orange
      - ○ Grapefruit
      - ○ Tomato
- Vitamin C toxicity
  - ▪ The body (for the average, healthy individual) can only hold and use 200 to 250 mg/day.
  - ▪ Greater than 2000 mg/day
    - ▪ Risk for kidney stones
    - ▪ Diarrhea

- Nausea
- Gastritis
- Special considerations
  - Anticoagulant drugs, such as warfarin (Coumadin), decrease action.
  - Some products may decrease levels of vitamin C.
    - Nicotine products
    - Oral contraceptives/estrogens
    - Tetracyclines
    - Barbiturates
    - Aspirin
  - Vitamin C may increase absorption of iron and lutein.

APPLICATION AND REVIEW

14. Which outcome is associated with a vitamin A deficiency?
    1. Hyperpigmentation of the skin
    2. Increased risk for infection
    3. Decreased mental alertness
    4. Respiratory failure
15. Which nutrient will need to be ingested in larger quantities by a client who is diagnosed as being obese?
    1. Sugar
    2. Starch
    3. Protein
    4. Vitamin D
16. What information should the nurse provide for an adult male client who consumes 2500 mg of vitamin C daily? **Select all that apply**.
    1. The body requires more vitamin C than is being consumed.
    2. This amount of daily vitamin C increases the risk for kidney stones.
    3. Body requirements are met when 150 mg of vitamin C are consumed daily.
    4. This amount of daily vitamin C increases the risk of developing muscle pain.
17. Which medical diagnosis places a client at an increased risk for ineffective vitamin D absorption?
    1. Obesity
    2. Celiac disease
    3. Gastroesophageal reflux disease
    4. Chronic obstructive pulmonary disease
18. A client is experiencing bleeding gums. Which statement made by the client indicates an understanding of dietary instructions provided by the nurse?
    1. "I've learned to enjoy a salad that contains tomatoes and broccoli."
    2. "Apple juice and some cheese is my favorite afternoon snack."
    3. "I really enjoy eating a bowl of fortified cereal at bedtime."
    4. "Dairy products are essential to my recovery."
19. A nurse should assess which client concerning dietary intake of vitamin D?
    1. A client who has reported fractures of three bones in the last 18 months
    2. A client who reports recently developing problems driving at night
    3. A client whose gums regularly bleed after brushing teeth
    4. A client who has developed several dark skin patches
20. A medical diagnosis of osteomalacia is likely to require the nurse to educate the client about which treatment modality?
    1. Weight-bearing exercise
    2. Vitamin A supplements
    3. Vitamin D supplements
    4. Iron injections

See Answers on pages 103–105.

ANSWER KEY: REVIEW QUESTIONS

1. **Answers: 1, 2, 3.**

   1, 2, 3 The utilization of foods by living organisms is essential for normal growth, reproduction, and health maintenance.

   4 Ineffective oxygenation is not a direct result of poor nutrient utilization. **5** Tumor formation is not a direct result of poor nutrient utilization.

   Client Need: Physiological Adaptation; **Cognitive Level:** Understanding; **Integrated Process:** Teaching and Learning

2. **Answers: 2, 3.**

   2 Human nutritional health requires macronutrients in large amounts. **3** Macronutrients provide the body with energy in the form of carbohydrates.

   1 Micronutrients have an impact on human health, especially in pregnant women and children. **4** Protein is found in egg whites. **5** Micronutrients include iron, copper, zinc, iodine, and fluoride.

   Client Need: Physiological Adaptation; **Cognitive Level:** Understanding; **Integrated Process:** Teaching and Learning.

3. **Answers: 1, 2, 3, 4.**

   1, 2, 3, 4 The predicted dietary energy intake average needed to maintain energy balance in a healthy adult within a certain age, gender, weight, height, and physical activity level.

   5 Allergies are not a consideration because they have little effect on energy needs.

   Client Need: Physiological Adaptation; **Cognitive Level:** Understanding; **Integrated Process:** Teaching and Learning.

4. **Answers: 2, 3.**

   2 Carbohydrates should comprise between 45% and 65% of one's daily diet. **3** Lipids (fats) should comprise 20% to 35% of one's daily diet.

   1 This client's diet is outside the accepted range on two of the nutrients considered. **4** The client's protein intake is too high and needs to be decreased. **5** The client is not eating a well-balanced diet; lipids and protein are not within recommended ranges.

   Client Need: Physiological Adaptation; **Cognitive Level:** Applying; **Nursing Process:** Implementation

5. **3** Marasmus is a condition triggered by the lack of energy-producing protein in the diet; it is associated with tuberculosis (TB).

   1 Bulimia is an eating disorder with a psychosocial foundation; it is not generally considered a comorbid condition associated with TB. **2** Rickets is a vitamin D deficiency; it is not generally considered a comorbid condition associated with TB. **4** Anorexia nervous is an eating disorder with a psychosocial foundation; it is not generally considered a comorbid condition associated with TB.

   Client Need: Physiological Adaptation; **Cognitive Level:** Understanding; **Integrated Process:** Teaching and Learning

6. **Answers: 1, 2, 3.**

   1, 2, 3 Kwashiorkor is a nutritional condition resulting from a severe protein deficiency. Signs and symptoms include a yellow-orange discoloration of hair and dermatosis (with skin ulcers and light patches).

   4, 5 These are not signs and symptoms of Kwashiorkor.

   Client Need: Physiological Adaptation; **Cognitive Level:** Analysis; **Nursing Process:** Assessment/Analysis

7. **4 Anorexia nervosa is a psychiatric disease characterized by a constant disturbance of eating habits and/or weight control negatives that result in significantly impaired physical health and psychosocial functioning. Physiologic stabilization of the client is the admission priority.**

   1 Although anxiety is believed to be the trigger for this condition, physiologic treatment for current disorders takes priority over psychosocial therapies. **2** Although family counseling is an appropriate intervention, physiologic treatment for current disorders takes priority over psychosocial therapies. **3** Whereas improving self-image is a focus of therapy for this condition, physiologic treatment for current disorders takes priority over psychosocial therapies.

   Client Need: Physiological Adaptation; **Cognitive Level:** Applying; **Nursing Process:** Planning

8. **1 Psychological features associated with anorexia nervosa include inflexible thinking. Being rigid about breakfast demonstrates that characteristic.**

    2 The client with anorexia nervosa would tend to wear clothing that covers the body to hide perceived imperfections. **3** The client with anorexia nervosa strives for perfection; such grades would not be acceptable. **4** Although hypothermia is a characteristic of anorexia nervosa, it is a physiologic, not psychological, characteristic.

    Client Need: Psychological Adaptation; **Cognitive Level:** Analysis; **Nursing Process:** Assessment

9. **Answers: 1, 3, 4.**

    1 Anorexia nervosa is commonly associated with several different psychiatric conditions including anxiety. **3** Anorexia nervosa is commonly associated with several different psychiatric conditions including substance abuse. **4** Anorexia nervosa is commonly associated with several different psychiatric conditions including depression.

    2 Anorexia nervosa is not commonly associated with hallucinations. **5** Anorexia nervosa is not commonly associated with paranoia.

    Client Need: Psychological Adaptation; **Cognitive Level:** Analysis; **Nursing Process:** Assessment

10. **Answers: 1, 3, 4.**

    1 Bulimia nervosa is characterized by recurrent episodes of binge eating followed by one or more compensatory behaviors that include compulsive exercise. **3** Bulimia nervosa is characterized by recurrent episodes of binge eating followed by one or more compensatory behaviors that include self-induced vomiting. **4** Bulimia nervosa is characterized by recurrent episodes of binge eating followed by one or more compensatory behaviors that include regular use of laxatives.

    2 The anorexic client will report feeling cold. **5** The anorexic client severely restricts food intake.

    Client Need: Physiological Adaptation; **Cognitive Level:** Understanding; **Integrated Process:** Teaching and Learning

11. **1 Psychiatric conditions associated with bulimia nervosa include acts of self-injury such ` hair pulling.**

    2 Hoarding is not a psychiatric condition associated with bulimia nervosa. **3** Compulsive lying is not a psychiatric condition associated with bulimia nervosa. **4** Kleptomania, the recurrent inability to resist urges to steal items that generally are not needed and that usually have little value, is not associated with bulimia nervosa.

    Client Need: Psychological Adaptation; **Cognitive Level:** Applying; **Nursing Process:** Assessment

12. **1 Anorexia nervosa is more prevalent among females living in westernized, post-industrialized societies such as America.**

    2, 3 Anorexia nervosa is more prevalent among females, especially those living in westernized, post-industrialized societies. **4** Although anorexia nervosa is more prevalent in females, it is diagnosed more often among females living in westernized, post-industrialized societies.

    Client Need: Psychosocial Adaptation; **Cognitive Level:** Analysis; **Nursing Process:** Assessment

13. **Answers: 1, 2, 3.**

    1, 2, 3 Physical and clinical signs and symptoms of bulimia nervosa include enamel erosion leading to oral cavities, arrhythmias, and calluses on the knuckles from the act of self-induced vomiting.

    4 Brittle hair is noted in clients diagnosed with anorexia nervosa. **5** Amenorrhea (absence of menses) is noted in clients diagnosed with anorexia nervosa.

    Client Need: Physiological Adaptation; **Cognitive Level:** Understanding; **Integrated Process:** Teaching and Learning

14. **2 Deficiency of vitamin A can result in the suppression of the immune system causing an increased risk for infection.**

    1 Hyperpigmentation of the skin is not associated with a vitamin A deficiency. **3** Mental alertness is not associated with a vitamin A deficiency. **4** A vitamin A deficiency is not known to cause respiratory failure.

    Client Need: Physiological Adaptation; **Cognitive Level:** Understanding; **Integrated Process:** Teaching and Learning

15. **4 Vitamin D is fat soluble and can be absorbed by fat cells. Obese individuals may need a higher intake of the vitamin to provide a sufficient available quantity.**

    1 Obesity does not present a sugar absorption problem. 2 Obesity does not present a starch absorption problem. 3 Obesity does not present a protein absorption problem.

    Client Need: Physiological Adaptation; **Cognitive Level:** Understanding; **Integrated Process:** Teaching and Learning

16. **2 Vitamin C is an essential micronutrient. Estimated average requirement for an adult male is 90 mg/day. Intake over 2000 mg/day increases the risk for the development of kidney stones.**

    1 The estimated average requirement for an adult male is 90 mg/day. 3 The estimated average requirement for an adult male is 90 mg/day. 4 The estimated average requirement for an adult male is 90 mg/day. A deficiency of vitamin C could result in muscle pain.

    Client Need: Physiological Adaptation; **Cognitive Level:** Applying; **Integrated Process:** Teaching and Learning

17. **2 Celiac disease is a condition that can interfere with the absorption of vitamin D.**

    1 Obesity is not known to interfere with the absorption of vitamin D. 3 Gastroesophageal reflex disease is not known to interfere with the absorption of vitamin D. 4 Chronic obstructive pulmonary disease is not known to interfere with the absorption of vitamin D.

    Client Need: Physiological Adaptation; **Cognitive Level:** Understanding; **Integrated Process:** Teaching and Learning

18. **1 Bleeding gums is a sign of a vitamin C deficiency. Sources of vitamin C include tomatoes and broccoli.**

    2 Neither cheese nor apple juice are good sources of vitamin C. 3 Cereals are fortified with vitamins A, B, and D, folic acid, iodine, and iron. 4 Dairy products are not considered to be good sources of vitamin C.

    Client Need: Physiological Adaptation; **Cognitive Level:** Applying; **Nursing Process:** Evaluation

19. **1 Vitamin D deficiency results in soft, brittle bones that fracture easily.**

    2 Night blindness is associated with a deficiency of vitamin A. 3 Bleeding gums are associated with a deficiency of vitamin C. 4 Protein deficiency is more likely responsible for the development of dark patches of skin.

    Client Need: Physiological Adaptation; **Cognitive Level:** Applying; **Nursing Process:** Assessment

20. **3 Osteomalacia is the softening of the bone caused by a severe deficiency of vitamin D.**

    1 Weight-bearing exercise is prescribed for osteoporosis to help prevent bone loss. 2 Osteomalacia is a result of a vitamin D deficiency; Vitamin A supplements would not benefit the client with osteomalacia. 4 Osteomalacia is a result of a vitamin D deficiency; iron injections would not benefit the client with osteomalacia.

    Client Need: Physiological Adaptation; **Cognitive Level:** Applying; **Nursing Process:** Planning

6 Infection

MICROBIOLOGY AND INFECTION OVERVIEW

- Microbiology is the study of microorganisms or microbes. These small living forms are visible only through a microscope.
- Microorganisms consist of viruses, bacteria, fungi, and parasites (protozoa).
- The process of infection includes
  - Colonization
  - Invasion
  - Multiplication
  - Dissemination

Microorganisms

- Microorganism classification
  - Morphologic characteristics
  - Life cycles
- Types of microorganisms (virus, bacteria, fungi, parasites)
  - Virus
    - Small obligate intracellular parasite
    - Requires a living host cell for replication
    - Most contain DNA
    - Simple microorganisms
    - Most common affliction of humans
    - During replication tend to mutate
      - Change slightly
    - Structure
      - Nucleic acid
      - Protein shell
      - Capsid
    - Classification
      - The format of the nucleic acid within the vision (RNA or DNA)
      - Whether it is single-stranded (ss) or double-stranded (ds)
      - If the virus uses reverse transcriptase (RT) for replication
    - Directly damage or destroy infected cells
      - May remain in a latent stage
      - Enter host cell and slowly replicate or do not replicate until later
    - Seven classifications
      - dsDNA
        - Herpes virus
        - Smallpox virus
      - ssDNA
        - Parvovirus

- dsRNA
  - Rotavirus
- ssRNA +sense
  - Hepatitis A and C viruses
  - Severe acute respiratory syndrome virus
  - Poliovirus
  - Rhinovirus
- ssRNA −sense
  - Ebola virus
  - Marburg virus
  - Influenza
  - Certain viruses that cause measles, mumps, rabies, Lassa virus, and hantavirus
- ssRNA +sense with RT
  - Human immunodeficiency virus (HIV)
- dsDNA with RT
  - Hepatitis B virus
- Bacteria
  - Prokaryotic cells
    - Simple, single-cell structure
      - Unicellular
    - Lack a nuclear membrane
    - Function metabolically
    - Can reproduce
  - Do not require living tissue to survive
  - Many bacteria are classified as nonpathogenic because they do not usually cause disease, in fact they often are beneficial.
  - Pathogens "germs" are the disease-causing bacteria.
  - Major groups of bacteria (based on cellular shape)
    - Bacilli
      - Rod-shaped
        - Vibrio
          - Curved rods
    - Spirals
      - Coiled shape
        - Spirochetes
        - Spirilla
    - Cocci
      - Spherical forms
  - Cells can be categorized by other characteristics
    - Diplo
      - Pairs
    - Strep(to)
      - Chains
    - Staph(ylo)
      - Irregular clusters
    - Tetras
      - Cells grouped in a packet or square of four cells

- Palisade
  - ○ Cells lying together with long sides parallel
- Pili and fimbriae are found on some bacteria. These tiny, hairlike projections are usually on gram-negative bacteria.
  - Assist in attachment
  - Facilitate transfer of genetic material between cells
- Certain bacteria secrete toxic substances
  - Exotoxins
    - ○ Produced by gram-positive bacteria
    - ○ Diffuse through body fluids
    - ○ Often interfere with nerve conduction
  - Endotoxins
    - ○ Present in gram-negative bacteria
    - ○ Released once the bacteria die
    - ○ May cause fever, weakness, and have serious effects on the circulatory system
- Superbugs
  - Drug-resistant bacteria
  - May lead to pandemic
- Fungi
  - Fungi are found everywhere
    - Animals
    - Plants
    - Humans
    - Foods
      - ○ Often growth can be seen on cheese, fruits, and bread
  - Fungi consist of single cells or chains of cells.
  - Hyphae
    - Long filaments of a fungus
    - Intertwine to form mycelium
      - ○ Visible mass
  - Fungi spores
    - Travel easily through air
    - Resistant to chemicals and temperature changes
    - Can stimulate allergic reaction in humans
  - Few fungi are pathogenic.
    - Causing infection in skin or mucous membranes
    - Most common contaminants of food and food surfaces
      - ○ Ability to grow on a wide range of environmental conditions
  - Mycosis is an infection from a fungus.
    - Damages tissue by secretion of enzymes and initiation of an inflammatory response
    - Eukaryotic microorganisms
    - Thick, rigid cell walls
    - May also grow as mold (aerobic), yeast (anaerobes), or dimorphic
    - Fungal cell composition is similar to the human cell.
    - Diagnosed by microscopic observation
  - Protozoa
    - Usually parasites
    - Complex eukaryotic organisms

- Unicellular
  - Commonly motile
  - Lack cell wall
  - Occur in many shapes
    - Within single life cycle
- How they live
  - Independently
  - On dead organic matter
  - In or on another living host
- Diseases caused by protozoan
  - Trichomoniasis
    - Distinguished by its flagella
    - Causes sexually transmitted infection to reproductive tract
    - Affects men and women
    - Attaches to mucous membranes
    - Causes inflammation
  - Malaria
    - Plasmodium species
    - Sporozoa
      - Nonmotile
    - Found in red blood cells
    - Transmitted by blood-sucking insects
      - Anopheles mosquito (female)
      - Global warming aids in extending the range of this mosquito and will increase the risk to larger population of people.
  - Amebic dysentery
    - Motile group
    - Ameboid movement
      - Extending part of their cytoplasm and flowing forward
      - How they engulf food.
  - *Entameba histolytica*
    - Large intestine
    - Causes amebic dysentery
      - Severe diarrhea
      - Potential liver abscesses
    - Form of *E. histolytica*
      - Trophozoite
        - Actively pathogenic
        - Secretes proteolytic enzymes
        - Forms cysts
        - Invades blood vessels and may spread to organs (e.g., liver)
    - Spread by fecal–oral route
    - Common in less developed countries
  - Giardia
    - Cause of gastrointestinal infections
    - Causes of giardia
      - Consumption of contaminated food/water
      - Person-to-person contact

- ○ Cyst forming
- ○ Excreted in feces
- ○ Can survive for a long period of time until ingested by host.
  - ■ Other agents of disease
    - ○ Helminths (worms)
      - ○ Worms, not microorganisms
      - ○ Parasites
      - ○ Multicellular
      - ○ Eukaryotic organisms
      - ○ Subgroups are determined based on physical characteristics
      - ○ Life cycles is three stages.
        - Ovum (egg)
        - Larva
        - Adult
      - ○ Often found in intestine

APPLICATION AND REVIEW

1. Which type of microorganism requires a living host to replicate?
   1. Bacteria
   2. Fungi
   3. Protozoa
   4. Viruses
2. The term pathogen is used to describe what microorganism?
   1. Viruses in the latent stage of their life cycle
   2. Fungi that are heat and chemical resistant
   3. Protozoa that live in or on a living host
   4. Disease-producing bacteria

See Answers on pages 125–127.

Resident Flora

- Found in many areas of the body (Table 6.1)
- Indigenous normal flora
  - Found in or on the human body
  - Semipermanent bases

TABLE 6.1   Location of Resident Flora

Resident Flora Present	Sterile Area
Skin	Blood, cerebrospinal fluid
Nose, pharynx	Lungs
Mouth, colon, rectum	
Vagina	Uterus, fallopian tubes, ovary
Distal urethra and perineum	Bladder and kidney

From Hubert, R. J., & VanMeter, K. C. (2018). *Gould's Pathophysiology for the Health Professions* (6th ed.). Philadelphia: Saunders.

- Resident microbiota (resident flora)
  - Found on the surface of the skin and under superficial cells
  - Permanent bases
- Most flora microbes are not pathogenic under normal circumstances.
- Flora causes disease when transferred to another location in the body.
- Opportunistic infection
  - If balance between flora is not maintained or the body's immune system is impaired.

APPLICATION AND REVIEW

3. What increases the risk of an individual developing an opportunistic infection?
   1. An impaired immune system
   2. Resident flora resides on the skin
   3. Indigenous flora exists in the gastrointestinal tract
   4. When resident and indigenous flora exist in equal amounts

See Answers on pages 125–127

Principles of Infection

- Transmission includes a chain of events that transfers the infecting organism from one person or organism to another.
  - Reservoir
    - Source of infection
      - Human
      - Animal
      - Contaminated food, water, soil, or equipment
  - Carrier
    - Carry, yet never develop infection
  - Direct transmission occurs when there is direct contact with infections from another individual.
    - Microbes may be in blood, body secretions, or lesion(s).
      - Physical contact
      - Ingestion
      - Inhalation
      - Placental transfer
    - An individual with a deficient immune system can become infected with opportunistic infections.
  - Indirect transmission occurs when there is contact with contaminated materials
    - Contaminated hands
    - Towels
    - Contaminated food
    - Sheets
    - Clothing
    - Toys
    - Bandages
  - Droplet transmission
    - Oral or respiratory
    - Secretions inhaled directly by another person or nearby objects transmit the pathogens indirectly.

- Aerosol transmission
  - Respiratory tract particles
  - Small particles remain suspended in air until inhaled by another person.
- Vector-borne transmission
  - Insect or animal serves as vector.
    - Mosquitos
    - Ticks
    - Mites
    - Lice
    - Snails
    - Blackflies
- Nosocomial infection transmission
  - Occurs in health care facilities
    - Hospitals
    - Clinics
    - Nursing homes
    - Dental offices
  - The Centers for Disease Control and Prevention (CDC) estimate that 10% to 15% of patients acquire an infection in the hospital.
  - Reasons for nosocomial infections
    - Large presence of microorganisms in environment
    - Contaminated instruments and equipment
    - Overcrowding
    - Transmission through health care providing staff
    - Presence of contagious diseases
    - Presence of medication-resistant microbes
  - Most frequent occurring nosocomial infections
    - Pneumonia
    - Gastrointestinal
    - Urinary tract
    - Bloodstream
    - Postsurgical
- Host resistance
  - Defense mechanism
  - Interferons
    - Signaling proteins released by human host cells
    - Cytokines (cell signaling molecules) are produced by white blood cells.
    - These proteins interfere with the production of new viral replication.
  - Certain factors may decrease host resistance.
    - Age
      - Infants and elderly
    - Genetic susceptibility
      - Any type of immunodeficiency
    - Malnutrition
    - Chronic disease
      - Cardiac disease
      - Cancer
      - Diabetes

- Severe physical or emotional stress
- Inflammation or trauma to skin or mucous
  - Invasive procedures
  - Insertion of catheter
  - Burns
- Inflammatory response that is impaired.

APPLICATION AND REVIEW

4. Which nursing interventions are implemented to minimize a client's risk for the indirect transmission of an infection? **Select all that apply**.
   1. Effective handwashing
   2. Using gloves to handle soiled linen
   3. Providing masks to visitors with coughs
   4. Substituting disposable cups for glass ones
   5. Encouraging the client to shower rather than tub bath
5. How can a vector-borne infection be transmitted?
   1. Drinking from a contaminated cup
   2. Being bitten by an infected tick
   3. Being cut with a dirty knife
   4. Eating spoiled food
6. Which nonhospitalized client is at greatest risk for being exposed to a nosocomial transmitted infection?
   1. A client diagnosed with influenza
   2. A client recovering from a fractured humerus
   3. A client having an impacted wisdom tooth extracted
   4. A client with a history of chronic exercised-induced asthma
7. The residents of a long-term care facility are at greatest risk for developing which nosocomial infections? **Select all that apply**.
   1. Otitis media
   2. Pneumonia
   3. Gastritis
   4. Sinusitis
   5. Cystitis
8. Which clients have a decreased resistance against infections? **Select all that apply**.
   1. A 3-month-old premature infant
   2. A 5-year-old child starting preschool
   3. An 18-year-old adult who smokes cigarettes
   4. A 40-year-old adult with a history of alcohol abuse
   5. A 65-year-old adult diagnosed with acute depression

See Answers on pages 125–127.

Virulence and Pathogenicity of Microorganisms
- Pathogenicity refers to the ability of microbes to cause disease.
- Nonpathogen microbes can turn into pathogens when introduced into another area of the body.
- Virulence refers to the degree of damage a microbe causes its host; this is based on several factors.
  - Invasive qualities
  - Toxic qualities
  - Adherence to tissue at receptor sites
  - Ability to avoid host defense
    - Frequent mutation allows microorganisms to avoid host defense.

Control of Transmission and Infection

- It is not feasible that health care professionals test every patient for infection prior to administering care.
- Avoiding transmission is dependent on
  - Infection control
  - Understanding transmission
  - Breaking transmission chain
- Standard precautions
  - Basic guidelines for health care professionals to follow when handling blood, body fluids, and waste
  - Applicable to all patients, regardless of apparent condition
- Techniques to reduce transmission
  - Adequate cleaning
  - Sterilization
  - Destruction of microorganisms using heat
    - Autoclaving
  - Time, packaging, and proper temperature are essential to destroy microorganisms effectively.
  - Disinfectants
    - Chemical solutions that destroy microorganisms on nonliving surfaces
      - Chemical solutions must have adequate exposure time and concentration mix.
  - Antiseptics
    - Chemical solutions that destroy microorganisms on living tissues
      - Isopropyl alcohol
- Factors that influence transmission of microorganisms
  - Communicability
    - Ability to spread
  - Immunogenicity
    - Ability to produce immune response
  - Infectivity
    - Ability to invade/multiply in host
  - Mechanism of action
    - How tissue is damaged
  - Pathogenicity
    - Ability of organism to cause disease and harm host
  - Portal of entry
    - Route of infection
      - Direct contact
      - Inhalation
        - Ingestion
        - Animal or insect bites
  - Toxigenicity
    - Ability to produce toxins or endotoxins
  - Virulence
    - Capacity to cause severe disease
      - Measles is low virulence
      - Rabies is high virulence

- Infections are also classified by prevalence and spread in the community.
  - Endemic
    - High and constant rate of infection in a specific population
  - Epidemic
    - Number of new infections in specific population exceeds the number normally observed.
  - Pandemic
    - Epidemic that spreads over large area (continental or worldwide)

APPLICATION AND REVIEW

9. What mechanism does autoclaving use to manage the transmission of disease-producing microorganisms?
   1. Chemical destruction of the microorganism on nonliving surfaces
   2. Chemical destruction of the microorganism on living surfaces
   3. Effective packaging as a barrier to microorganism growth
   4. Use of heat to destroy the microorganism
10. Which situations is an example of an endemic?
    1. Malaria in sub-Saharan Africa
    2. Tuberculosis (TB) in the northern hemisphere
    3. Acquired immunodeficiency syndrome (AIDS) worldwide
    4. Severe acute respiratory syndrome (SARS) in Britain and Ireland

See Answers on pages 125–127.

Physiology of Infection

- Onset and development (Fig. 6.1)
  - Onset is the first appearance of the signs or symptoms of an infection.
  - Development of microorganisms is dependent on
    - Microorganisms gaining entry to the body
    - Finding a hospitable site
    - Establishing a colony
    - Reproducing
  - Incubation period
    - Time from exposure to clinical appearance
    - Timeline can vary depending on characteristics of organism
    - Can last from days to months
  - Prodromal period
    - Early symptoms stage
    - Fatigue, loss of appetite, headache
  - Acute period
    - Full development of disease
    - Clinical manifestations reach peak
    - Length
      - Dependent on virulence of pathogen and host resistance
  - Convalescent period
    - Recovery
    - Signs and symptoms subside and body returns to normal state.

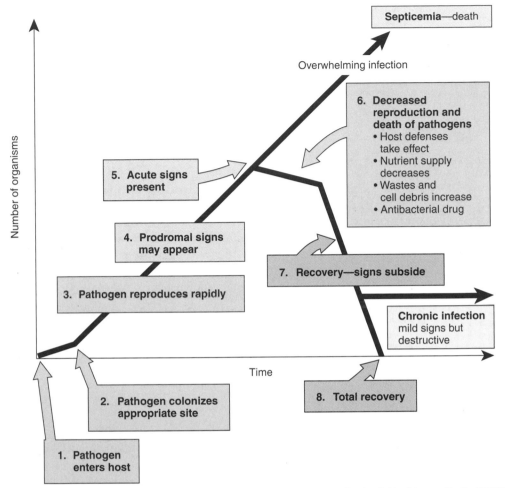

FIG. 6.1   Onset and possible courses of infection. (From Hubert, R. J., & VanMeter, K. C. [2018]. *Gould's pathophysiology for the health professions* [6th ed.]. Philadelphia: Saunders.)

- Patterns of infection vary depending on characteristics or location.
  - Local infection
    - Infection is restricted to specific location.
  - Focal infection
    - Spread from specific (local) infection to other tissues
  - Systemic infection
    - Several sites become infected, often through the circulatory system.
      - Septicemia
        - Cause of sepsis
          - Microorganisms multiply in the blood.
          - Toxic inflammatory condition
      - Bacteremia
        - Bacteria in the blood

- Toxemia
  - Toxins in the blood
- Viremia
  - Viruses in the blood
- Mixed infections
  - A range of infections concurrently established at the same site
- Acute infections
  - Rapidly appearing
  - Severe symptoms
  - Short lived
- Chronic infections
  - Less severe symptoms
  - Persist for longer period of time
- Primary infections
  - Initial infection
- Secondary infections
  - Follows primary
  - Caused by a different microbe
  - Often opportunistic pathogens
- Subclinical infections
  - No apparent symptoms
  - May persist for longer period of time
- Signs and symptoms of infection
  - Local signs of infection
    - Inflammation
      - Pain
      - Swelling
      - Redness
      - Warmth
    - Viral compared with bacterial
      - Viral
        - Clear exudates
      - Bacterial
        - Purulent exudates
        - Pus
  - Systemic signs and symptoms of infection
    - Fever
    - Fatigue
    - Weakness
    - Headache
    - Nausea
  - May present as clinical or subclinical
    - Clinical
      - Measurable signs and symptoms
    - Subclinical
      - No signs or symptoms although infection is present
  - Effects may be acute or chronic
    - Secondary to immune and inflammatory responses

- Consequences of toxins
- Injury to infected cells
- Most symptoms are caused by the individual's own inflammatory response.
- Initial signs and symptoms
  - Fever
    - Beneficial adaptive host-defense response
    - Hypothalamus is the central thermostat for the body.
    - Body temperature being regulated at higher than normal level
    - Pyrogens, when introduced or released into the blood, produce fever.
  - Fatigue
  - Malaise
  - Weakness
  - Loss of concentration
  - Body aching
  - Loss of appetite
- Clinical manifestations vary depending on pathogen, organ system affected, and intensity of inflammatory response.
- Methods of diagnosis
  - Many microbes can be grown in a laboratory in a Petri dish. This environment is appropriate for the growth of specific microbial groups.
  - Culture and staining techniques
    - Uses specific specimens
      - Sputum
  - Testing to identify infection
    - Blood test
      - Bacterial infections
        - Leukocytosis
          - Increase in white blood cells
      - Viral infections
        - Leukopenia
          - Reduction of leukocytes in the blood
      - Acute infection
        - Increase in neutrophils
      - Chronic infection
        - Increase in lymphocytes and monocytes.
    - Rapid diagnostic test (RDT)
      - Based on metabolic and serologic characteristics
      - Quick and accurate identification
      - Easy to perform
    - Radiologic examination
      - Identify site of infection
      - May aid in identification of organism
  - Drug sensitivity test
    - Kirby-Bauer method (KB test)
      - Antibiotic testing
      - Uses antibiotic disks to test whether bacteria are susceptible to certain antibiotics.

- Minimum inhibitory concentration (MIC) method
  - Incubation technique
  - Test to determine the lowest concentration of a drug that is needed to inhibit the growth of a microorganism
- Viruses will grow only in living host.

Infectious Illnesses

- Influenza
  - Respiratory transmission
  - Viral infection
    - May affect upper and lower respiratory tracts
  - ssRNA virus
    - Myxovirus group
      - Transmitted via aerosol and body fluids
      - Usually sudden, acute onset
        - Fever
        - Chills
        - Malaise
        - Headache
        - General muscle aching
        - Sore throat
        - Unproductive or dry cough
        - Nasal congestion
  - Several variant forms
  - Virus undergoes antigen shifts which allow them to evade vaccine protection.
  - Virus can survive at room temperatures for up to 2 weeks.
  - Heat and some disinfectants (ethanol and detergents) can destroy a virus.
  - Three subgroups of the influenza virus
    - Type A
      - Most prevalent
      - Difficult to control
        - Undergoes frequent mutations
        - Limits ability to develop long-term immunity
          - As new strands emerge, immunization through vaccines become complicated.
        - Cause epidemics and pandemics which tend to occur in cycles
    - Type B
      - Found only in humans (unlike type A)
      - May be less severe symptoms
      - Can cause outbreaks, but occur less frequently than influenza A outbreaks
    - Type C
      - Mild symptoms
        - Has potential to lead to more severe infections
          - Bronchitis
          - Pneumonia
      - In North America 5% to 20% of the population is affected annually.
      - All three strands have potential to lead to secondary complications.
        - Pneumonia

- Epidemiologists predict serious future pandemics.
- Influenza vaccination
  - Specifically designated each year
  - Monitored by the World Health Organization (WHO)
  - Administration
    - Intranasal spray
      - Live vaccine
    - Intramuscular injection
      - Inactivated or killed
      - Remains effective from 2 to 4 months
- Measles, mumps, and rubella (MMR)
  - Measles
    - Signs and symptoms
      - Fever
      - Rash
      - Cough
      - Runny nose
      - Watery, red eyes
      - Potential complications
        - Diarrhea
        - Ear infection
        - Pneumonia
        - Brain damage
        - Death
  - Mumps
    - Signs and symptoms
      - Fever
      - Headache
      - Body aches
      - Fatigue
      - Loss of appetite
      - Swollen salivary glands
      - Potential complications
        - Deafness
        - Swelling of testicles or ovaries
        - Inflammation of brain/surrounding tissue
        - Inflammation of spinal cord
        - Death (rarely)
  - Rubella
    - Signs and symptoms
      - Fever
      - Sore throat
      - Rash
      - Headache
      - Itchy, red eyes
    - Potential complications
      - During pregnancy could potentially cause miscarriage or serious birth defects to the baby

- MMR vaccine
  - Children should get two doses.
    - First dose at 12 to 15 months
    - Second dose at 4 to 6 years of age
- Methicillin-resistant *Staphylococcus aureus* (MRSA)
  - Gram-positive bacteria
  - Accounts for 80% of *S. aureus* infections
  - Carries an extra chromosomal gene for resistance
  - Small proteins bind to the target and prevent treatment with the antibiotic.
  - Can be caused by overuse of antibiotics and not completing regimen
- Herpes (simplex, zoster)
  - Virus that causes infection for life of host
    - May have dormant stages
  - Herpes simplex virus (HSV)
    - HSV-1
      - Oral herpes
        - Cold sores
    - HSV-2
      - Genital herpes
  - Herpes zoster
    - Varicella zoster virus (VZV)
      - Chickenpox
        - Initial infection
      - Shingles
        - When signs and symptoms occur after initial infection with chickenpox
        - Usually occurs as an individual ages or with immunosuppression
- Mononucleosis
  - Infectious mononucleosis
    - Called mono or kissing disease
- Epstein-Barr virus (EBV)
  - Virus that causes mono
  - Herpes virus family
    - Human herpes virus 4 (HHV-4)
  - Prevalent in high school and college aged population
  - Once infected, will most likely develop immunity, very unlikely to get it again
  - Spreads through saliva
  - Self treatable
  - Signs and symptoms
    - High fever
    - Swollen lymph glands
    - Sore throat
    - Fatigue
    - Body aches
  - Resolves within days to weeks
- Lyme disease
  - Boreliosis
  - Tick-borne illness
    - *Borrelia burgdorferi* bacterium

- Transmitted to humans by a bite
- Carried by deer ticks
  - Signs and symptoms
    - Rash
      - Often bulls-eye pattern
    - Flu-like signs and symptoms
      - Fever
      - Chills
      - Headache
      - Fatigue
      - Joint pain
      - Weakness to limbs
  - Resolves within days to weeks
- Rabies
  - Zoonotic infection
  - Spread by animal bite
    - Carried in saliva of infected animal
      - Bats
      - Coyotes
      - Foxes
      - Skunks
      - Raccoons
  - Signs and symptoms
    - Fever
    - Headache
    - Excess salivation
    - Muscle spasms
    - Paralysis
    - Altered mental status
    - Once symptoms appear, nearly always fatal
- Respiratory syncytial virus (RSV)
  - Highly contagious
  - Spreads through droplets
    - Can live on surfaces
  - Common among children
  - Most common cause of bronchitis
  - Signs and symptoms
    - Mild, cold-like
      - Stuffy or runny nose
      - Sore throat
      - Mild headache
      - Cough
      - Fever
      - General malaise
  - Usually resolves within 1 to 2 weeks
- Salmonellosis
  - Bacteria

- Caused by ingested substances (food, water) which may be contaminated by small amounts of human feces
- Most common among children
  - Individuals with compromised immune systems are more likely to have severe cases.
- Signs and symptoms
  - Diarrhea
  - Fever
  - Chills
  - Abdominal pain
- Resolves within days to weeks
- Toxoplasmosis
  - *Toxoplasma gondi* parasite
    - Found in cat feces and contaminated food
    - Causes serious complications with pregnant women
    - One of the world's most common parasites
  - Spreads easily
  - Signs and symptoms
    - Muscle pain
    - Fever
    - Headache
  - Resolves within months
- Vancomycin-resistant enterococcus (VRE)
  - Gram-positive bacteria that is resistant to the antibiotic vancomycin
  - Spread from one person to another
    - Often spread in health care environments
      - Nosocomial infection
    - Casual contact or through contaminated objects
- *Clostridium difficile*
  - Opportunistic infection
  - Most common risk factor is prolonged antibiotic therapy.
  - Antibiotic use can cause alterations in the microbiome, which can cause overgrowth of opportunistic microorganisms.
  - A genus anaerobic gram-positive bacteria that creates some of the most powerful toxins known
  - Spores
    - Can live on hard surfaces for as long as 5 months
      - Proper disinfection is necessary to prevent spread.
  - Signs and symptoms
    - Watery diarrhea
      - 10+ times a day
    - Abdominal pain
    - Fever
    - Bloating
    - Potentially could lead to pseudomembranous colitis
      - Destructive inflammatory disease of large intestine
      - Life-threatening
  - Usually resolves (with antibiotic treatment) within a week or two

APPLICATION AND REVIEW

11. A client is suspected of having rabies. For which clinical indicators should the nurse assess the client? **Select all that apply.**
    1. Hyperactivity
    2. Altered mental status
    3. Headache
    4. Excessive salivation
    5. Muscle spasms

12. A nurse in a public health clinic is teaching clients how to prevent toxoplasmosis. What should the nurse instruct the clients to avoid?
    1. Contact with cat feces
    2. Working with heavy metals
    3. Ingestion of freshwater fish
    4. Excessive radiation exposure

13. Which client would be at highest risk to develop a vancomycin-resistant enterococcus (VRE) infection?
    1. A resident of a long-term care facility
    2. A client diagnosed with pneumonia
    3. An immunosuppressed child
    4. A pregnant client

14. What intervention should individuals be taught to minimize the risk of developing salmonellosis?
    1. The use of masks when in direct contact with a contagious individual
    2. Avoiding contact with wild animals, including bats
    3. Proper handwashing, especially after toileting
    4. Use anti-tick repellant when outdoors

15. Which statement demonstrates the nurse's understanding of the characteristic clinical manifestation of Lyme disease?
    1. "The cervical lymph nodes feel like solid rocks."
    2. "The client's rash resembles a bulls-eye pattern."
    3. "Older clients develop a shingles-like rash."
    4. "The client presents with itchy, red eyes."

16. Which client requires special care when determining the risk for complications associated with an exposure to the rubella virus?
    1. A teenage adolescent demonstrating depression
    2. An older adult diagnosed with gastroesophageal reflux disease (GERD)
    3. A young adult with asthma
    4. A client who is pregnant

17. Which statement, if made by an older client, demonstrates an understanding of an appropriate strategy for avoiding the development of Methicillin resistant *Staphylococcus aureus* (MRSA) infection?
    1. "I'll take all the antibiotic medication I've been prescribed."
    2. "If I get another infection, I know that I'll need methicillin to get better."
    3. "I'll need to stay away from my grandchildren when they get an infection."
    4. "Getting a parasitic infection will certainly increase my risk of developing MRSA."

18. Which statement, if made by a parent, demonstrates an understanding regarding the measles, mumps, and rubella (MMR) vaccination?
    1. "My child will need the first dose of the vaccine between 8 and 12 months of age."
    2. "My child will only need a rubella booster before going to school."
    3. "I'm pleased that the vaccination doesn't require a booster shot."
    4. "The second dose is required between 4 and 6 years of age."
19. Which assessment findings support the possibility that the client has contracted influenza? **Select all that apply**.
    1. Oral temperature of 100,6° F
    2. Requested "something for nausea"
    3. Client reports "feeling achy all over"
    4. Client claims an acute onset of symptoms
    5. Requested pain medication to relieve headache
20. Which statement, if made by the parent of a child diagnosed with measles, demonstrates an understanding of the possible complications? **Select all that apply**.
    1. "I'll encourage fluids if diarrhea is a problem."
    2. "It's a bad sign if my child develops a red rash."
    3. "A runny nose means my child's condition is worsening."
    4. "If my child reports having an ear ache, I'll call the clinic."
    5. "Pneumonia is a really bad problem that can come with the measles."

See Answers on pages 125–127.

ANSWER KEY: REVIEW QUESTIONS

1. **4 A virus requires a living host cell for replication to occur.**
   1 Bacteria do not require a living host to reproduce. 2 Fungi do not require a living host to reproduce. 3 Protozoa do not require a living host to reproduce.
   Client Need: Physiological Adaptation; **Cognitive Level:** Understanding; **Nursing Process:** Assessment/Analysis
2. **4 Many bacteria are classified as nonpathogenic because they do not usually cause disease, in fact they often are beneficial, but those that are disease-causing are referred to as pathogens.**
   1 The term pathogen is not used to refer to viruses in the latent stage of their life cycle. 2 The term pathogen is not used to refer to fungi that are heat and/or chemical resistant. 3 The term pathogen is not used to refer to protozoa that live in or on a living host.
   Client Need: Physiological Adaptation; **Cognitive Level:** Understanding; **Nursing Process:** Assessment/Analysis
3. **1 Opportunistic infections can occur if balance between flora is not maintained or the body's immune system is impaired.**
   2 Resident flora normally resides on the skin. 3 Indigenous flora does normally exist in the gastrointestinal tract. 4 When resident and indigenous flora exist in equal amounts, the individual is generally considered to be healthy.
   Client Need: Physiological Adaptation; **Cognitive Level:** Understanding; **Nursing Process:** Assessment/Analysis
4. **Answers: 1, 2, 4.**
   1 Indirect transmission occurs when there is contact with contaminated materials such as contaminated hands. 2 Indirect transmission occurs when there is contact with contaminated materials such as soiled linen. 4 Indirect transmission occurs when there is contact with contaminated materials such as contaminated glassware.
   3 Direct transmission occurs when there is direct contact with infections from another individual such as the inhalation of pathogens via droplet or aerosol transmission. 5 When done appropriately, a tub bath is no more likely to spread an infection as is a shower.
   Client Need: Physiological Adaptation; **Cognitive Level:** Applying; **Nursing Process:** Planning/Implementation

5. **2 Vector-borne infections are transmitted through contact with an infected animal or insect.**
   1 Coming into contact with a contaminated object, such as a cup, is an example of indirect transmission. **3** Coming into contact with a contaminated object, such as a dirty knife, is an example of indirect transmission. **4** Eating contaminated food is an example of indirect transmission.
   Client Need: Physiological Adaptation; **Cognitive Level:** Analysis; **Nursing Process:** Assessment/Analysis

6. **3 Nosocomial infection transmission occurs in health care facilities where there is a significant presence of pathogens. A client experiencing an invasive procedure at a dental office is at risk for such an infection.**
   1 The primary factor associated with the exposure to a nosocomial infection is time spent in a health care facility where there is a significant presence of pathogens and not a specific infection. **2** The primary factor associated with the exposure to a nosocomial infection is time spent in a health care facility where there is a significant presence of pathogens and not a specific injury. **4** Although chronic illness can increase the risk for developing an infection, the primary factor associated with the exposure to a nosocomial infection is time spent in a health care facility where there is a significant presence of pathogens and not a specific disease process.
   Client Need: Physiological Adaptation; **Cognitive Level:** Analysis; **Nursing Process:** Assessment/Analysis

7. **Answers: 2, 3, 5.**
   2 Pneumonia is a frequently occurring nosocomial infection. **3** Gastritis is a frequently occurring nosocomial infection. **5** Cystitis is a frequently occurring nosocomial infection.
   1 Otitis media is not a frequently occurring nosocomial infection. **4** Sinusitis is not a frequently occurring nosocomial infection.
   Client Need: Physiological Adaptation; **Cognitive Level:** Understanding; **Nursing Process:** Assessment/Analysis

8. **Answers: 1, 5.**
   1 Age affects host resistance, making the premature infant at risk for infections. **5** Age and emotional stress affect host resistance, making the 65-year-old diagnosed with depression at risk for infections.
   2 The 5-year-old starting preschool has an increased risk of exposure to infections, but no host-related risk factors. **3** The 18-year-old smoker has an increased risk of exposure to infections associated with smoking, but no host-related risk factors. **4** The 40-year-old with a history of alcoholism has an increased risk of exposure to infections associated with alcohol abuse, but no host-related risk factors.
   Client Need: Physiological Adaptation; **Cognitive Level:** Analysis; **Nursing Process:** Assessment/Analysis

9. **4 Autoclaving is a means of destroying microorganisms using heat.**
   1 Disinfecting uses chemicals to destroy microorganisms on nonliving surfaces. **2** Antiseptics destroy microorganisms on living surfaces. **3** Autoclaving does not use effective packaging as a barrier to microorganism growth.
   Client Need: Physiological Adaptation; **Cognitive Level:** Understanding; **Nursing Process:** Assessment/Analysis

10. **1 An endemic is a high and constant rate of infection in a specific population, such as the presence of malaria in sub-Saharan Africa.**
    2 The occurrence of TB in the northern hemisphere is an example of a pandemic—an epidemic which spreads over a large area. **3** AIDS worldwide is an example of a pandemic—an epidemic which spreads over a large area. **4** SARS in Britain and Ireland is an example of an epidemic—a number of new infections in a specific population that exceed the number normally observed.
    Client Need: Physiological Adaptation; **Cognitive Level:** Understanding; **Nursing Process:** Assessment/Analysis

11. **Answers: 2, 3, 4, 5.**
    2 Memory is affected by this disease. **3** A throbbing headache is a clinical indicator of rabies. **4** Rabies, an acute infectious disease affecting the central nervous system, causes excessive salivation. **5** Painful muscle spasms are a characteristic of rabies.
    1 Hyperactivity is not an expected clinical indicator of rabies.
    Client Need: Physiological Adaptation; **Cognitive Level:** Applying; **Nursing Process:** Assessment/Analysis

12. **1** *Toxoplasma gondii,* **a protozoan, can be transmitted by exposure to infected cat feces or by ingestion of undercooked, contaminated meat.**

    2 Toxoplasmosis is not related to heavy metals. **3** *T. gondii* is a parasite of warm-blooded animals; fish are not considered a source of contamination. **4** Toxoplasmosis is not related to radiation.
    Client Need: Health Promotion and Maintenance; **Cognitive Level:** Application; **Integrated Process:** Teaching/Learning; **Nursing Process:** Planning/Implementation

13. **1 VRE is a gram-positive bacterium that is resistant to the antibiotic vancomycin: it is spread from one person to another in health care environments.**

    2 Pneumonia does not increase the risk of developing VRE. **3** Neither immunosuppression nor age are primary risk factors for VRE. **4** Pregnancy does not increase the risk of developing VRE
    Client Need: Physiological Adaptation; **Cognitive Level:** Analysis; **Nursing Process:** Assessment/Analysis

14. **3 Salmonellosis is a bacterial disease caused from the ingestion of food/water that has been contaminated with human feces. Proper, effective handwashing is vital to the control of this disease.**

    1 Salmonellosis does not spread by droplets, so masks are not effective. **2** Rabies is contracted from the bite of an infected bat. **4** Lyme disease is associated with the bite of a deer tick.
    Client Need: Health Promotion and Maintenance; **Cognitive Level:** Applying; **Nursing Process:** Teaching/Learning

15. **2 The classic rash pattern associated with Lyme disease is the bulls-eye pattern.**

    1 Lyme disease is not generally associated with swollen lymph glands. **3** Older clients develop shingles when exposed to herpes zoster. **4** Rubella is characterized by red, itchy eyes.
    Client Need: Physiological Adaptation; **Cognitive Level:** Analysis; **Nursing Process:** Evaluation/Outcomes

16. **4 During pregnancy rubella could potentially cause miscarriage or serious birth defects.**

    1 Neither age, gender, nor mental health issues place clients at an increased risk for rubella-related complications. **2** Neither age nor GERD places clients at an increased risk for rubella-related complications. **3** Neither age nor asthma places clients at an increased risk for rubella-related complications.
    Client Need: Health Promotion and Maintenance; **Cognitive Level:** Analysis; **Nursing Process:** Assessment/Analysis

17. **1 MRSA can be caused by the overuse of antibiotics and/or not completing the antibiotic treatment as prescribed.**

    2 MRSA is resistant to methicillin. **3** Although avoiding contact with infected individuals is an effective strategy to avoid being infected, it does not directly reduce the risk of developing MRSA. **4** A parasitic infection does not trigger MRSA.
    Client Need: Health Promotion and Maintenance; **Cognitive Level:** Analysis; **Nursing Process:** Evaluation/Outcomes

18. **4 The MMR vaccine is given in two doses; first dose at 12 to 15 months of age and the second dose at 4 to 6 years of age.**

    1 The MMR vaccine is given in two doses; first dose at 12 to 15 months of age. **2** The MMR vaccine (not just a rubella booster) is given in two doses; first dose at 12 to 15 months of age and the second dose at 4 to 6 years of age. **3** The MMR vaccine is given in two doses; first dose at 12 to 15 months of age and the second dose at 4 to 6 years of age.
    Client Need: Health Promotion and Maintenance; **Cognitive Level:** Analysis; **Nursing Process:** Evaluation/Outcomes

19. **Answers: 1, 3, 4, 5.**

    1 Fever is a characteristic of influenza. **3** General muscle aching is a characteristic of influenza. **4** Influenza signs and symptoms are sudden and acute in nature. **5** A headache is a characteristic of influenza.
    2 Nausea is not generally associated with influenza.
    Client Need: Physiological Adaptation; **Cognitive Level:** Applying; **Nursing Process:** Assessment/Analysis

20. **Answers: 1, 4, 5.**

    1 Diarrhea and accompanying dehydration is a possible complication of measles. **4** An ear ache is a possible complication of measles and generally requires medical attention. **5** Pneumonia is a serious complication of measles.
    2 A red rash is a sign associated with measles. **3** A runny nose and cough are signs and symptoms of measles.
    Client Need: Physiological Adaptation; **Cognitive Level:** Analysis; **Nursing Process:** Evaluation/Outcomes

7

Immune System Disorders

OVERVIEW

Stress

- Factor that creates a significant change in the body or environment
  - Physical, psychological, or a combination of both
  - Real or anticipated
  - Short term or long term
  - Examples: anxiety, fever, pain, cold temperature exposure, fear, infection, happy occasion
  - Occurs when the person's status is altered by the reaction to a stressor
- Stressors are perceived and responded to differently by individuals.
  - The same stressor may cause a mild stress response in one individual and cause significant illness in another.
  - Major or prolonged stress can cause disrupted intellectual function and memory.
  - Stressors are a normal part of life.
  - Stimulate growth and development
- Stress adaptation
  - General adaptation syndrome
    - "Fight or Flight"
    - Described by Seyle in 1946
    - Alarm
    - The body becomes mobilized if there is perceived threat.
      - Hypothalamus, sympathetic nervous system, and adrenal glands are activated.
    - Resistance
    - Hormonal levels are elevated.
    - Marked increase in adrenocorticotropic hormone (ACTH) secretion followed by a great increase in cortisol secretion
    - Body systems function at peak performance levels.
- Stress: Body responses
  - Central nervous system (CNS) arousal
  - Strong emotional response
  - Facial or verbal expressions
  - High anxiety level
  - Increased circulation
  - Increased blood pressure and heart rate increase
  - Increased oxygenation
  - Bronchodilation increases ventilation
  - Gluconeogenesis in the liver
  - Lipolysis
  - Protein catabolism in muscle
  - Decreased inflammatory and immune responses

- Decreased cortisol in early and late stages of stress response
  - Exhaustion
- Body is unable to respond further or is damaged by the increased demands.

APPLICATION AND REVIEW

1. What information should be included in a discussion concerning stress? **Select all that apply**.
   1. Stress must be eliminated from one's life to achieve health
   2. Sources of stress can be either physical or psychological
   3. People can respond to similar stressors quite differently
   4. Major stress can affect a person's cognitive function
   5. Stress can be either real or imagined
2. Which components of the human body are activated in response to a threat of physical or emotional harm? **Select all that apply**.
   1. Adrenal glands
   2. Hypothalamus
   3. Central nervous system
   4. Sympathetic nervous system
   5. Parasympathetic nervous system
3. Which assessment data support the presence of the "Fight or Flight" stress response? **Select all that apply**.
   1. Pallor
   2. Tachypnea
   3. Tachycardia
   4. Hypertension
   5. Facial expression of fear

See Answers on pages 143–145.

Components of the Immune System

- Antigens (immunogens)
  - Foreign substances or human cell surface antigens that are unique in each human
  - Composed of complex proteins or polysaccharides, or a combination of molecules such as glycoproteins
  - Activate the immune system to produce specific antibodies
  - The antigens representing self are present on an individual's plasma membranes.
  - Antigen molecules are coded by a group of genes inherited from the parents.
    - Major histocompatibility complex (MHC) located on chromosome 6
    - The huge number of possible gene combinations inherited from the parents makes it unlikely that two people would ever have the same antigens (except identical twins).
    - Human MHC is known as human leukocyte antigen (HLA).
      - These antigens are used to provide the closest match for a tissue transplant.
    - Immune system can tolerate self-antigens; no immune response is initiated against the person's own cells.
    - Autoimmune diseases are exceptions; the immune system does not recognize self from non–self and attacks its own cells, structures, or organs.
- Immunoglobulins (Table 7.1)
  - Immunoglobulins are made of proteins and each has a unique sequence of amino acids that are attached to a common base.
  - Bind to specific matching antigens and destroy them
  - The specificity of antigen for antibody (like a key opening a lock) is significant when considering the development of immunity to various diseases.

TABLE 7.1	Functions of Immunoglobulin
Ig	**Function**
IgA	• Found in tears, saliva, mucus, and in colostrum • Provides protection for the newborn child • Guards against viruses and bacteria
IgD	• Antigen receptor for B cells • Activates B cells
IgE	• Binds to mast cells in skin and mucous membranes • Associated with allergens • Causes release of histamine and other chemicals—the allergic response • Results in inflammation
IgG	• Most common antibody in the blood • Made in both primary and secondary immune responses • Activates complement • Antibacterial, antiviral, and antitoxin antibodies • Crosses the placenta to create passive immunity in the newborn
IgM	• Bound to B lymphocytes in circulation • First to increase in an immune response • Activates complement • Forms natural antibodies • Guards against viruses and bacteria • Involved in ABO blood type incompatibility

Ig, Immunoglobulin.

- Found in the general circulation
- Form the globulin portion of the plasma proteins and lymphoid structures
- There are five types of immunoglobulins.
- Autoantibody
  - Antibodies against self-antigen
  - Attacks the body's own tissues and organs
- Thymus
  - Located below the sternum
  - Contains lymph tissue
  - Produces T cells which are important for cell-mediated immunity
  - Very large in childhood until puberty, then begins to atrophy.
  - Produces the peptide hormones thymosin and thymopoietin which promote the growth of peripheral lymph tissue
  - Lymphoid tissue in bone marrow
    - Lymphocytes that are to become B cells are in the bone marrow.
  - Lymphocytes are exposed to hormones and cytokines that cause them to proliferate and differentiate into B cells.
- Immune cells (Table 7.2)
  - White blood cells (WBCs)
    - Granulocytes
      - Neutrophils, eosinophils, and basophils
      - Have a single nucleus and granules in the cytoplasm
      - Each has quite different actions and are activated by different stimuli

TABLE 7.2 Functions of Immune Cells

Immune Cells	Immune Cell Function
Neutrophils	<ul><li>Produced in the bone marrow</li><li>Most numerous granulocyte</li><li>Phagocytes</li><li>Fight against bacteria and fungi</li><li>Migrate to site of infection and accumulate</li><li>First to arrive</li><li>Worn out neutrophils become pus</li><li>55%–65% of circulating WBCs</li></ul>
Immature neutrophils	<ul><li>Known as bands</li><li>Once all neutrophils are used, the bone marrow releases the bands.</li><li>Normally <1% in blood</li></ul>
Eosinophils	<ul><li>Respond to allergic reaction</li><li>Accumulate in loose connective tissue</li><li>Ingest antigen-antibody complexes</li><li>Kill parasites</li><li>0.3%–7% of circulating WBCs</li></ul>
Basophils	<ul><li>Granules in cytoplasm secrete histamine in response to inflammatory and immune stimuli.</li><li>Histamine makes the blood vessels more permeable and lets fluid into the tissues.</li><li>Less than 2% of circulating WBCs</li></ul>

Lymphocytes	<ul><li>Smallest WBC</li><li>Derive from stem cells in bone marrow</li><li>Termed immunocompetent cells</li><li>20%–43% of circulating WBCs</li><li>Three types
	1. T lymphocytes
	  a. Attack infected cells
	  b. Mature in the thymus
	2. B lymphocytes
	  a. Produce antibodies against specific antigens
	  b. Mature in the bone marrow
	3. Natural killer cells
	  a. Provide immune protection and resistance infection</li></ul>

Monocytes/ macrophages	<ul><li>Largest WBC</li><li>Respond to inflammation</li><li>Phagocytic</li><li>1%–9% of circulating WBCs</li><li>When outside the bloodstream, monocytes become tissue macrophages (called histiocytes)
	1. Roam around freely in the body
	2. Concentrate in the liver, spleen, and lymph nodes and fight foreign organisms
	3. Stimulated by inflammation
	4. Part of the reticuloendothelial system
	  a. Defend against infection
	  b. Efficient phagocytes
	  c. Dispose of cell breakdown products
	  d. Promote healing</li></ul>

Continued

TABLE 7.2	Functions of Immune Cells—cont'd
Immune Cells	**Immune Cell Function**
Mast cells	• Not blood cells • Accumulate in connective tissue • Lungs, intestine, and skin • Have receptor sites for immunoglobulin E. • Present in an allergic reaction

T cells	• Come from stem cells
	• Cell-mediated immunity
	  1. Protect against bacteria, viruses, and fungi by deactivating the antigen; provide resistance against tumor and transplanted cells
	  2. T cells move more directly to destroy invaders.
	• Incompletely differentiated cells held in reserve in the bone marrow and travel to the thymus
	  1. Become more differentiated
	  2. Develop cell membrane protein receptors
	  3. Recognize antigens and directly destroy the invading antigens
	  4. Fight against virus-infected cells, fungal protozoa, cancer, and foreign cells (transplant)

Helper T cells	• Helper CD4-positive T cell • Facilitate the immune response • Initiate B cells to make antibodies

Killer T cells	• CD8-positive T-killer cell destroys the target cell by binding to the antigen
	• Release damaging enzymes or chemicals
	  1. Monokines and lymphokines
	    a. Destroy foreign cell membranes
	    b. Cause an inflammatory response
	    c. Attract macrophages to the site
	    d. Stimulate the proliferation of more lymphocytes and stimulate hematopoiesis

Memory T cells	• Remain in the lymph nodes for years • Ready to activate an immune response
B cells	• Also known as B lymphocytes • Humoral immunity 1. Antigens stimulate B cells to differentiate into plasma cells and produce antibodies that will circulate to disable bacteria and viruses before they can enter the host cells • Produce antibodies and immunoglobulins • Mature in the bone marrow and then go to spleen and lymphoid tissue
Plasma cells	• Antibody-producing plasma cell or a B memory cell
Helper B cells	• Provide for repeated production of antibodies • Produced in humoral immune responses • Natural killer
Natural killer lymphocytes	• Lymphocytes distinct from the T and B lymphocytes • Destroy tumor cells, infected cells, and cells infected with viruses • No prior exposure and sensitization

WBC, white blood cell.

- Agranulocytes are lymphocytes and monocytes.
  - Possess a nucleus
  - Do not have specific granules
- Immune system mediators and their functions (Table 7.3)
- First line of defense
  - Innate immunity
    - Epithelium of skin and linings of the respiratory, gastrointestinal (GI), and genitourinary tracts
    - Pathogens attempt to penetrate; they are removed by physical means.
      - Sloughed off with dead skin cells
      - Low temperature of the skin inhibits pathogens.
      - Microorganisms grow best at about 98.6° F and skin is usually less than that.

TABLE 7.3	Functions of Immune Systems Mediators

Immune System Mediator	Immune System Mediator Functions

Complement	• Complement proteins are inactive in the bloodstream.
	• Complement system is activated when tissue has been injured or there is an antigen-antibody complex.
	• Combines cell-mediated and humoral immunity
	• Phagocytic neutrophils, macrophages to the site
	• Made of 25 enzymes that work with antibodies by helping with phagocytosis and destroying bacterial cells
	• When the complement system is activated, the first complement goes to work and activates other complements.
	• There is a carefully controlled sequence of the complements referred to as the *complement cascade*.
	• The cascade leads to the creation of a membrane attack complex.
	• The complex inserts itself into the membrane of the target cell and allows fluids and molecules both in and out of the cell.
	• Eventually the target cell bursts.
	• The complement cascade by-products
	  1. Produce an inflammatory response
	    a. From the release of mast cells and basophils
	  2. Stimulate and attract neutrophils which help with phagocytosis
	  3. Coat the target cell with C3b which is an inactive fragment of complement protein C3
	    a. Attracts phagocytes

Histamine	• Secreted from the cytoplasmic granules of basophils in response to inflammatory and immune stimuli • Makes blood vessels more permeable and allows fluids to pass from the capillaries into body tissues

Kinins	• Plasma protein system
	• Interacts with coagulation system
	• Bradykinin
	  a. Final product of kinin system
	  b. Causes dilation of blood vessels
	  c. Increases vascular permeability
	  d. Works with prostaglandins to cause pain
	  e. Causes smooth muscle cell contraction

Continued

TABLE 7.3   Functions of Immune Systems Mediators—cont'd

Immune System Mediator	Immune System Mediator Functions
Prostaglandins	• Lipoprotein • Modify hormone responses • Encourage the inflammatory response • Open the airways
Leukotrienes	• Lipoprotein • Active when there are allergic or inflammatory responses

Cytokines	• Provide communication between macrophages and lymphocytes
	• Induce and regulate many inflammatory and immune responses
	• Can be proinflammatory or antiinflammatory whether they induce or inhibit inflammatory response
	• Several types of cytokines
	  1. TNF
	    a. Secreted by macrophages and other cells
	    b. Induces many proinflammatory effects on the vascular endothelium and macrophages
	    c. In large amounts, TNF
	      1. Induces fever as an endogenous pyrogen
	      2. Increases production of inflammation-related serum proteins in the liver
	      3. Causes muscle wasting
	      4. Causes intravascular thrombosis with severe infection and cancer
	      5. High levels of TNF can cause shock and death from gram-negative bacterial infections.
	  2. Transforming-growth factor
	    a. Produced by many cells in response to inflammation
	    b. Induces cell division and differentiation of other cell types
	  3. Colony-stimulating factor
	    a. Stimulates bone marrow to initiate maturation of healthy new cells, including lymphocytes
	  4. Interferons
	    a. Protect against viral infections
	      1. Do not kill viruses directly
	      2. Induce antiviral proteins and protect other cells
	    b. Modulate the inflammatory response
	  5. Interleukins
	    a. Produced by macrophages and lymphocytes when stimulated by other cytokines
	    b. More than 30 have been identified
	    c. Interleukins
	      1. Alter the adhesion on many types of cells
	      2. Enhance or suppress inflammation
	      3. Induce the proliferation and maturation of leukocytes in the bone marrow
	      4. Attract leukocytes to inflammation
	      5. Develop an acquired immune response

Chemotactic factors	• Attract phagocytic cells to the site of inflammation

TNF, Tumor necrosis factor.

- ▪ Removed by coughing and sneezing
- ▪ Mucus and cilia in the respiratory tract mobilize pathogens and move them upward; they are expectorated.
- ▪ Expelled from the stomach
- ▪ Low pH of the stomach inhibits microorganisms (most microorganisms need a neutral environment to grow).
- ▪ Flushed through the urinary system
  - Biophysical factors
    - ▪ Epithelial cells produce and secrete substances that protect against infection.
      - ▪ Mucus, tears, and saliva have lysozymes that attack the cell walls of gram-positive bacteria.
      - ▪ Contain antimicrobial peptides that can kill or inhibit the growth of disease-causing microorganisms
    - ▪ Sebaceous glands
      - ▪ Secrete lactic acid and fatty acids that can kill bacteria and fungi by creating an acidic environment that is not conducive to bacterial growth
    - ▪ Glycoproteins (collectins)
      - ▪ Produced and secreted from the lungs
      - ▪ Include surfactant proteins and mannose-binding lectin
      - ▪ Collectins help cells of the innate immune system to recognize and kill invading microorganisms.
    - ▪ Human microbiome
      - ▪ The human body's skin and mucous membranes are colonized with many different kinds of organisms known as normal flora.
      - ▪ Eyes, upper and lower GI tracts, upper respiratory tract, urethra, and vagina are all colonized by microorganisms that are unique to the location.
      - ▪ Microorganisms in a microbiome do not cause disease.
  - Mutualistic relationship that benefits both the organisms and the body
    - ▪ Benefits of the microbiome
  - Enzymes that hasten digestion
  - Antibacterial factors that prevent colonization of pathogenic microorganisms
  - Metabolites that are usable (vitamins B and K)
  - Induces growth of gut-associated lymphoid tissue
  - Develops both local and systemic adaptive immunity
  - *Brain-gut axis* is the two-way communication between the brain and the GI tract which is influenced by the microbiome of the GI tract and plays an integral part in cognitive function, behavior, pain, and stress response.
    - ▪ Antibiotics have the potential to alter the microbiome.
  - Loss of protective effect
  - Allows for the overgrowth of pathologic microorganisms
  - *Clostridium difficile*
  - *Candida albicans*
    - ▪ Microbiome contains microorganisms that are considered opportunistic.
  - If the body's defenses are down, the opportunistic microorganisms can take over and cause significant disease.
- Second line of defense
  - Inflammatory response
    - ▪ Responds to cell or tissue injury

- Occurs in tissues with blood supply
- Rapidly initiates humoral and cellular immunity
  - Helps prevent damage
  - Destroys the invading microorganisms
  - Begins the adaptive immune response
  - Initiates the healing process
- Cardinal signs of inflammation
  - Redness
  - Swelling
  - Warmth
  - Pain
  - Loss of function
- Microscopic signs of inflammation
  - Vasodilation (heat and redness)
  - Increased permeability of vessels and tissues (swelling)
  - Red blood cells (RBCs) rush to the site of injury (redness and warmth)
  - WBCs migrate to the site.
- Benefits of inflammation
  - Prevents infection
- Extra fluid in the area of injury dilutes any invading microorganisms.
- Activation of plasma protein system
- Complement system
- Clotting system
- Kinin system
- Phagocytes
- Remove cellular debris
  - Prevents further tissue damage
  - Controls the inflammatory response
  - Fluid and debris that have accumulated during the inflammatory response are drained via the lymph system.
  - Facilitates acquired immunity
- Third line of defense (this information is explained in more depth earlier in this outline)
  - Adaptive immunity (acquired immunity)
    - Antigen-specific immune response
      - The antigen is processed and recognized.
      - Cells will have memory for that antigen in the future.
  - Lymphocytes are responsible for both the induction and expression of adaptive immunity.
    - There are two major classes of lymphocytes
      - B cells
      - T cells
  - Humoral immunity
    - In response to an invading antigen, B cells divide and differentiate into plasma cells. Each plasma cell then makes and secretes a large amount of antigen-specific immuno-globulins into the blood stream.
  - Cell-mediated immunity
    - Protects the body against bacteria, viruses, and fungi by deactivating the antigen
    - Macrophages process the antigen and then it is presented to the T cells.
    - T cells may become sensitized and destroy the antigen.

- Other T cells release lymphokines, which activate macrophages that destroy the antigens.
- T cells go on to do surveillance for specific antigens.
- Passive immunity
  - Resistance to a disease or toxin where the resistance occurs without the immune system producing antibodies
  - Provides a barrier that prevents harmful substances from gaining access to the organism
  - Antibodies can also be passed from one organism to another.
  - Natural and artificial passive immunity
    - The passing of antibodies from mother to baby via the umbilical cord
    - Injected immunoglobulins to protect when there has been an exposure like hepatitis A

APPLICATION AND REVIEW

4. What component of the immune system is responsible for the production of antibodies?
   1. Antigens
   2. Glycoproteins
   3. Polysaccharides
   4. Immunoglobulins
5. What type of antigen is used to identify compatible organ donors?
   1. Self-antigens
   2. Non–self-antigens
   3. Incomplete antigens
   4. Human leukocyte antigen (HLA)
6. Which client is receiving the greatest benefit from the protection provided by immunoglobulin A (IgA)?
   1. Newborn client
   2. Older adult client
   3. Unconscious client
   4. Immunosuppressed client
7. Where are T cells produced?
   1. Bone marrow
   2. Sternum
   3. Thymus
   4. Liver
8. Which client statements support diagnosis condition of inflammation? **Select all that apply**.
   1. "It is hard to move my shoulder since I fell."
   2. "The skin around the cut on my hand is really red."
   3. "There is a greenish drainage when I blow my nose."
   4. "My ankle is swollen since I sprained it two days ago."
   5. "My elbow is really sore since I played tennis yesterday."
9. A nurse is caring for a client with an impaired immune system. Which blood protein associated with the immune system is important for the nurse to consider?
   1. Albumin
   2. Globulin
   3. Thrombin
   4. Hemoglobin

See Answers on pages 143–145.

Immune System Disorders

- Hypersensitivity
  - An exaggerated or inappropriate immune response that can lead to hypersensitivity disorder
  - Type I anaphylactic
    - Immediate
    - IgE mediated

- Types
  - Systemic anaphylaxis
  - Seasonal allergic rhinitis
  - Reaction to insect stings
  - Some food and medication reactions
  - Urticaria (hives)
- Type II cytotoxic
  - Cytolytic disorders; complement-dependent toxicity
  - Types
    - Goodpasture syndrome
    - Autoimmune hemolytic anemia
    - Transfusion reactions
    - Hemolytic disease of the neonate
    - Myasthenia gravis
- Type III immune complex disease reactions
  - Types
    - Reactions associated with infections like Hepatitis B and bacterial endocarditis
    - Autoimmune disorders such as systemic lupus erythematosus (SLE)
    - Follows some drug and serum treatments
- Type IV delayed (cell-mediated) hypersensitivity
  - Types
    - Latex sensitivity
    - Tuberculin reactions
    - Sarcoidosis
    - Transplanted organs

APPLICATION AND REVIEW

10. Which client is **most** directly impacted by the function of immunoglobulin E (IgE)?
    1. A client requiring a blood transfusion
    2. A client experiencing a reaction to a bee sting
    3. A client whose immune system has been activated
    4. A client who has been exposed to a bacterial infection
See Answer on pages 143–145.

Autoimmune Disorders

- Systemic lupus erythematosus (SLE)
  - Most common autoimmune disorder
  - May have a genetic predisposition
  - Body produces a large number of autoantibodies against self-antigens.
  - Affects nucleic acids, erythrocytes, coagulation proteins, phospholipids, lymphocytes, platelets, and more
  - Most individuals with SLE have antibodies against nuclear antigens
  - Some symptoms of SLE come from a Type III hypersensitivity reaction.
  - DNA/anti-DNA complexes in the kidneys can cause severe inflammation and kidney damage.
  - Other tissues are also at risk.
    - Brain

- Lungs
- Heart
- Spleen
- GI system
- Skin
- Other problems with SLE are caused by type II hypersensitivity reaction
  - Destruction of RBCs (anemia) and lymphocytes (lymphopenia)
- SLE Characteristics
  - More common in females
  - Blacks are affected more often
  - SLE is a chronic autoimmune disease that can affect almost any organ system.
  - Presentation and course are highly variable, ranging from indolent to fulminant.
  - Signs and symptoms of SLE may wax and wane. Individuals with SLE may have remission of disease.
  - Flares are not uncommon.
  - Difficult to diagnose
  - Fever, joint pain, and rash in a woman of childbearing age should be investigated as SLE.
  - Myriad of signs and symptoms
    - Constitutional (fatigue, fever, arthralgia, weight changes)
    - Musculoskeletal (arthralgia, arthropathy, myalgia, arthritis, avascular necrosis)
    - Dermatologic (malar rash, photosensitivity, discoid lupus)
    - Renal (acute or chronic renal failure, acute nephritic disease)
    - Neuropsychiatric (seizure, psychosis)
    - Pulmonary (pleurisy, pleural effusion, pneumonitis, pulmonary hypertension, interstitial lung disease)
    - Gastrointestinal (nausea, dyspepsia, abdominal pain)
    - Cardiac (pericarditis, myocarditis)
    - Hematologic (anemia, leukopenia, lymphopenia, or thrombocytopenia)
- Diagnosis
  - Combination of clinical findings and laboratory evidence
  - Presence of 4 of the 11 American College of Rheumatology (ACR) criteria yields a sensitivity of 85% and a specificity of 95% for SLE.
  - The following are the ACR diagnostic criteria in SLE, presented in the "SOAP BRAIN MD" mnemonic
    - Serositis
    - Oral ulcers
    - Arthritis
    - Photosensitivity
    - Blood disorders
    - Renal involvement
    - Antinuclear antibodies
    - Immunologic phenomena (e.g., dsDNA; anti-Smith [Sm] antibodies)
    - Neurologic disorder
    - Malar rash
    - Discoid rash
- Laboratory tests
  - Compete blood count (CBC) with differential

- Serum creatinine
- Urinalysis with microscopy
- Erythrocyte sedimentation rate (ESR) or C-reactive protein (CRP) level
- Complement levels
- Liver function tests
- Creatinine kinase assay
- Spot protein/spot creatinine ratio
- Autoantibody tests
- Imaging studies
  - Joint radiography
  - Plain chest x-ray; chest computed tomography (CT) scan
  - Echocardiography
  - Brain magnetic resonance image or magnetic resonance angiography (MRI/MRA)
  - Cardiac MRI/MRA
  - Procedures
    - Arthrocentesis
    - Lumbar puncture
    - Renal biopsy
- Immunodeficiency
  - Absent or depressed immune response
  - Primary immunodeficiency
    - When the cause of this deficiency is hereditary or genetic, it is called a primary immunodeficiency disease (PIDD).
    - Researchers have identified more than 300 different kinds of PIDD.
    - In the most common PIDDs, different forms of cells or proteins are missing or do not function.
    - There is a pattern of repeated infections, severe infections, and/or infections that are unusually hard to cure.
    - These infections may attack the skin, respiratory system, ears, brain, spinal cord, or the urinary or GI tracts.
    - Severe T-cell or combined immune deficiencies typically present in infancy. However, some antibody deficiencies may present in older children or adults. In milder forms, it often takes a pattern of recurrent infections before PIDD is suspected.
    - Important signs that may indicate a PIDD include
      - Recurrent, unusual, or difficult-to-treat infections
      - Poor growth or loss of weight
      - Recurrent pneumonia, ear infections, or sinusitis
      - Multiple courses of antibiotics or intravenous antibiotics necessary to clear infections
      - Recurrent deep abscesses of the organs or skin
      - A family history of PIDD
      - Swollen lymph glands or an enlarged spleen
      - Autoimmune disease
  - Secondary immunodeficiency
    - Occurs when the immune system is compromised owing to an environmental factor
    - Examples of these outside forces include human immunodeficiency virus (HIV), chemotherapy, severe burns, or malnutrition.

- Acquired immunodeficiency syndrome (AIDS)
  - Environmental risk factors for AIDS
    - Sexual contact with a person who has HIV (with or without the use of condoms)
    - Exposure to contaminated blood or contaminated needles or syringes
    - Blood transfusion before 1986 or out of the US
    - Transplacental transmission
    - Mother who has HIV infection can transfer it to infant during breastfeeding.
    - Transfer from HIV donor
  - Stages of HIV (CDC 2017 classification)
    - Stage 1: Acute HIV infection
      - Flu-like signs and symptoms within 2 to 4 weeks after infection with HIV; may last for a few weeks; body's natural response to infection
      - Large amount of virus in the blood; very contagious even if unaware of infection or not experiencing signs and symptoms
      - HIV screening
        - Fourth-generation antibody/antigen test or a nucleic acid test (NAT)
        - Individuals who have been exposed to HIV, through sex or drug use and have flu-like symptoms, should seek medical care and receive a screening test for HIV.
    - Stage 2: Clinical latency (HIV inactivity or dormancy)
      - Also called asymptomatic HIV infection or chronic HIV infection
      - HIV is still active but reproduces at very low levels.
      - May not have any signs or symptoms
      - Without treatment for HIV, this period can last a decade or longer, but some may progress through this phase faster.
      - With treatment for HIV, individuals may be in this stage for several decades.
      - Individuals are contagious and can still transmit HIV to others during this phase.
      - Individuals who take antiretroviral agents to treat HIV are usually virally suppressed (having a very low level of virus in the blood) and are much less likely to transmit HIV.
      - At the end of this phase, an individual's viral load increases and the CD4 cell count decreases. As this happens, the individual may begin to develop signs and symptoms.
    - Stage 3: AIDS
      - AIDS is the most severe phase of HIV infection.
      - Individuals with AIDS have suppressed immune systems and develop an increasing number of severe illnesses, called opportunistic illnesses.
      - Without treatment, individuals with AIDS typically survive about 3 years.
      - Common signs and symptoms of AIDS
        - Chills, fever, sweats
        - Swollen lymph glands
        - Weakness
        - Weight loss
      - Diagnostic criteria for AIDS
        - CD4 cell count drops below 200 cells/mm.
        - Individuals develop certain opportunistic illnesses.
        - Individuals with AIDS can have a high viral load and be very infectious.

APPLICATION AND REVIEW

11. Which clients are at risk for developing acquired immunodeficiency syndrome (AIDS)? **Select all that apply.**
    1. A 5-year-old diagnosed with hemophilia
    2. A 20-year-old with a history of intravenous drug use
    3. A 2-month-old whose mother was human immunodeficiency virus (HIV) positive at the time of birth
    4. A 60-year-old who had a blood transfusion as a teenager
    5. A 32-year-old who engages in protected sex with a partner who is HIV positive

12. What assessment data support the possibility that a client has been recently infected by the HIV virus?
    1. Received a blood transfusion after a recent auto accident
    2. Engaged in unprotected sex with an intoxicated person
    3. Is currently experiencing flu-like signs and symptoms
    4. Has a slowly declining CD4 cell count

13. A nurse is caring for a client who expresses concern about recent sexual exposure to HIV. Which response by the nurse would be appropriate?
    1. "It will require having a primary health care provider arrange to test your CD4 cell count."
    2. "Talk to your primary health care provider about a nucleic acid test (NAT)."
    3. "One of the autoantibody tests will be prescribed by your primary health care provider."
    4. "Your primary health care provider will prescribe a test to evaluate your viral load."

14. A client who is HIV positive is concerned about transmitting the virus to others. Which response by the nurse is best?
    1. "Eat well, exercise appropriately, and make healthy lifestyle choices."
    2. "Adhere to your prescribed antiviral medication therapy regimen."
    3. "Protected sex is not necessary when your viral count is low."
    4. "Avoid direct contact with others when your CD4 count begins to fall."

15. Which sign or symptom is most indicative of the progression from HIV positive to AIDS?
    1. Increasing weakness
    2. Swollen lymph glands
    3. Continued weight loss
    4. A CD4 count of 190 cells/mm

16. Which statement made by a client who was exposed to HIV demonstrates a need for additional information about the onset of the disease?
    1. "My exposure was about 3 weeks ago so it's too early to have symptoms."
    2. "I'm told that flu-like symptoms are the first indication of infection."
    3. "I'm scheduled for an HIV screening test."
    4. "My CD4 count won't be affected this early."

17. Which client diagnosed with AIDS is **most** likely to transmit the human immunodeficiency virus?
    1. A client who has a high viral load
    2. A client who has a CD4 count below 200 cells/mm
    3. A client who has contracted a classic opportunistic illness
    4. A client who has night sweats and swollen lymph glands

18. Which client has the greatest potential for transmitting HIV?
    1. A client diagnosed in stage 1 of the infection process
    2. A client in the latency phase of the disease
    3. A client with a negative NAT result
    4. A client with a high CD4 count
19. Which conditions place clients at risk for secondary immunodeficiency from an outside force? **Select all that apply.**
    1. A series of chemotherapy treatments
    2. Third degree burns to 10% of the body
    3. Current treatment for chronic hypertension
    4. A diagnosis of HIV
    5. A diagnosis of a gastrointestinal disorder that affects food absorption

ANSWER KEY: REVIEW QUESTIONS

1. **Answers: 2, 3, 4, 5.**

   2 Stress can be either physical, psychological, or a combination of both. **3** The same stressor may cause a mild stress response in one person and cause significant illness in another. **4** Major or prolonged stress can cause disrupted intellectual function and memory. **5** Stress can be either real or anticipated as being real.

   1 Stress is a normal part of life; it cannot and should not be removed entirely.
   Client Need: Physiological Adaptation; **Cognitive Level:** Understanding; **Integrated Process:** Teaching and Learning

2. **Answers: 1, 2, 4.**

   1, 2, 4 The hypothalamus, sympathetic nervous system, and adrenal glands are activated.

   3, 5 Neither the central or parasympathetic nervous systems are activated by stress.
   Client Need: Physiological Adaptation; **Cognitive Level:** Understanding; **Integrated Process:** Teaching and Learning

3. **Answers: 2, 3, 4, 5.**

   2 A physiological response associated with "Fight or Flight" is increased respirations. **3** A physiological response associated with "Fight or Flight" is increased heart rate. **4** A physiological response associated with "Fight or Flight" is increased blood pressure. **5** A psychological response associated with "Fight or Flight" is a sense of fear.

   1 A physiological response associated with "Fight or Flight" is increased circulation resulting in a reddish skin color not pallor.
   Client Need: Physiological Adaptation; **Cognitive Level:** Understanding; **Integrated Process:** Teaching and Learning

4. **1 Antigens activate the immune system to produce specific antibodies.**

   2, 3 Antigens are composed of polysaccharides and glycoproteins. **4** Immunoglobins bind to specific matching antigens and destroy them.
   Client Need: Physiological Adaptation; **Cognitive Level:** Understanding; **Integrated Process:** Teaching and Learning

5. **4 HLA antigens are used to provide the closest match for a tissue transplant.**

   1, 2, 3 None of the other options are used to identify compatible organ donor tissue.
   Client Need: Physiological Adaptation; **Cognitive Level:** Understanding; **Integrated Process:** Teaching and Learning

6. **1 IgA provides the newborn with protection against viral and bacterial infections for a finite period.**

   2, 3, 4 None of the other clients are as directly benefited from IgA as is the newborn.
   Client Need: Physiological Adaptation; **Cognitive Level:** Analysis; **Nursing Process:** Analysis

7. **3 T cells are produced by the thymus.**

   1 Bone marrow produces neutrophils and lymphocytes. **2, 4** T cells are not produced in any of the locations mentioned.
   Client Need: Physiological Adaptation; **Cognitive Level:** Understanding; **Integrated Process:** Teaching and Learning

8. **Answers: 1, 2, 4, 5.**

   1, 2, 4, 5 The cardinal signs of inflammation are redness, swelling, warmth, pain, and loss of function.

   3 A greenish discharge is associated with an infection.

   Client Need: Physiological Adaptation; **Cognitive Level:** Analysis; **Nursing Process:** Analysis

9. **2 The gamma-globulin fraction in the plasma is the fraction that includes the antibodies.**

   1 Albumin helps regulate fluid shifts by maintaining plasma oncotic pressure. **3** Thrombin is involved with clotting. **4** Hemoglobin carries oxygen.

   Client Need: Physiological Adaptation; **Cognitive Level:** Understanding; **Integrated Process:** Teaching and Learning

10. **2 IgE causes the release of histamine and other chemicals triggering an allergic response.**

    1 IgM is associated with ABO blood type incompatibility. **3** IgG is made because of immune response. **4** IgM guards against both viral and bacterial invasions.

    Client Need: Physiological Adaptation; **Cognitive Level:** Analysis; **Nursing Process:** Analysis

11. **Answers: 2, 3, 4, 5.**

    2 Risks for AIDS include exposure to contaminated blood or syringes. **3** Risks for AIDS include placental transmission. **4** Risks for AIDS include blood transfusion prior to 1986. **5** Risks for AIDS includes any sexual contact with an HIV-positive partner.

    1 Transfusions are not a risk if received after 1986.

    Client Need: Physiological Adaptation; **Cognitive Level:** Analysis; **Nursing Process:** Analysis

12. **3 Within 2 to 4 weeks after infection with HIV, individuals may experience a flu-like illness, which may last for a few weeks.**

    1 A blood transfusion before 1986 is considered a risk factor but does not support possible infection. **3** Unprotected sex is considered a risk factor but does not support possible infection. **4** In the second phase of infection a person's viral load starts to go up, and the CD4 cell count begins to go down.

    Client Need: Physiological Adaptation; **Cognitive Level:** Applying; **Nursing Process:** Assessment

13. **2 To know whether someone has acute infection, either a fourth-generation antibody/antigen test or an NAT is necessary.**

    1 A CD4 cell count will not be affected in the acute stage of the infection. **3** Systemic lupus erythematosus (SLE) is associated with the autoantibody tests. **4** Viral load will not be affected in the acute stage of the infection.

    Client Need: Physiological Adaptation; **Cognitive Level:** Analysis; **Integrated Process:** Teaching and Learning

14. **2 People who are on antiviral medications and stay virally suppressed (having a very low level of virus in their blood) are much less likely to transmit HIV.**

    1 Although good advice, a healthy lifestyle will not be sufficient to minimize the risk of transmission. **3** Protection should be used in all sexual encounters to reduce the risk of transmission of HIV. **4** A low viral load has a greater impact on minimizing the risk for transmission.

    Client Need: Physiological Adaptation; **Cognitive Level:** Analysis; **Integrated Process:** Teaching and Learning

15. **4 Individuals are diagnosed with AIDS when their CD4 cell count drops below 200 cells/mm.**

    1, 2, 3 Although these are signs and symptoms of AIDS, none are as definitive as a CD4 cell count below 200 cells/mm.

    Client Need: Physiological Adaptation; **Cognitive Level:** Analysis; **Nursing Process:** Analysis

16. **1 Within 2 to 4 weeks after infection with HIV, an individual may experience a flu-like illness, which may last for a few weeks.**

    2 Within 2 to 4 weeks after infection with HIV, an individual may experience a flu-like illness, which may last for a few weeks. **3** To know whether someone has acute infection, either a fourth-generation antibody/antigen test or an NAT test is necessary. **4** At the end of phase 2, an individual's viral load starts to go up, and the CD4 cell count begins to go down.

    Client Need: Physiological Adaptation; **Cognitive Level:** Analysis; **Nursing Process:** Evaluation

17. **1 Clients with AIDS and a high viral load are very infectious.**

    2, 3 Clients are diagnosed with AIDS when their CD4 cell count drops below 200 cells/mm or if they develop certain opportunistic illnesses; those characteristics are not necessarily associated with infectiousness. **4** Night sweats and swollen lymph glands are common symptoms associated with AIDS; those characteristics are not necessarily associated with infectiousness.

    Client Need: Physiological Adaptation; **Cognitive Level:** Analysis; **Nursing Process:** Analysis

18. **1 When clients have acute HIV infection (stage 1), they have a large amount of virus in their blood and are very contagious.**

    2 Clients who are in the clinically latent stage (stage 2) can still transmit HIV to others, although clients who are on antiviral therapy and stay virally suppressed (having a very low level of virus in their blood) are much less likely to transmit HIV. **3** A negative NAT result would indicate no HIV is present. **4** A high CD4 count is less relevant to infection transmission than a high viral count.

    Client Need: Physiological Adaptation; **Cognitive Level:** Analysis; **Nursing Process:** Analysis

19. **Answers: 1, 2, 4, 5.**

    1, 2, 4, 5 Examples of these outside forces include HIV, chemotherapy, severe burns, or malnutrition. **3** Neither hypertension nor the classic medication therapy increases the risk for secondary immunodeficiency.

    Client Need: Physiological Adaptation; **Cognitive Level:** Analysis; **Integrated Process:** Teaching and Learning

8

Neurologic System Disorders

OVERVIEW

Central Nervous System

- Anatomy Review
- Skull: protective bony covering of the brain
  - Composed of eight bones
  - The cranial and facial bones are connected by sutures, which are relatively immovable joints consisting of fibrous tissue.
  - Galea aponeurotica is a thick fibrous tissue that overlies the cranium between the frontal and occipital muscles.
  - Subgaleal space has venous connections with the dural sinuses.
    - With increased intracranial pressure (ICP), the blood can be shunted to the space reducing the pressure on the brain.
    - The skull contains a number of cavities, or fossae, as well as foramina (openings) and canals through which nerves and blood vessels pass.
      - The largest opening, the foramen magnum, is located in the occipital bone at the base of the skull, where the spinal cord emerges.
- Meninges: membranes surrounding the brain
  - Dura mater (meaning hard mother)
    - Outer most layer
    - Two layers of membrane with venous sinuses between them
      - Periostium is the outermost layer.
      - Inner dura mater forms rigid membranes that support and separate various brain structures.
      - Subdural space lies between the dura and the arachnoid.
        - Between the dura mater and the brain is the epidural space.
    - Arachnoid
      - Spongy, web-like structure that follows the contours of the cerebral structures.
      - Subarachnoid space lies between the arachnoid and the pia mater, contains cerebral spinal fluid (CSF).
        - Pia mater
          - Adheres to the contours of the brain and spinal cord
          - Supports blood vessels in the brain
          - Choroid plexuses produce CSF.
- Cerebrospinal fluid and ventricular system
  - CSF is a clear, odorless fluid that is similar to plasma and interstitial fluid.
  - The intracranial and spinal cord float in CSF and protect the brain from jolts and blows.
    - Between 125 and 150 mL of CSF are in the ventricles and subrachnoid space.
    - Approximately 600 mL of CSF is produced every day.
    - The choroid plexuses in the lateral, third, and fourth ventricles produce most of the CSF.
    - CSF exerts pressure in the brain and spinal cord and changes with position changes.

- Blood–brain barrier
  - Protective mechanism that provides impermeable capillaries in the brain
  - The endothelial cells of the capillaries are tightly joined together by tight junctions.
  - Barrier limits the passage of potentially damaging materials into the brain and controls the delicate but essential balance of electrolytes, glucose, and proteins in the brain.
  - Similar blood–CSF barrier at the choroid plexus to control the constituents of CSF
  - The blood–brain barrier can be a disadvantage because it does not allow the passage of many essential drugs into the brain.
  - Lipid-soluble substances, including alcohol, pass freely into the brain.
- Brain
  - Cerebrum
    - Largest brain structure
    - Contains 70% of the neurons and supporting cells of the brain
    - Right and left hemispheres
      - Separated by the corpus callosum
      - Massive bundle of fibers crossing the brain
      - Principal means of communication between the hemispheres
  - Cerebral cortex
    - The outermost layer of the cerebrum; it consists of gray matter with six different layers of tissue
    - Each layer of tissue communicates with different parts of the brain.
  - Four lobes of the cerebrum
    - Frontal lobe: motor cortex and association areas; prefrontal cortex involved in complex thought; ethical behavior; morality
    - Parietal lobe: somatosensory cortex; association areas
    - Occipital lobe: visual cortex; association areas
    - Temporal lobe: hearing; equilibrium; emotion; memory
- Limbic structures
  - Contains the amygdala, fornix, hippocampus, and parts of the thalamus
  - Encircles the brain stem and is responsible for short-term memory, emotions, and olfaction
- Basal ganglia
  - Includes the caudate, putamen, subthalamic nucleus, nucleus accumbens, globus pullidus, and substantia nigra
  - It is a loop circuit that begins and ends in the cortex and is responsible for initiation, coordination, and execution of movement.
  - Lesions of the basal ganglia cause unwanted movements at rest.
    - Resting tremor
    - Dystonia (painful muscle contractions)
    - Chorea (involuntary dance-like movements)
    - Broca and Wernicke areas: interpretation and expression of language
- Diencephalon
  - A connecting structure between the upper brain stem (midbrain) and the cerebral hemispheres.
  - The third ventricle also crosses the diencephalon.
  - Cranial nerves I (olfactory) and II (optic) originate in the diencephalon.
  - Structures of the diencephalon
    - Thalamus
      - Relay center from the spinal cord, cerebellum, and basal ganglia to the cerebral cortex

- Involved in the execution of motor activities
- Creates the constant background electrical activity seen on electroencephalogram (EEG)
- Connection between thalamus and brain stem are necessary to maintain consciousness.
  - Connections between thalamus and the limbic and cortex are necessary for the expression of those qualities considered to be human (emotion, language, creativity, and complex thought).
- Hypothalamus
  - Lies just below the thalamus on top of the diencephalon
  - Extends downward to form the pituitary gland (hypophysis)
  - The posterior pituitary gland is an extension of the nerve tissue of the hypothalamus, whereas the anterior pituitary gland is derived from glandular tissue.
  - Neurons in the hypothalamus regulate the secretion of anterior pituitary hormones by releasing and inhibiting hormones.
  - Is the regulatory center for the autonomic nervous system and basic body functions
    - Sleep
    - Sex drive
    - Body temperature
    - Appetite
  - Responsible for homeostasis of life-sustaining functions, including cardiovascular, respiratory, metabolic, fluid and electrolyte, and stress responses
    - Responds to sensors of blood pressure, osmolarity, blood oxygen concentration, carbon dioxide level, serum pH, and temperature
  - Epithalamus: contains the pineal gland
  - Pineal gland: regulates the circadian rhythms in response to light-dark cycles
  - Ventral thalamus: contains the basal ganglia also known as the subthalamic nucleus
- Cerebellum
  - Located in the posterior fossa behind the pons
  - Separated from the cerebrum by the tentorium cerebelli
  - Uses feedback from the spinocerebellar tracks, which travel uncrossed from the spinal cord, to monitor movements that are happening and sends output via the thalamus to adjust the movements
  - Maintains balance and posture
  - Receives information from the proprioceptors in muscle and joints and from the vestibular apparatus in the inner ear about the position of the head in space
  - Lesions of the cerebellum result in uncoordinated movements (ataxia) and cerebellar deficits occur ipsilateral to the side where the lesion is.
    - Cerebellar lesions can be caused by toxins, alcohol, stroke, tumor, multiple sclerosis, and paraneoplastic syndrome.
    - Unable to do finger to nose and heel to shin tasks
    - Difficulty with rapid alternating movements (RAM)
    - Intention tremor (no tremor when still; tremor when trying to move)
    - Imbalance
    - Nystagmus and vertigo

- Brain stem
  - Stalk of neural tissue that lies between the upper spinal cord and the diencephalon
  - Most important task is the transmission of impulses between the brain and spinal cord
  - Divided into three parts
    - Midbrain
    - Medulla
    - Pons
  - The medulla and pons house the centers for regulating cardiovascular and respiratory functions.
  - The reticular activating neurons that maintain consciousness and alertness go through the brain stem to reach the thalamus.
  - Cranial nerves III to XII originate from the nuclei in the brain stem.
- Midbrain contains the
  - Cerebral peduncles, which are motor tracks to the spinal cord
  - Superior and inferior colliculi, which control head and eye movements
  - Red nucleus, which is part of a major motor tract
  - Cranial nerve III (oculomotor) emerges from the midbrain and is susceptible to compression when pressure in one of the cerebral hemispheres is elevated.
  - Increased intracranial pressure (from injury, ischemia, edema, tumor, etc.) is commonly manifested by dysfunction of cranial nerve III resulting in abnormal pupil size and poor reactivity to light.
  - Cranial nerve IV (trochlear) also emerges at the level of the midbrain.
- Pons (which means bridge)
  - Connects the midbrain to the medulla
  - Dorsal pons consists of
    - Reticular formation fibers
    - Ascending sensory tracts
    - Descending motor tracts
      - Two respiratory centers that work with the respiratory center in the medulla
  - Ventral pons
    - The corticospinal tract, which is responsible for voluntary motor control, passes through the ventral pons on its way to the motor cortex in the spinal cord.
  - Medulla oblongata
    - Lower third of the brain stem
    - Continuous with the spinal cord
    - Contains the centers that regulate cardiac, vascular, and respiratory systems
    - Contains the centers that coordinate swallowing, vomiting, coughing, and sneezing
    - Site of decussation (crossing over) of the sensory (dorsal column) and motor (corticospinal) tracts such that innervation of one side of the body is connected to the contralateral cerebral hemisphere.
    - Motor tracts that do not cross over are called extrapyramidal tracts.
    - Dysfunction of the extrapyramidal tracts causes problems with balance, posture, and gait.
  - Spinal cord
    - Extends from the base of the skull (foramen magnum) to the first or second lumbar vertebrae

- Extends several inches past the lumbar vertebrae in order to provide a reservoir for CSF and a place for the lumbar and sacral spinal nerves to exit
- Allows nervous impulses between the brain and 31 pairs of spinal nerves that innervate sensory organs and muscle cells of the body
- Mediates spinal reflexes necessary to maintain posture, protective responses to pain, urination, and muscle tone
- Gray matter of the spinal cord allows for the integration and processing of nerve impulses.
- White matter contains bundles of myelinated axons that form tracts up and down the cord.
  - Contains afferent (sensory) and efferent (motor) fibers that are organized into transmitting and communicating fibers that run between the two sides of the spinal cord.
  - There are two types of descending tracts.
  - Pyramidal (corticospinal) conduct impulses concerned with voluntary movements from the motor cortex (upper motor neurons) to the lower motor neurons in the anterior horn at the appropriate level of the spinal cord. Most of these tracts cross in the medulla.
  - Extrapyramidal tracts carry impulses that modify and coordinate voluntary movement and maintain posture.
- Lower motor neurons can receive both stimulatory and inhibitory input from upper neurons and from interneurons in the spinal cord. This interaction decides where the activity will occur, either spinal nerves or skeletal muscles.
  - Tracts in the spinal cord are somatotropically organized so that the innervation of a particular body region is connected to a specific region in the cerebral cortex.
  - A cross-section of the spinal cord looks like a butterfly of gray matter surrounded by white matter.
    - There are three horns (bumps).
      - Ventral horn (motor neurons)
      - Dorsal horn (sensory neurons)
      - Lateral horn (sympathetic neurons)
    - The horns contain neuron body cells, synapses, and small unmyelinated interneurons.
- Interneuron is a neuron that transmits impulses between other neurons, especially as part of a reflex arc.
  - The white matter is divided into columns that contain tracts of nerve fibers traveling to and from the brain.
- Dorsal (posterior) column
- Anterior column
- Lateral columns
  - Some of the columns convey signals from one level of the spinal cord to another and are important in reflex responses and postural adjustments.
- Vertebral column
  - Formed by interlocking sections of bone separated and cushioned by intervertebral disks
  - At the lateral aspect of the intersection of two vertebrae there is an opening (intervertebral foramen) where the spinal nerves exit the cord.

APPLICATION AND REVIEW

1. What is the primary function of the subgaleal space when considering intracranial pressure (ICP)?
   1. It is a source of cerebrospinal fluid (CSF)
   2. It is a component of the blood–brain barrier
   3. It provides a place for the shunting of blood
   4. It is the primary storage site for cerebrospinal fluid
2. What is the primary disadvantage associated with the blood–brain barrier?
   1. It tends to exacerbate an existing increase in ICP.
   2. It interferes with the entry of lipid-soluble substances into the brain.
   3. It interferes with the passage of some medications into the brain.
   4. It can be a barrier to the free flow of cerebrospinal fluid.
3. What client statement focuses on a characteristic that is a result of frontal lobe function?
   1. "I have trouble remembering names and faces."
   2. "I've worn a hearing aid since I was in my 50s."
   3. "I don't think cheating is acceptable regardless of the situation."
   4. "I've been experiencing visual problems since I fell and hit my head."
4. Which sign or symptom would the nurse expect in a client diagnosed with a lesion of the basal ganglia?
   1. Hand tremors when eating
   2. Nausea and vomiting
   3. Generalized seizures
   4. Memory loss
5. Which statement, if made by the nurse, demonstrates an understanding of the function of the hypothalamus?
   1. "The client is very sensitive to odors."
   2. "I'll try to spend more time orienting the client to the unit."
   3. "I'll be sure to ask whether the client needs an extra blanket"
   4. "The blinds need to be drawn to protect the client from the sunlight."

See Answers on pages 169–170.

Peripheral Nervous System

- Cranial nerves (Table 8.1)
- Spinal nerves
  - There are 31 pairs of spinal nerves that emerge from the spinal cord.
  - Carry motor and sensory fibers to and from the organs and tissues of the body
  - Named and numbered by their location in the vertebral column where they exit
    - Cervical nerves (C1 to C8)
    - Thoracic nerves (T1 to T12)
    - Lumbar (L1 to L5)
    - Sacral (S1 to S5)
  - The areas of sensory innervation of the skin by any specific spinal nerve is called a dermatome.
    - The assessment of the sensory awareness using the dermatomes helps determine the level of injury to the spinal cord.
  - Divide into two sections as they make contact with the spinal cord
    - Ventral (anterior) root
      - Contain efferent (motor) neurons that come from the lower motor neurons in the anterior horn and travel to the spinal nerve to skeletal muscles

TABLE 8.1 Cranial Nerves: Their Origins and Function

Cranial Nerve	Origin	Function
I Olfactory	Nasal mucous membranes	Smell
II Optic	Retina	Vision
III Oculomotor	Midbrain	Movement of eyeball, eyelid, constriction of the pupil
IV Trochlear	Lower midbrain	Lateral eye movements
V Trigeminal		
Ophthalmic	Forehead, eyes	Sensation from forehead, eye, scalp
Maxillary	Upper jaw, lip	Sensation from cheek, upper lip
Mandibular	Lower jaw area	Sensation from chin and lower jaw; motor chewing
VI Abducens	Lower pons	Lateral eye movements
VII Facial	Pons	Taste from anterior tongue; control of facial muscles
VIII Vestibulocochlear	Cochlear Inner ear	Hearing Equilibrium
IX Glossopharyngeal	Medulla	Taste from posterior tongue; secretion of saliva; swallowing
X Vagus	Medulla	Monitors oxygen, carbon dioxide, and pH levels; senses blood pressure; inhibits cardiac action and extensive gastrointestinal activities
XI Spinal accessory	Medulla and cervical cord	Voice production, movement of head and shoulders
XII Hypoglossal	Medulla	Movements of the tongue during speech and swallowing

- Dorsal (posterior) root
  - Carry afferent (sensory) information from somatic receptors to neurons in the posterior horn
  - The cell bodies of sensory afferents collect together in the dorsal root ganglion.
  - Autonomic nerves also travel in the spinal cord and exit and enter the cord by way of the ventral and dorsal roots.
- Reflexes
  - Automatic, rapid, involuntary response to a stimulus
  - There is a sensory stimulus from a receptor that is conducted from an afferent nerve fiber to a synapse at the level of the spinal cord that leads to an efferent impulse to be conducted along a peripheral nerve to elicit the response.
  - Connecting neurons or interneurons transmit the sensory information to the brain to initiate an immediate assessment and appropriate response.
- Neurons
  - The basic units of the nervous system
  - In the central nervous system (CNS) and peripheral nervous system (PNS)
  - Neurons need glucose and oxygen for metabolism.
  - Receive and transmit electrochemical nerve impulses
  - Neurons are protected by glial cells.

- Astroglia (astrocytes) provide a link between neurons and capillaries for physical and metabolic support.
- Contribute to the blood–brain barrier
- Axons and dendrites extend from the central cell body of the neuron and transmits signals.
- Each neuron has many dendrites and one axon.
  - Dendrites
    - The receptor site that then conducts impulses toward the cell body.
  - Cell body
    - Contains the nucleus
  - Axons
    - Conduct nerve impulses away from cell bodies
    - Have terminal branches and are covered in myelin sheath
      - Myelin sheath is produced by Schwann cells which are phagocytic cells separated by gaps called the nodes of Ranvier.
      - Regeneration of neurons
        - Neurons do not undergo cell division.
        - If a cell body is damaged, the neuron dies.
        - If the cell body is alive, axons might be able to regenerate.
        - The section distal to the injury degenerates because it lacks nutrients and is removed by macrophages and Schwann cells.
        - The Schwan cells attempt to form a new tube at the end of what is left of the axon.
        - This process can be successful; however, interference from surrounding tissues is not uncommon.
      - Conduction of impulses
        - A stimulus increases the permeability of the neuronal membrane.
        - Depolarization occurs when sodium ions flow inside a cell, which generates an action potential when threshold is reached.
      - Positive electrical charge inside the membrane results in increased permeability of the adjacent area, and the impulse moves along the membrane.
        - Repolarization (recovery) occurs as potassium ions move out and the normal permeability of the cell is restored.
        - In myelinated fibers, this action potential occurs only at the nodes of Ranvier, which allows impulses to move rapidly (salutatory conduction).
        - Larger axons conduct more rapidly than smaller ones.
        - The synapse is the connection between two or more neurons.
        - Synapse
          - The release of neurotransmitters from vesicles in the synaptic buds of the axons
      - When the impulse originates in the presynaptic neuron, the impulse goes to the vesicles where the neurotransmitters are stored in the synaptic bouton.
      - Once the impulse is released, the neurotransmitters diffuse across the synaptic cleft (space between neurons) and bind to specific receptor sites on the plasma membrane of the postsynaptic neuron.
      - May stimulate or inhibit a postsynaptic neuron
      - Brain synapses can change in strength and numbers throughout a lifetime; this is known as neuroplasticity.

APPLICATION AND REVIEW

6. Which sign or symptom would be expected in a client with cranial nerve VIII dysfunction?
   1. Difficulty with speech
   2. Problems with swallowing
   3. Recurrent falls
   4. Low blood pressure
7. Which set of spinal nerves would be assessed when a client reports neck pain?
   1. Cervical nerves (C–)
   2. Thoracic nerve (T1–T12)
   3. Lumbar nerves (L1–L5)
   4. Sacral nerves (S1– S50)

See Answers on page 169–170.

Autonomic Nervous System

- Consists of sympathetic and parasympathetic nervous systems which usually have antagonistic effects providing homeostasis
- Provides motor and sensory innervation to smooth muscle, cardiac muscle, and glands
- Motor nerve fibers have two neurons and a ganglion.
  - The preganglionic fiber is located in the brain or spinal cord.
  - This axon then synapses with a second neuron in the ganglion outside the CNS and the postganglionic fiber continues to an organ or tissue.
    - Sympathetic nervous system (SNS)
      - Also known as the thoracolumbar nervous system
      - Increases the general activity in the body
        - Cardiovascular
        - Respiratory
        - Neurologic
      - Responsible for the flight or fight (stress) response
      - Preganglionic fibers of the sympathetic nerves arise from the thoracic and lumbar segments of the spinal cord.
        - The ganglia are located in two chains (trunks) on either side of the spine.
        - Preganglionic fibers synapse with postganglionic fibers to other ganglia in the chain.
        - Acetylcholine is the neurotransmitter released in preganglionic fibers, which are called cholinergic fibers.
        - Most SNS postganglionic fibers release norepinephrine, also called adrenaline (adrenergic fibers).
        - The postganglionic fibers to sweat glands and blood vessels in skeletal muscles are cholinergic.
    - Parasympathetic nervous system (PNS)
      - Also known as craniosacral nervous system, it dominates the digestive system and aids in recovery after the sympathetic activity
      - Location of PNS preganglionic fibers
        - Cranial nerves (CN) III, VII, IX, X at the brain stem level and the sacral spinal nerves
        - CN X: The vagus nerve provides extensive innervation to the heart and digestive tracts.
        - Ganglia are scattered and located close to the target organ, and the neurotransmitter at both preganglionic and postganglionic synapses is acetylcholine.

- ○ Two cholinergic receptors
  - ○ Nicotinic
    - Stimulated by acetylcholine and are located in all postganglionic cholinergic neurons in the PNS and SNS
  - ○ Muscarinic
    - Located in all effector cells and may be stimulated or inhibited by acetylcholine depending on the organ

Central Nervous System Abnormalities

- Hydrocephalus
  - Excess CSF accumulates within the skull, compressing the brain tissue and blood vessels.
  - CSF accumulates because more is produced than is absorbed, often because of obstruction to the flow at some point.
  - In some instances, production of CSF is normal, but there is a reduction in the amount reabsorbed.
  - Sometimes called "water on the brain"
  - Because the cranial sutures have not yet closed, the infant's head enlarges beyond the normal size as the amount of fluid increases.
  - Two types of hydrocephalus
    - Noncommunicating or obstructive
      - Hydrocephalus occurs when the flow of CSF through the ventricular system is blocked, usually at the aqueduct of Sylvius or the foramen magnum.
      - Results from a fetal development abnormality, such as stenosis or a neural tube defect
      - Associated with myelomeningocele or Arnold-Chiari malformation
      - Obstruction leads to increased fluid in the ventricles of the brain, which gradually enlarges the ventricles and compresses the blood vessels and brain tissue.
    - Communicating hydrocephalus
      - Absorption of CSF through the subarachnoid villi is impaired, resulting in increased pressure of CSF in the system.
      - The presence of pliable sutures in the skull of an infant allows the skull to expand in the early stages of hydrocephalus.
      - If left untreated, the brain tissue is permanently damaged.
      - Without pliable skull sutures, the ICP in older children and adults increases more rapidly than infants and the amount of brain damage depends on the rate at which pressure increases and the time that elapses before relief occurs.
      - Brain damage may result in major physical disability and intellectual impairment.
  - Etiology
    - Combination of genetic and environmental factors
    - There is a familial incidence.
    - Environmental factors include exposure to radiation, gestational diabetes, and deficits of vitamin A or folic acid.
    - Folic acid supplements are recommended before conception and for the first 6 weeks of pregnancy as a preventive measure.
      - Research has shown that such supplementation reduces the incidence of myelomeningocele.
    - Stenosis or atresia (the absence of a canal or opening) at the connecting channels between the ventricles or a thickened arachnoid membrane that occurs prior to birth is the most common cause of hydrocephalus.

- Obstruction may also develop at any age from tumors, infection, or scar tissue.
- Meningitis can cause obstructive hydrocephalus during the acute infection or lead to fibrosis in the meninges, impairing absorption.
- Signs and symptoms
  - Depends on the age of the individual
  - Newborn to 24 months of age
    - Infants with open sutures will have an increase in head size and the fontanels may bulge early in the process.
    - Recording head size is a standard procedure from birth until 2 years of age and is usually done during routine examinations.
    - As hydrocephalus worsens, the scalp veins may dilate.
    - Eyes show the "sunset sign," where the white sclera is visible above the colored iris.
    - Pupil response to light is sluggish.
    - Infant may be listless, irritable, and difficult to feed.
    - With increasing ICP the infant may have a high-pitched or shrill cry when moved or picked up.
    - Early diagnosis is imperative to avoid brain damage.
  - Children, adolescents, and adults
    - Once the anterior fontanel closes around 2 years of age, the head cannot enlarge and the classic signs of increased ICP develop as the volume of CSF expands.
    - Severe headache
    - Nausea and vomiting
    - Decreasing memory
    - Difficulty in coordination
    - Impaired balance
    - Urinary incontinence
      - Depending on the underlying cause, there may be other symptoms.
- Diagnosis
  - Computed tomography (CT) or magnetic resonance imaging (MRI) scan can locate the obstruction or abnormal flow and determine the size of the ventricles.
- Spina bifida
  - The neural tube develops during the fourth week of gestation, beginning in the cervical area and progressing toward the lumbar area.
  - Spina bifida occurs when there is a failure of the posterior spinous processes on the vertebrae to fuse, which may permit the meninges and spinal cord to herniate, resulting in neurologic impairment.
  - Many vertebrae can be involved and the lumbar area is the most common location.
  - Types of spina bifida
    - Spina bifida occulta
      - Spinous processes fail to fuse.
      - Herniation of the spinal cord and meninges does not happen.
      - The defect is usually not visible, although there may be a sacral dimple or a tuft of hair at the site of the defect.
      - Diagnosed by routine x-ray examination or when mild neurologic signs manifest owing to tension on the cord during a growth period
    - Meningocele
      - Spinal processes fail to fuse and there is herniation of the meninges at the site of the defect.

- Meninges and CSF create a sac on the surface of the infant's back.
- Transillumination of the sac confirms the absence of nerve tissue in the sac.
- There is usually no neurologic impairment.
- Infection or rupture of the sac may lead to neurologic damage.
  - Myelomeningocele
    - Herniation of the spinal cord and nerves along with the meninges and CSF
    - There may be considerable neurologic impairment with damage to the spinal cord.
    - The location and extent of the herniation determine how much function is lost.
    - Hydrocephalus is common in myelomeningocele.
- Diagnosis
  - Alpha-fetoprotein (AFP) leaks from the spinal defect, resulting in an elevated level in maternal blood at 16 to 18 weeks' gestation.
  - Amniocentesis detects the presence of AFP that has leaked into the amniotic fluid surrounding the fetus.
  - Prenatal ultrasound
- Cerebral palsy (CP)
  - Pathophysiology
    - Group of disorders with some degree of motor impairment
    - There is abnormal fetal formation of functional brain areas, infection, or brain damage in the perinatal period.
    - Damage usually occurs in other areas of the brain which makes for a clinical presentation that is variable, depending on the specific areas affected and the severity of the trauma.
    - Damage occurs before, during, or shortly after birth.
    - The damage is nonprogressive.
  - Epidemiology
    - There are about 500,000 individuals with CP in the United States.
    - Approximately 10,000 new cases of pediatric CP each year
  - Etiology
    - Single or multiple factors may be implicated in the development of CP.
    - Hypoxia or ischemia happens prenatally, perinatally, or postnatally and is the major cause of brain damage.
    - Causes of hypoxia
      - Placental complications
      - Difficult delivery
      - Vascular occlusion or hemorrhage
      - Aspiration
      - Respiratory impairment in the premature infant
      - Hyperbilirubinemia from problems such as prematurity or Rh blood incompatibility
      - Kernicterus: accumulation of bilirubin in the blood that crosses the blood–brain barrier and damages the neurons
      - Infection or metabolic abnormalities
  - Signs and symptoms
    - Occasionally there are signs of CP at birth.
    - A delay in motor development or abnormal muscle tone may not be present for several months or years.
    - Newborn reflexes that do not go away when expected is an early sign of CP (Moro reflex).

- CP is classified either on the basis of area affected (e.g., quadriplegia or diplegia) or on the basis of the motor disability.
- Spastic paralysis
  - Most common
  - Damage to the pyramidal tracts (diplegia) or the motor cortex (hemiparesis), or from general cortical damage (quadriparesis)
  - Signs include hyperreflexia (excessive reflex response).
  - Infant may have crossed straight legs with scissoring motions when help up off surface.
  - Children may maintain straight-legged posture with scissoring or persist with toe-walking.
- Dyskinetic disease
  - Damage to the extrapyramidal tract, basal nuclei, or cranial nerves
  - Manifested by athetoid or choreiform involuntary movement
  - Loss of coordination with fine movements
- Ataxic CP
  - Damage to the cerebellum
  - Loss of balance and coordination
  - Increased muscle tone or resistance to passive movement
  - Excessive reflex responses
  - Unilateral use of the hands or feet
  - Asymmetric body movements
  - Writhing movements or facial grimaces may indicate athetoid CP.
- Motor dysfunction may cause persistent tongue-thrusting and feeding difficulties that can interfere with nutrition and growth.
- Resting posture or when held is very abnormal
- Other findings with CP
  - Intellectual function may or may not be a concern.
  - One-third of individuals with CP will likely have normal intelligence, one-third will have mild intellectual impairment, and one-third will have severe cognitive dysfunction.
  - Communication and speech difficulties
  - Hearing loss
  - Seizures
    - Most common are generalized tonic-clonic type.
  - Visual problems
    - Astigmatism
    - Strabismus
  - Learning disabilities and behavioral problems
    - Attention deficit disorder
    - Spatial disorientation
    - Hyperactivity
- Meningitis
  - Inflammation of the covering of the brain and spinal cord caused by infection or toxins
  - Caused by virus, bacteria, fungi, parasites, or toxins
    - Each cause may have own presentation
    - Can be acute, subacute, or chronic
    - Bacterial meningitis is the most common cause.
      - Follows an upper respiratory infection

- Epidemiology
  - More common in children but can happen at any age
- Pathophysiology
  - Bacterial meningitis
    - Involves the pia mater, arachnoid, subarachnoid space, the ventricles, and the CSF
    - 1 in 100,000 persons are affected annually.
    - Common pathogens
    - Increase in drug resistance
      - More common in young children and individuals over 40 years of age
      - Associated with ear infection, sinusitis, pneumonia, and immunocompromised state
      - Spread by respiratory droplets, contact with infected saliva, and contaminated surfaces
      - Signs and symptoms of bacterial meningitis
        - Infectious signs
          - Fever
          - Increased heart rate
          - Chills
        - Meningeal signs
          - Severe throbbing headache
          - Severe photophobia
          - Nuchal rigidity
          - Kernig sign is positive when the thigh is flexed at the hip and an attempt to straighten the leg at the knee is met with resistance.
          - Brudzinski sign is positive when an attempt to flex the patient's neck causes involuntary flexion of the hip and knees.
        - Neurologic signs
          - Decreased level of consciousness
          - Delirium
          - Unconsciousness
          - Death
- Cranial nerve palsies
  - Focal neurologic dysfunction
  - Focal seizures
  - Ataxia
  - Hemiparesis/hemiplegia
  - Projectile vomiting and papilledema (increased ICP)
  - Specifically, with meningococcus
  - Petechiae or purpura on skin and mucus membranes
  - Can progress to tissue death and the need for amputation
    - Diagnosis
      - Physical examination
        - Lumbar puncture for evaluation of CSF
        - Viral polymerase chain reaction; bacterial and viral cultures
        - Blood cultures
    - Complications
      - Septic shock
      - Purpura fulminans
      - Disseminated intravascular coagulation (DIC)

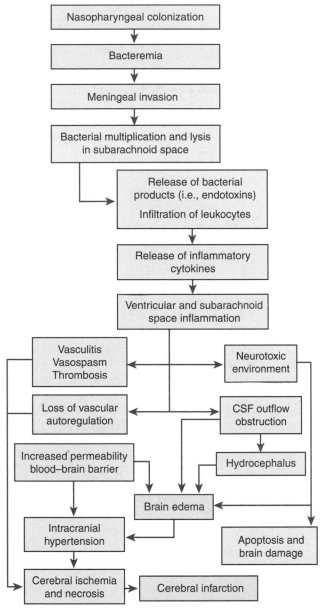

FIG. 8.1 Pathogenesis of meningitis. (Adapted from Cohen, J., & Powderly, W.G. [2004]. *Infectious diseases* [2nd ed.]. Edinburgh: Mosby.)

- ■ Limb damage
- ■ Multiple organ failure
- ■ Prevention
  - ■ Haemophilus influenza, pneumococcal, and meningococcal vaccines in childhood, adolescence, and adulthood
- • Viral meningitis (aseptic or nonpurulent meningitis)
  - • Enterovirus, arboviruses, and herpes simplex

- Enter nervous system by crossing the blood–brain barrier, by direct spread long peripheral nerves, or through the choroid plexus epithelium
- Similar, but milder symptoms than bacterial meningitis
- Fungal meningitis
  - Less common, more chronic
  - Usually occurs in person who are immunocompromised
  - Onset subtle and happens over days or weeks
  - Creates a granulomatous reaction forming a mass in the meninges at the base of the brain
  - May extend into brain tissue producing thrombi, infarction, and hydrocephalus
  - Meningeal fibrosis
  - Cranial nerve dysfunction
  - Communicating hydrocephalus
  - Dementia
- Seizure disorder
  - Abnormal electric discharges of the neurons in the brain which trigger convulsive movements, an interruption of sensation, and a change in the level of consciousness
  - Seizures do not generally affect intelligence.
  - Epidemiology
    - Affects all people of all ages, races, and ethnic backgrounds
    - More common in childhood and in the elderly
    - Approximately three million individuals have been diagnosed with seizure disorders.
  - Pathophysiology
    - The electric activity at the neuron level of the brain increases the reactivity of the neuronal membrane.
    - Hypersensitive neurons begin to fire abnormally.
  - Causes
    - Hypoglycemia (low blood sugar)
    - Hyponatremia (low sodium level)
    - Fever or hyperthermia
    - Low oxygen level
    - Medications
    - Medication or drug withdrawal
    - Head trauma
    - Infection
    - Tumor
    - Stroke
    - Structural abnormalities in the brain
    - Continued sensory stimulation
    - Other causes
  - Once the seizure activity starts it spreads to the adjacent brain areas most likely to produce seizures.
    - Midbrain
    - Thalamus
    - Cerebral cortex
      - Eventually the discharges lessen and the seizure should stop.
- Generalized seizures
  - Abnormal electrical activity spreads across both sides of the brain.

- Loss of consciousness
- Uncontrollable muscle spasms
  - Tonic and clonic movements
- Partial seizures
  - Complex partial
    - Starts in one hemisphere of the brain and then spreads to both hemispheres
    - May stare into space and be unaware of the present
    - There may be purposeless movements (lip smacking, hand flapping).
  - Simple partial
    - Begins in one hemisphere of the brain
    - One part of the body may have involuntary movements.
    - No loss of consciousness
    - Signs and symptoms
      - Auras (precede the epileptic event)
      - Smell
      - Nausea
      - Sinking feeling in the stomach
      - Dreamy feeling
      - Unusual taste
      - Visual disturbance (flashing light)
      - Seizures
      - Tonic movements
      - Stiffening followed by muscle contractions
      - Clonic movements
      - Jerking and twitching movements
      - Bite or chew on tongue
      - Incontinence
      - Purposeless movements
      - Change in level of awareness
      - Blank stare
      - Loss of muscle tone
  - Status epilepticus
    - Life threatening emergency that requires prompt recognition and immediate treatment to avoid neuronal damage and cell death in the brain.
    - Seizure lasting longer than five minutes or two seizures that occur without total recovery between seizures.
    - Refractory status epilepticus is defined as clinical or electrographic evidence of seizure following the administration of an initial benzodiazepine and a secondary antiepileptic drug.
    - Convulsive status epilepticus: rhythmic jerking movements of the arms and legs
      - Convulsive syncope
        - Repetitive decerebrate or decorticate posturing
        - Involuntary movement disorders
        - Psychogenic nonepileptic spells (pseudo-seizures)
      - Non-convulsive status epilepticus: electrographic evidence of seizure without motor findings
      - Aggression
      - Automatisms

- Blinking
- Crying
- Delirium
- Delusions
- Echolalia
- Facial twitching
- Laughter
- Nausea/ vomiting
- Eye deviation contralateral to the lesion
- Perseveration
- Psychosis
- Tremulousness
- Aphasia
- Amnesia
- Catatonia
- Staring
- Normal brain function means that there is balance between inhibition and excitation of the neurons.
- Neurotransmitters inhibit or excite neurons.
  - γ-Aminobutyric acid (GABA) is the most common inhibiting neurotransmitter.
  - Glutamate is the most common excitatory neurotransmitter.
  - During status epilepticus there is a failure of inhibitory GABA causing the seizure to be self-sustaining and resistant to medications.
  - Resistance to benzodiazepine medication occurs at 10 to 45 minutes after the onset of the status epilepticus.
- Seizures, both convulsive and non-convulsive, cause intense metabolic demands on the brain that require increased blood flow to the brain.
- When the metabolic demands cannot be met because of the ongoing seizure leading to neuronal damage and cell death.
- During status epilepticus, homeostasis cannot be maintained and causes a shift of intracellular calcium to enter the mitochondria, which then lose their membrane potential.
- Risk factors for status epilepticus
  - History of seizures regardless of age
  - Structural causes
    - Tumors
    - Stroke
    - Traumatic brain injury
  - Infectious causes
    - Virus
    - Fever
  - Metabolic derangements
    - Hyponatremia
    - Hypo/ hypercalcemia
    - Hypoglycemia
    - Hepatic encephalopathy
    - Hypomagnesemia
  - Drug toxicity

- Diagnosis
  - Electroencephalogram (EEG)
  - Other radiologic procedures depending on the presumed cause
- Cerebral vascular accident (Stroke)
  - Pathophysiology
    - Ischemic stroke
      - Approximately 87% of all strokes are ischemic in nature.
      - There is an obstruction within a blood vessel in the brain.
      - Atherosclerosis is the underlying cause
        - Cerebral thrombosis
          - Blood clot that forms at the clogged area of the blood vessel
        - Cerebral embolism
          - A blood clot that forms in another part of the body (usually the heart or larger blood vessels in the chest and neck)
          - The clot travels via the circulatory system until it gets to a blockage or small vessel that it cannot pass.
          - Atrial fibrillation can cause clots to form in the heart that can travel to the brain.
  - Hemorrhagic stroke
    - Less common kind of stroke
    - More likely to result in death
      - Intracerebral hemorrhage
        - The most common hemorrhagic stroke
        - Blood vessel in the brain ruptures and blood leaks into the brain tissue
        - Causes brain cell death and the affected part of the brain stops working
        - Aging blood vessels and high blood pressure are the most common cause of this type of stroke.
      - Subarachnoid hemorrhage
        - Bleeding between the brain and the subarachnoid space
          - Most common is a ruptured aneurysm.
          - Arteriovenous malformation
          - Bleeding disorder
          - Head injury
          - Blood thinners
    - Sudden impairment of cerebral circulation
    - Diminished oxygen supply to the brain
    - Five minutes (or less) of ischemia causes irreversible nerve cell damage leading to loss of function.
    - A central area of necrosis develops, surrounded by an area of inflammation.
    - Serious damage or necrosis of brain tissue
  - Epidemiology
    - It is estimated that a stroke occurs every 45 seconds in the United States.
    - Approximately 700,000 strokes are experienced annually; about 500,000 are first strokes and 200,000 are recurrent strokes.
    - Account for more than 1 of 15 deaths in the United States
    - Strokes are considered a major cause of disability.
  - Risk factors
    - Hypertension
    - Cardiac disease

- History of transient ischemic attacks (TIAs)
- Diabetes
- Hyperlipidemia
- Cigarette smoking
- Increased alcohol intake
- Obesity or sedentary lifestyle
- Use of hormonal contraception
  - Signs and symptoms
    - Sudden transient weakness, numbness, or tingling in the face, an arm or leg, or on one side of the body
    - Temporary loss of speech, failure to comprehend, or confusion
    - Sudden loss of vision
    - Sudden severe headache (subarachnoid hemorrhage)
    - Unusual dizziness or unsteadiness; immediate medical treatment may prevent permanent brain damage.
    - The National Institutes of Health has developed a diagnostic stroke scale that is designed to assist with rapid diagnosis of a cerebral vascular accident in an emergency situation. The stroke scale includes commands to determine capacity for speech, level of consciousness, motor abilities, and assessment of eye movements. The scale also identifies areas of damage based on resulting dysfunction.
- Multiple sclerosis (MS)
  - Pathophysiology
    - Theorized to be an autoimmune response of the nervous system
    - Genetic factors may be involved.
    - Other causes include malnutrition, trauma, anoxic injury toxins, vascular lesions, and anorexia nervosa any of which can destroy the myelin sheath.
    - Progressive demyelination of the white matter of the brain and spinal cord
    - Widespread neurologic dysfunction
    - Most common structures involved are optic and oculomotor nerves, cerebellum, and spinal nerve tracts.
    - Disease with exacerbations and remissions
    - Scattered demyelinating lesions prevent normal neurologic conduction.
    - Once the myelin is destroyed, neurologic tissue in the white matter of the CNS proliferates forming hard yellow plaques of scar tissue which damages the underlying axon fiber, disrupting nerve conduction.
  - Etiology: unknown
  - Epidemiology
    - Estimated incidence runs from 30 to 100 per 100,000 individuals in the United States.
    - Second most common cause of disability in the United States; motor vehicle accidents are the first.
  - Risk factors
    - Female gender
    - Residence in northern urban area
    - Higher socioeconomic groups
    - Family history of MS
  - Signs and symptoms
    - Paresthesias in the extremities or face
    - Excessive fatigue and dizziness

- Gait disturbance and imbalance
- Heat intolerance
- Blurred vision or diplopia
- Scotoma: a spot in the visual field
- Emotional lability
- Dysphagia
- As the number of plaques increases with each exacerbation, progressive weakness and paralysis extending to the upper limbs, loss of coordination, and bladder, bowel, and sexual dysfunction occur.
- Chronic fatigue is common.
- Sensory deficits worsen with a loss of position sense in the upper body, face, and legs.
  - Diagnosis
    - No definitive test for MS
    - Long delay may precede the diagnosis
    - History of exacerbations and remissions
    - Involvement of multiple focal areas
    - Progression and absence of other neurologic diagnostic criteria are often the basis for an initial diagnosis of MS.
    - MRI studies are best for diagnosis and monitoring.
    - Lumbar puncture: elevated protein, gamma globulin, and lymphocytes levels in the CSF
- Parkinson's disease
  - Pathophysiology
    - Parkinson's disease affects the extrapyramidal system, which influences initiation, modulation, and completion of movement.
    - The extrapyramidal system includes the corpus striatum, globus pallidus, and substantia nigra in the midbrain.
    - Normally, dopamine input from the substantia nigra to the corpus striatum excites the direct pathway and inhibits the indirect pathway, which allows for cortical excitation without abnormal movements.
    - In Parkinson's disease, there is a loss of dopamine from the substantia nigra which leads to decreased activity from the direct pathway and increased activity in the indirect pathway. This means there is decreased activity in the cortex and increased inhibition of the cortex.
  - Etiology: unknown
  - Epidemiology
    - Affects more males than females
  - Signs and symptoms
    - Gait and movement disturbances
    - Progressive muscle rigidity
    - Uniform rigidity (lead pipe)
    - Jerky rigidity (cogwheel)
    - Loss of muscle movement (akinesia)
    - Unable to move
    - Unilateral "pill rolling" resting tremor
    - Involuntary tremors
    - Mask-like facial expression
    - Head bobbing

- Myasthenia gravis
  - Pathophysiology
    - Disease of the neuromuscular junction
    - Autoantibodies are produced against the acetylcholine receptors on muscle cells.
    - Antibodies block the receptor so that the acetylcholine cannot bind and stimulate muscle contraction.
  - Etiology
    - Idiopathic
    - Secondary to tumor of the thymus (thymoma)
  - Signs and symptoms
    - Progressive skeletal muscle weakness
    - Abnormal fatigue
    - Inability to maintain arm abduction for more than a brief period
    - Facial muscle weakness and fatigue (clinical hallmark)
    - Ptosis (droopy eyelids)
    - Rapid fatigue of eyelids with prolonged upward gaze
    - Dysphagia (difficulty swallowing)
    - Dysarthria (trouble speaking)
    - No associated pain or sensory deficits, which helps when making the diagnosis
  - Complications of myasthenia gravis
    - Myasthenic crisis
      - Too many receptors are destroyed by the immune system
      - Remaining receptors are not able to provide muscle contractions which leads to severe muscle weakness.
      - Symptoms
        - Muscles weak
        - Normal oral secretions
        - Tachycardia
        - Pupils normal or dilated
        - Skin is faint and cold
      - Diagnosis is made by giving the patient edrophonium (Tensalon) and if the patient improves they should be given edrophonium, neostigmine, or pyridostigmine.
    - Cholinergic crisis
      - Too much cholinergic activity caused when enzymes that break down acetylcholine are deactivated
      - Can occur when taking neostigmine or pyridostigmine
      - Overstimulation of the neuromuscular junctions leads to overactivation of the receptors that leaves them unable to stimulate and causes increased muscle weakness
      - Symptoms
        - Muscles weak and fasciculations
        - Increased oral secretions
        - Bradycardia
        - Pupils constricted
        - Skin is warm and flushed
        - Diagnosis is made by giving the patient edrophonium (Tensalon) and if the patient gets worse they should be given atropine.
  - Diagnostic testing
    - Electromyography, which demonstrates fatigue during repetitive stimulation

- Detection of the acetylcholine receptor antibody in the blood
- Edrophonium (Tensilon) can be used for diagnosis of myasthenia gravis because it competitively inhibits the binding sites of acetylcholinesterase, which increases the life of acetylcholine in the synapse. It can give the person with myasthenia gravis fast improvement of weakness that is, unfortunately, only temporary.

APPLICATION AND REVIEW

8. The nurse explains to a client that the signs and symptoms being experienced are related to a loss of dopamine production in the brain. Which neurologic disorder is the client most likely experiencing?
   1. Parkinson's disease
   2. Myasthenia gravis
   3. Multiple sclerosis
   4. Seizure disorder
9. Which assessment alerts the nurse to suspect increasing intracranial pressure (ICP) in an infant diagnosed with hydrocephalus?
   1. Sunken eyes
   2. Projectile vomiting
   3. Depressed fontanels
   4. Narrowing pulse pressure
10. A client is prescribed a medication to block acetylcholinesterase. Which neurologic disorder is this client most likely experiencing?
    1. Parkinson's disease
    2. Myasthenia gravis
    3. Multiple sclerosis
    4. Seizure disorder
11. A client is admitted to the hospital with a diagnosis of myasthenia gravis. For which common early clinical finding should the nurse assess the client?
    1. Tearing
    2. Blurring
    3. Ptosis
    4. Nystagmus
12. A nurse is caring for a 3-year-old child with bacterial meningitis. Which signs and symptoms would the nurse expect? **Select all that apply.**
    1. Vomiting
    2. Headache
    3. Impaired balance
    4. Negative Kernig sign
    5. Bradycardia
13. Which behaviors are characteristic of a 2-month-old infant who is diagnosed with communicating hydrocephalus? **Select all that apply.**
    1. Dilated scalp veins
    2. Brisk pupil response
    3. Shrill high-pitched cry
    4. High degree of irritability
    5. White sclera noted above pupils
14. Which statement, if made by a parent, assures the nurse that the parent understands the diagnostic test used for meningitis?
    1. "My child will have a myelogram today."
    2. "Complete blood counts will be done."
    3. "A lumbar puncture is not comfortable but is needed."
    4. "Spinal x-rays will be painless but helpful in diagnosis."
15. What is a classic characteristic of myasthenia gravis?
    1. Unilateral 'pill rolling' tremors
    2. Profound intolerance to heat
    3. Facial muscle drooping
    4. Facial grimacing

See Answers on pages 169–170.

ANSWERS TO REVIEW QUESTIONS

1. **3 Subgaleal space has venous connections with the dural sinuses; when increased ICP occurs, the blood can be shunted to the space reducing the pressure on the brain.**

   1 The subgaleal space has no role in the production of cerebrospinal fluid (CSF). **2** The subgaleal space has no role in the blood–brain barrier which is a protective mechanism that provides impermeable capillaries in the brain. **4** The brain's ventricles and subarachnoid space holds between 124 and 150 mL of CSF normally.

   Client Need: Physiological Adaptation; **Cognitive Level:** Understanding; **Integrated Process:** Teaching and Learning

2. **3 The blood–brain barrier can be a disadvantage because it does not allow the passage of many essential drugs into the brain.**

   1 The blood–brain barrier has no role to play in increasing ICP. **2** The blood–brain barrier allows for the free passage of lipid-soluble substances. **4** The blood–brain barrier plays no role in the flow of CSF.

   Client Need: Physiological Adaptation; **Cognitive Level:** Understanding; **Integrated Process:** Teaching and Learning

3. **3 The frontal lobe is located in the motor cortex and association areas; prefrontal cortex is involved in complex thought; ethical behavior; morality.**

   1 Memory is a function of the temporal lobe. **2** Hearing is a function of the temporal lobe. **4** Visual function is the function of the occipital lobe.

   Client Need: Physiological Adaptation; **Cognitive Level:** Analysis; **Nursing Process:** Analysis

4. **1 Lesions of the basal ganglia cause unwanted movements at rest; such hand tremors can infer with independent eating.**

   2, 3, 4 Lesions of the basal ganglia are not associated with nausea and vomiting, seizures, or memory loss.

   Client Need: Physiological Adaptation; **Cognitive Level:** Applying; **Nursing Process:** Planning

5. **3 The hypothalamus is involved in regulating body temperature; the client may be sensitive to the cold.**

   1 The hypothalamus is not associated with the sense of smell. **2** The hypothalamus is not associated with memory. **4** The hypothalamus is not associated with photosensitivity.

   Client Need: Physiological Adaptation; **Cognitive Level:** Analysis; **Nursing Process:** Analysis

6. **3 CN VIII (vestibulocochlear) is associated with equilibrium, making falls precautions appropriate.**

   1 Speech is associated with CN XII (hypoglossal). **2** Swallowing is associated with CN IX (glossopharyngeal). **4** Blood pressure regulation is associated with CN X (vagus).

   Client Need: Physiological Adaptation; **Cognitive Level:** Applying; **Nursing Process:** Planning

7. **1 The first 8 vertebrae with cervical nerves 1 to 8 are found in the cervical or neck area.**

   2 The thoracic nerves are from T1 to T12 in the thoracic area. **3** L1 to L5 are in the lumbar region. **4** S1 to S5 are in the sacral region.

   Client Need: Physiological Adaptation; **Cognitive Level:** Applying; **Nursing Process:** Assessment

8. **1 Signs and symptoms of Parkinson's disease are related to a loss of dopamine production in the brain.**

   2, 3, 4 Signs and symptoms of myasthenia gravis, MS, and seizure disorder are not related to a loss of dopamine production.

   Client Need: Physiological Adaptation; **Cognitive Level:** Understanding; **Integrated Process:** Teaching and Learning

9. **2 Increased ICP exerts pressure on the vomiting center in the brain, resulting in projectile vomiting unrelated to feeding.**

   1 The eyeballs will show signs of increased fluid volume in the skull and will be pushed forward, pulling the lids taut. **3** The fontanels will show signs of increased fluid volume in the skull and therefore will bulge. **4** In adults, increased ICP causes a widening pulse pressure (the systolic pressure is increased and the diastolic pressure is the same or decreased). This is rarely seen in infants and children.

   Client Need: Physiological Adaptation; **Cognitive Level:** Applying; **Nursing Process:** Assessment

10. **2 Clients with myasthenia gravis will be prescribed a medication to block acetylcholinesterase, which can reduce signs and symptoms of the disorder.**

    1, 3, 4 Parkinson's disease, MS, and seizure disorder are not related to acetylcholinesterase production.
    Client Need: Physiological Adaptation; **Cognitive Level:** Understanding; **Integrated Process:** Teaching and Learning

11. **3 With myasthenia gravis, ptosis (or drooping of the eyelids) occurs related to muscle weakness.**

    1, 2, 4 Tearing, blurring, and nystagmus are not clinical manifestations associated with myasthenia gravis.
    Client Need: Physiological Adaptation; **Cognitive Level:** Understanding; **Integrated Process:** Teaching and Learning

12. **Answers: 1, 2, 3.**

    1 Increased ICP can precipitate vomiting because of its effect on the chemoreceptor trigger zone in the medulla. **2** Because the cranial sutures are closed by this age, increased pressure can cause headache. **3** Impaired balance (ataxia) results from increased pressure in the cranium.

    4 A positive (not negative) Kernig sign occurs related to meningeal irritation. **5** Tachycardia (not bradycardia) is expected with bacterial infections.
    Client Need: Physiological Adaptation; **Cognitive Level:** Understanding; **Integrated Process:** Teaching and Learning

13. **Answers: 1, 3, 4, 5.**

    1 As the hydrocephalus worsens, the infant may start to have scalp veins that become dilated. **3** The condition is characterized by a shrill high-pitched cry. **4** The infant is lethargic, but irritable. **5** The eyes show the "sunset sign," in which the white sclera is visible above the colored pupil.

    2 Pupil response to light is sluggish.
    Client Need: Physiological Adaptation; **Cognitive Level:** Understanding; **Integrated Process:** Teaching and Learning

14. **3 A culture of CSF obtained via a lumbar puncture can reveal the presence of the causative microorganism (e.g., pneumococcus, tubercle bacillus, meningococcus, or streptococcus).**

    1 A myelogram is used to detect the presence of abnormalities through injection of a contrast medium into the subarachnoid space; it does not identify the causative microorganism. **2** A complete blood count assesses the child's general health, but not the cause of the meningitis. **4** Spinal x-rays assess the structure of the spine, but will not identify the causative microorganism
    Client Need: Physiological Adaptation; **Cognitive Level:** Analysis; **Nursing Process:** Evaluation

15. **3 A classic clinical hallmark of myasthenia gravis is facial muscle weakness that includes ptosis.**

    1 Parkinson's disease presents with hand tremors referred to as 'pilling rolling.' **2** MS presents with heat intolerance. **4** Ataxic cerebral palsy is characterized by facial grimacing.
    Client Need: Physiological Adaptation; **Cognitive Level:** Applying; **Nursing Process:** Planning

PAIN OVERVIEW

- Pain is an unpleasant but protective mechanism of defense for the human body.
- Pain provides a warning that the body may be experiencing damage.
- Pain can be related to a variety of factors including, but not limited to, physical and emotional factors.
- Pain is a subjective symptom of distress or disease.

Etiology of Pain

- Pain can occur for a variety of reasons including
  - Inflammation or infection of tissues
  - Lack of oxygen supplied to tissues
  - Stretching of tissues caused by tumors or excess fluid accumulation
  - Mechanical trauma from burns or other injuries

Transmission of Pain Impulses

- The normal or typical pain response in the human body is known as nocioception.
- Pain sensation is transmitted by nociceptors.
  - Nociceptors are free nerve endings located throughout the body in varying concentrations.
  - They are part of the peripheral nervous system that sends messages to the central nervous system for interpretation.
  - They respond to a variety of stimuli including
    - Chemical
    - Thermal
    - Physical
  - There are two primary types of nociceptors involved in pain perception.
    - A delta fibers
      - Covered in a myelin sheath
      - Transmit pain quickly
      - Typically transmit acute pain
      - Sensation may be described as sharp and/or sudden.
    - C fibers
      - Lack a myelin sheath
      - Transmit pain that is dull or diffuse
      - Often associated with chronic pain
- Nociception occurs in four stages.
  - Transduction
    - Noxious stimulus triggers nociceptors in the periphery.
    - Injury to the tissue can be caused by naturally occurring chemicals in the body including
      - Prostaglandin
      - Histamine
      - Bradykinin
      - Leukotrienes

- Other causes of injury could include exposure to excessive cold or heat and stretching or pressure from mechanical sources.
- Transmission
  - Stimulated message moves from the source of injury up the spinal cord.
- Perception
  - The meaning of pain is processed in the cerebral cortex.
- Modulation
  - Reactions from the central nervous system (CNS) that serve to increase or decrease pain
  - The process may be mediated by neurotransmitters including
    - Excitatory neurotransmitters
      - Prostaglandins
      - Bradykinin
      - Histamine
      - Tumor necrosis factor (TNF)
    - Inhibitory neurotransmitters
      - Gamma-aminobutyric acid (GABA)
      - Glycine
      - Possible influence of serotonin
    - Endogenous opioids
      - Endorphins
      - Enkephalins
      - Dynorphins
      - Endomorphins

Characteristics of Pain

- Pain is a subjective symptom, but physical and emotional signs and cues may alert the provider that the patient is experiencing pain.
- These cues can include
  - Changes in vital signs (increased pulse and blood pressure)
  - Anxiety and fear
  - Restlessness and agitation
  - Diaphoresis
  - Pallor
  - Guarding of part of the body
  - Grimacing
  - Crying

Classifications/Types of Pain

- Acute pain
  - Considered protective because it causes individuals to try to remove themselves from a noxious stimulus
  - Characterized by a sudden onsct
  - Time limited, usually lasting from a few seconds up to about 3 to 6 months
  - Often associated with changes in vital signs, anxiety, and associated symptoms such as vomiting and sweating
  - Classified based on tissue from where pain originates
    - Somatic pain
      - Pain arises from connective tissue and skin.

- Visceral pain
  - Pain arises from internal organs.
- Referred pain
  - Pain arises in one area, but sensation is felt in a different area.
- Chronic pain (Table 9.1)
  - Often more difficult to treat than acute pain
  - Lasts longer than expected or past healing time of injury
  - Severity may not correlate with severity of original injury/illness
  - May be difficult to locate a cause for pain on a diagnostic scan, such as a computed tomography (CT) scan or magnetic resonance imagery (MRI)
  - May be accompanied by depression and feelings of anger

TABLE 9.1 Common Chronic Pain Conditions

Condition	Description
Persistent low back pain	Most common chronic pain condition Results from poor muscle tone, inactivity, muscle strain, or sudden, vigorous exercise
Myofascial pain syndromes	Second most common chronic pain condition Pain results from muscle spasm, tenderness, and stiffness Examples include myositis, fibrositis, myofibrositis, myalgia, and muscle strain—conditions that involve injury to the muscle and fascia As the disorder progresses, pain becomes increasingly generalized
Chronic postoperative pain	Chronic pain that can occur with disruption or cutting of sensory nerves
Cancer pain	Can be pain attributed to advance of disease, associated with treatment, or attributed to coexisting disease entities
Deafferentation pain	Painful condition resulting from damage to a peripheral nerve Common types include severe burning pain triggered by various stimuli, such as cold, light touch, or sound, and reflex sympathetic dystrophies (occur after peripheral nerve injury and are characterized by continuous, severe, burning pain associated with vasomotor changes and muscle wasting)
Hyperesthesias	Increased sensitivity and decreased pain threshold to tactile and painful stimuli Pain is diffuse, modified by fatigue and emotion, and mixed with other sensations May result from chronic irritations of central nervous system areas
Hemiagnosia	Loss of ability to identify source of pain on one side of the body Painful stimuli on that side produce discomfort, anxiety, moaning, agitation, and distress but no attempt to withdraw from the stimulus Associated with stroke
Phantom limb pain	Pain experienced in amputated limb after stump has completely healed; may be immediate or occur months later Influenced by emotions or sympathetic stimulation Trigger points—small hypersensitive regions in muscle or connective tissues that, when stimulated, produce pain in a specific area
Complex regional pain syndrome	Chronic pain usually associated with limb injury, surgery, or fractures Characterized by autonomic and neuroinflammatory features and pain out of proportion to expected pain

From McCance, K. L., & Huether, S. E. (2018). *Pathophysiology: The biologic basis for disease in adults and children* (8th ed.). St. Louis: Elsevier.

- May be neuropathic pain
  - Excessive pain response in the absence of illness/injury
  - Characterized by terms such as burning, tingling, and/or shooting
  - Patient may experience
    - Hyperalgesia
      - Excessive sensitivity to stimuli
    - Allodynia
      - Pain caused by something that is typically not pain inducing
- Phantom pain
  - Pain that occurs where tissue has been amputated.
  - The patient continues to feel pain despite the loss of the tissue.
  - The pathology of this type of pain likely relates to the hyperactivity of severed nerves and lack of normal inhibitory processes.

APPLICATION AND REVIEW

1. A client experiencing abdominal pain, shares with the nurse, "I don't understand why my stomach has to hurt so much." How should the nurse respond to address the client's need for information?
   1. "I can see that the pain is really a problem for you."
   2. "Let's talk about how you can better cope with pain."
   3. "I can see about getting you additional pain medication."
   4. "The pain is a way to let you know something is wrong with your stomach."
2. A client is reporting pain in the lumbar region. A nurse demonstrates an understanding of the triggers for pain when asking which assessment question?
   1. "When did your back pain start?"
   2. "How would you rate your back pain on a scale of 1 to 10?"
   3. "Is there anything that seems to make your back pain worse?"
   4. "Do you remember doing anything to stretch your back muscles?"
3. Which characteristics apply to the delta fiber type of nociceptors? **Select all that apply.**
   1. Covered by a myelin sheath
   2. Associated with chronic pain
   3. Transmits pain sensations quickly
   4. Transmits diffuse pain sensations
   5. Pain is typically described as sharp
4. What event occurs during the transduction stage of the nociception pain process?
   1. Pain sensations are triggered in the periphery.
   2. Pain messages move from the site of injury to the spinal cord.
   3. The cerebral cortex processes the pain message for meaning.
   4. Gama-aminobutyric acid (GABA) is released to help mediate the existence of pain sensations.
5. What nonverbal cues would alert the nurse to the possibility a client is experiencing pain in the lumbar region? **Select all that apply.**
   1. An increase in blood pressure
   2. Resists getting out of bed
   3. Restlessness while sleeping
   4. Ruddy skin color on face
   5. Shivering

6. Which statement supports the possibility that a client is experiencing acute rather than chronic pain? **Select all that apply**.
   1. "The pain came on so quickly."
   2. "I've had this pain for 3 weeks now."
   3. "Nothing seems to help manage this pain."
   4. "I'm sure this pain is causing me to be depressed."
   5. "The pain is responsible for the increase in my blood pressure."
7. What term is used to accurately describe pain that occurs where tissue has been amputated?
   1. Hyperalgesia
   2. Allodynia
   3. Phantom
   4. Referred

See Answers on pages 187–189.

SPECIAL SENSES

Overview of the Eye

- The eye is the organ of vision.
- The eye is protected by the bony orbit around it and the eyelids and eyelashes that cover it anteriorly.
- Cranial nerves III, IV, and VI control the movement of the eye and cranial nerve II transmits sensory input from the eye to the vision center in the brain.
- The eye contains three primary layers.
  - The outer layer is composed of two structures.
    - The sclera is the white part of the eye ball.
    - The cornea is located anterior to the sclera and is responsible for refracting light as it enters the eye.
  - The middle layer is known as the choroid.
    - This is a darkly pigmented and highly vascular layer of the eye.
    - This layer contains the ciliary body, which changes the shape of the lens to focus visual input on the back of the eye.
    - The iris is the colored ring surrounding the pupil.
    - The pupil, the center of the eye, is the area through which light passes into the eye.
    - The lens works with the cornea to bend and change light as it enters the eye.
  - The inner layer of the eye is the retina.
    - There are two kinds of photoreceptor cells in the retina.
      - Rods assist with vision at night.
      - Cones assist with color vision.
        - Cones are red, blue, and green; deficits in these receptors may account for color blindness.
- The eye contains two cavities that are separated by the lens and ciliary body.
  - The area between the lens and retina is known as the posterior cavity.
    - The posterior cavity is filled with vitreous humor.
    - Vitreous humor functions to maintain the shape and size of the eye and hold the retina in place.
  - The space between the cornea and the lens is the anterior cavity; it is composed of the anterior and posterior chambers.
    - Aqueous humor fills the anterior chamber.
    - The function of aqueous humor is to provide nutrients to the cornea and lens.

- The exposed part of eye is covered by a protective lining called the conjunctiva.
  - The palpebral conjunctiva is clear; covers the eyelids.
  - The bulbar conjunctive covers the eyeball itself.

Abnormalities of Eye Function

- Abnormalities caused by structural defects/abnormal movements
  - Hyperopia
    - Known as farsightedness
    - Causes an image to be focused behind the retina
    - Creates difficulty seeing near objects
    - Corrected with lenses
  - Myopia
    - Known as nearsightedness
    - Image is focused too far in front of the retina.
    - Creates difficulty seeing at a distance
    - Corrected with lenses
  - Presbyopia
    - Caused by a loss of elasticity in the lens
    - Occurs with aging
    - Causes the same types of deficits as hyperopia
  - Astigmatism
    - Abnormality in the curve of the cornea or lens
    - Light rays do not focus in a singular fashion on the retina.
    - May accompany presbyopia, myopia, or hyperopia
    - Can be corrected with lenses
  - Strabismus
    - Caused by abnormal extraocular muscles movements
    - Symptoms may include diplopia (double vision).
    - Can lead to amblyopia in children
      - Amblyopia should be corrected early in childhood to prevent permanent visual damage.
  - Nystagmus
    - Abnormal eye movements that can be jerky or rhythmic in nature.
    - Movements are involuntary.
    - Can have a variety of etiologies including
      - Intoxication with drugs and/or alcohol
      - Neurologic diseases
      - Disruptions in cerebellar function
  - Ptosis
    - Upper eyelid paralysis
    - May result from damage to cranial nerves that paralyze extraocular eye muscles
- Infections of the eye
  - Conjunctivitis
    - Inflammation of the conjunctival lining of the eye
    - Also known as "pink eye"
    - Causes may be bacterial, viral, chemical, or allergic in nature
    - Bacterial and viral forms can be spread by contamination from hands and other objects.

- Common symptoms include
  - Sensitivity to light (photophobia)
  - Redness
  - Pain
  - Swelling
  - Itching
  - Tearing/watery discharge
- Antibiotic treatment is required for bacterial forms.
- Trachoma
  - Most common cause of blindness worldwide
  - The organism *Chlamydia trachomatis* causes infection.
  - Bacteria enters the eye owing to poor hygiene and/or transmission by flies carrying bacteria into the eye.
  - Those affected report eyes feeling irritated and "scratchy," but no drainage is present.
  - A key diagnostic finding is pearl-like follicles on the upper eyelid.
  - Without antibiotic treatment, the eyelids become scarred and the cornea can be abraded.
- Keratitis
  - Irritation, inflammation, and/or infection of the corneal lining
  - May be caused by viruses, bacteria, or chemical/mechanical trauma
  - Risk factors include wearing contact lens and traumatic injury of the cornea.
  - Symptoms include sensitivity to light and pain.
    - Pain is owing to the cornea being innervated with many pain receptors.
  - If untreated, erosion and scarring of the cornea can lead to visual deficits.
  - Treatment may include antibiotics if the cause is bacterial contamination.
  - Prevention of keratitis includes proper care of contact lens and wearing protective lens to prevent chemical and mechanical trauma.
- Blepharitis
  - Inflammation and/or infection of the eyelids
  - Causative organism is often staphylococcus
  - Signs and symptoms include
    - Edema
    - Lacrimation
    - Redness
    - Itching
- Hordeolum
  - Infected sebaceous gland in the eyelid
  - Commonly known as a stye
- Chalazion
  - Inflammation of the Meibomian glands of the eyelid
  - Not infectious
- Glaucoma
  - Caused by increased amount of aqueous humor in the eye
  - Intraocular pressure will be increased.
    - Normal intraocular pressure should be between 12 and 20 mm Hg.
  - Considered to be a leading cause of blindness in adults
  - Risk factors for glaucoma can include genetic predisposition.
  - Prolonged increased intraocular pressure can lead to the death of retinal tissue and degeneration of the optic nerve.

- Untreated glaucoma can lead to blindness over a period of years but severely increased intraocular pressure can cause loss of sight within hours or days.
- The condition may initially be asymptomatic, which makes routine screening and early detection crucial.
- Continued elevation in intraocular pressure can lead to eye pain and eventually loss of peripheral vision.
- There are several types of glaucoma.
  - Open-angle
    - Risk factors can include being nearsighted
    - Obstructed flow of aqueous humor at Schlemm canal
  - Narrow-angle
    - Iridiocorneal is narrowed creating a blockage of aqueous humor out of the anterior chamber.
  - Acute-angle closures
    - Same pathology as narrow-angle glaucoma
    - Occurs suddenly with acute rise in the pressure in the eye
    - Signs and symptoms include
      - Severe pain
      - Redness of the eye
      - Visual changes
  - Chronic-angle closures
    - Similar pathology to acute-angle closures
    - Closure will be progressive and permanent
  - Secondary
    - Obstruction of the iridocorneal angle that occurs secondary to another condition.
    - Causes could include
      - Inflammation of the middle layer of the eye
      - Bleeding in the eye
      - Tumors in the eye
      - Lens rupture
  - Congenital
    - Present from birth owing to malformations of eye structures including
      - Trabecular meshwork
- Treatment may be pharmacological or surgical depending on the type of glaucoma.
  - Surgical treatment may be needed in acute forms of glaucoma to prevent vision loss.
  - Chronic glaucoma may be treated with beta-adrenergic blocking agents, which decrease the production of aqueous humor in the eye.
- Cataracts
  - Deficit in light transmission through the eye caused by clouding of the lens
  - Altered transport of nutrients and metabolic changes are causes of cataracts.
  - Risk factors include
    - Age (more common with advanced age)
    - Metabolic disorders, such as diabetes
    - Excess sun exposure
    - Maternal infection can lead to congenital cataracts.
    - Iris pigment imprinting on the lens following trauma to the eye

- Symptoms include
  - Changes in visual acuity
  - Decreased ability to perceive colors
  - Blurring vision
- Treatment includes removal of damaged lens and replacement with an artificial one.
- Macular degeneration
  - A leading cause of blindness in older adult population
  - Vision loss is irreversible.
  - Risk factors include
    - Age
    - Family history of macular degeneration
    - Smoking
    - High blood pressure
    - History of cataract surgery
  - Symptoms include
    - Loss of central vision
    - Peripheral vision unaffected
    - Depth perception decreased
  - Types of macular degeneration
    - Dry/atrophic form
      - Most common form of macular degeneration
      - Buildup of lipfuscin and drusen causes inflammation in the retina.
      - Retinal cells are gradually destroyed.
      - Vision loss is slower and progressive.
      - Treatment may include nutrition therapy.
        - Ensure adequate amounts of antioxidants and zinc
    - Wet/exudative form
      - Abnormal blood vessels develop in the retina.
      - Leaking of blood and/or serum into the retina
      - Scarring and loss of photoreceptors
      - Vision loss is more severe and occurs faster.
      - Treatment may include
        - Photodynamic therapy to seal new leaky vessels in the retina
        - Medications to slow growth of new vessels in the retina
- Retinal detachment
  - Condition where the retina is separated from the choroid layer
  - Vitreous humor flows behind the retina, producing more separation between the choroid layer and the retina.
  - Leads to lack of nutrition for the retinal cells
  - Eventually the retinal cells die from lack of nutrition.
  - Risk factors include
    - Age
    - Severe myopia (nearsightedness)
    - Scar tissue in the eye
  - Signs and symptoms include
    - Floaters or flashes of light in the visual field
    - Initially painless

- Blind spot develops and enlarges over time.
- Called a "dark curtain" across the visual field
  - Treatment is surgical reattachment of the retina in relation to the choroid layer to restore nutrient supply to the tissues.
- Color blindness
  - X-linked recessive genetic disorder
  - Males are affected most often.
  - Occurs in about 6% to 8% of the population
  - Those affected most commonly have difficulty distinguishing red and green shades.
  - Some affected can only see shades of white, gray, and black.

Overview of the Ear

- The ear is the organ of hearing.
- Cranial nerve VIII assists with hearing and balance functions.
- The ear is composed of three distinct sections.
  - External ear is composed of two structures
    - Pinna
      - External portion of the ear that is visible
    - External auditory canal
  - Middle ear
    - Separated from the external ear by the tympanic membrane
    - Contains three bones known as ossicles
      - Tympanic membrane vibrations are transmitted to the inner ear by movement of the bones in the middle ear.
      - Malleus
      - Incus
      - Stapes
        - Presses against the oval window between the middle and inner ear cavities
    - Connects to nasopharynx via the Eustachian tube
      - Eustachian tube equalizes pressure on both sides of the tympanic membrane.
      - Opens with swallowing and yawning
  - Inner ear
    - Also known as the labyrinth
    - Two major parts
      - Cochlea
        - Contains the organ of Corti
          - Organ of Corti contains hearing receptors
      - Semicircular canals/vestibule
        - Contain the receptors for equilibrium
- Process of normal hearing
  - Tympanic membrane vibration begins after sound waves enter the external ear and strike the membrane.
  - Tympanic membrane vibrations cause the bones of the middle ear to vibrate in turn.
  - The stapes moves against the oval window, starting movement of fluids in the cochlea (endolymph and perilymph).
  - Movement of these fluids stimulates the hair cells and membranes in the organ of Corti.

- Nerve impulses are generated by the organ of Corti.
- The temporal lobe receives and interprets the nerve impulses.
- Hearing loss
  - There are two main types of hearing loss.
    - Sensorineural
      - Damage is related to malfunction of the organ of Corti or cranial nerve VIII
      - Possible causes include
        - Head trauma
          - Injury to temporal lobe
          - Injury to cranial nerve VIII
        - Neurologic disorders
        - Damage to structures caused by medications such as
          - Furosemide
          - Ibuprofen
          - Aspirin
          - Vancomycin
          - Neomycin
          - Streptomycin
        - Damage to structures caused by infectious illnesses such as
          - Herpes
          - Influenza
          - Rubella
        - Damage related to loud noise impairing hair cell function in the inner ear
          - Injury may be from prolonged exposure or from exposure to sudden and excessively loud sounds.
    - Conductive
      - Blockage of sound in either the external or middle ear
      - Possible causes include
        - Excess wax in the external canal
        - Foreign body in the external canal
        - Abnormal function/movement of ossicles or tympanic membrane owing to adhesions and/or scarring
- Other forms of hearing loss
  - Presbycusis
    - Age-related hearing changes (Table 9.2)
    - May be caused by accumulated environmental exposures coupled with genetic predisposition
    - Tends to cause problems with hearing high frequency sounds first
      - Negatively impacts an individual's ability to understand conversational speech
  - Functional hearing loss
    - No cause can be found for the deficit.
    - Hypothesized to be related to emotional trauma or psychological issues
  - Congenital deafness
    - May be hereditary
    - Can also be related to prenatal injury
    - Early intervention is key for the infant's development.
      - Deafness may disrupt speech and social interactions.

TABLE 9.2 Changes in Hearing Caused by Aging	
Changes in Structure	**Changes in Function**
Cochlear hair cell degeneration	Inability to hear high-frequency sounds (presbycusis, sensorineural loss); interferes with understanding speech; hearing may be lost in both ears at different times
Loss of auditory neurons in spiral ganglia of organ of Corti	Inability to hear high-frequency sounds (presbycusis, sensorineural loss); interferes with understanding speech; hearing may be lost in both ears at different times
Degeneration of basilar (cochlear) conductive membrane of cochlea	Inability to hear at all frequencies, but more pronounced at higher frequencies (cochlear conductive loss)
Decreased vascularity of cochlea	Equal loss of hearing at all frequencies (strial loss); inability to disseminate localization of sound
Loss of cortical auditory neurons	Equal loss of hearing at all frequencies (strial loss); inability to disseminate localization of sound

From McCance, K. L., & Huether, S. E. (2019). *Pathophysiology: The biologic basis for disease in adults and children* (8th ed.). St. Louis: Elsevier.

Abnormalities of Ear Function

- Infections of the ear
  - Otitis externa
    - Inflammation and/or infection of the external portion of the ear
    - May involve the pinna and/or the external auditory canal
    - May be caused by bacteria including
      - *Staphylococcus aureus*
      - *Escherichia coli*
      - Pseudomonas
    - Signs and symptoms may include
      - Pain
      - Edema
      - Itching
      - Possible hearing loss owing to conduction issues
      - Possible obstruction of the external auditory canal
    - Exposure to moisture is a common cause.
      - Is also known as swimmer's ear owing to an association with moisture
  - Otitis media
    - Inflammation and infection of the middle section of the ear
    - Can occur in any age, but is most commonly seen in infants and children
    - Risk factors include
      - Enlarged tonsils and adenoids
      - History of allergies
      - History or current diagnosis of sinusitis
      - Cleft palate
      - Bottle feeding for infants
    - Signs and symptoms can include
      - Pain
        - Pain may be relieved suddenly if the tympanic membrane ruptures.

- ▪ Elevated temperature
- ▪ Abnormalities in the appearance and function of the tympanic membrane
- ▪ Irritability, especially in young infants and children
- ▪ Pulling or tugging on the ear lobe
- ▪ Condition can be acute or chronic in nature.
- Other disorders of the ear
  - Otosclerosis
    - ▪ Excess bone formation in the middle ear
    - ▪ Sound conduction is blocked because the stapes become fused to the oval window.
    - ▪ More common in young females
    - ▪ Appears to be genetic in nature
  - Meniere's disease
    - ▪ Disease process affecting the inner ear (specifically the labyrinth)
    - ▪ Typically affects one side
    - ▪ Excess production of endolymph stretches membranes in the inner ear and disrupts function of hair cells.
    - ▪ Symptoms include
      - ▪ Vertigo
      - ▪ Tinnitus
      - ▪ Hearing loss on the affected side
    - ▪ Repeated episodes or attacks cause permanent damage in the inner ear.
    - ▪ Possible triggers for attacks
      - ▪ Excessive stress
      - ▪ Changes in weather and barometric pressure
      - ▪ Use of tobacco, alcohol, and caffeine
      - ▪ High levels of sodium in the diet
- Symptoms associated with ear dysfunction
  - Vertigo
    - ▪ Feeling that one is spinning or that the room is spinning
    - ▪ Causes balance changes and increases fall risk
    - ▪ Associated symptoms can include nausea and vomiting.
  - Tinnitus
    - ▪ Excessive noise in the ear
    - ▪ Often characterized as "ringing in the ear"

APPLICATION AND REVIEW

8. A nurse is caring for a client with glaucoma. What information should the nurse include in a teaching program for this client?
   1. Total blindness is inevitable.
   2. Lost vision cannot be restored.
   3. Use of both eyes usually is restricted.
   4. Surgery will help the problem only temporarily.
9. What is the focus of the assessment the nurse should perform to monitor for possible signs and symptoms associated with trauma to cranial nerve III?
   1. Photophobia
   2. Color blindness
   3. Eye movement
   4. Intraocular pressure

10. The nurse is preparing a discussion on eye disorders treated primarily with corrective lens. This information should be presented to clients with which medical diagnosis? **Select all that apply**.
    1. Ptosis
    2. Myopia
    3. Hyperopia
    4. Nystagmus
    5. Astigmatism

11. The nurse is providing the parent of a child diagnosed with conjunctivitis with information on how to avoid the cross contamination of others in the family. What statement by the parent indicates an understanding of preventive strategies?
    1. "I'll be sure everyone washes their hands frequently."
    2. "This eye problem is a result of a bacterial or viral infection."
    3. "If someone else get a pinkish eye, we'll get treatment immediately."
    4. "Giving everyone a vitamin C pill daily will help keep the problem under control."

12. A nurse is caring for a client who reports scratchy eyes after returning from a trip to Africa. The diagnosis of trachoma has been suggested by the primary care provider. The nurse demonstrates an understanding of the signs and symptoms of this eye disorder when asking which assessment question?
    1. "Have you noticed any white, pearly lumps on your eyelids?"
    2. "Can you describe the eye drainage you've been experiencing?"
    3. "Was the water supply safe in the areas you visited during your trip?"
    4. "Did you ever experience an animal bite or a scratch during your trip?"

13. A client is being diagnostically evaluated for glaucoma. What response should the nurse provide to the client when the results show intraocular pressure at 14 mm Hg?
    1. "The results indicate you have open angle glaucoma."
    2. "Your intraocular pressure is low and will need further evaluation."
    3. "The results are inconclusive and so you will need to be retested in 3 months."
    4. "Your intraocular pressure is within the accepted normal range ruling out glaucoma."

14. A client diagnosed with glaucoma has not been compliant with treatment. What report by the client alerts the nurse to a potentially dangerous symptom of long-term elevated intraocular pressure.
    1. "My right eye has started to be painful."
    2. "I use to see dark flecks but that has stopped recently."
    3. "I have a dark spot in the center of my field of vision."
    4. "My eyes are so much more watery than they ever were."

15. A client has been diagnosed with a small, benign tumor in the right eye. What form of glaucoma is the client now at risk for developing?
    1. Chronic angle
    2. Acute angle
    3. Congenital
    4. Secondary

16. Which client is at greatest risk for developing cataracts?
    1. A 62-year-old diagnosed with a closed head concussion
    2. A 64-year-old diagnosed with hyperopia since age 40
    3. A 65-year-old diagnosed with bilateral ptosis
    4. A 60-year-old diagnosed with diabetes type 2

17. What client has a risk factor for the development of macular degeneration? **Select all that apply**.
    1. A client with a baseline blood pressure of 110/64 mm Hg.
    2. A client with a history of cigar smoking over the last 30 years
    3. A client who underwent bilateral cataract removal 2 years ago
    4. A client who takes a prescribed antihistamine for seasonal allergies

18. What intervention will the nurse implement to support the treatment of dry/atrophic macular degeneration?
    1. Identify foods that are good natural sources of zinc
    2. Encourage the client to wear sunglasses when outdoors
    3. Discourage the client from bending down from the waist
    4. Educate the client on the benefits of photodynamic therapy
19. A client is experiencing dizziness. What structures of the ear will be the focus of a physical assessment?
    1. Cochlea
    2. Eustachian tubes
    3. Semicircular canals
    4. Tympanic membranes

See Answers on pages 187–189.

OTHER SPECIAL SENSES

- Taste
  - Also known as gustation
  - Can be impaired when sense of smell is impaired
  - Cranial nerves VII and IX are involved in transmitting taste sensations.
  - Taste buds are found all over the tongue and different types of taste buds respond to different flavors.
  - Primary taste sensations include
    - Salty
    - Bitter
    - Sweet
    - Sour
    - Savory
  - Causes of changes in sensation of taste include
    - Infections of the mouth and/or respiratory system
    - Injury to the head and/or cranial nerves VII or IX
    - Administration of medications
    - Change in function owing to normal aging
  - Alterations in taste include
    - Hypogeusia
      - This is a decrease in ability to taste.
    - Ageusia
      - This is the inability to taste.
- Smell
  - Also known as olfaction
  - Can be impaired when sense of taste is impaired
  - Cranial nerves I and trigeminal branch of cranial nerve V control sense of smell.
  - Alterations in smell include
    - Hyposmia
      - Decreased sense of smell
    - Anosmia
      - Loss of the sense of smell
    - Olfactory hallucinations
      - Sensation of smelling something that is not actually there to be smelled

- Parosmia
  - Abnormal or altered sense of smell
- Touch
  - The sensation of touch is based several factors including the location and intensity of stimulus.
  - Alterations in the sensation of touch can occur owing to disruptions anywhere from the local receptors in the skin to the cerebral cortex.
  - The sensation of touch typically evokes and is accompanied by an affective/emotional response.
  - Spinothalamic tract contains neurons that transmit sensation of light touch along with pain and temperature.
  - Neurons that transmit the sensations of localized touch, position, and vibratory sensations arise from the posterior column.
- Proprioception
  - Understanding of the position of one's body in space
  - Based on sensory data from the periphery being transmitted through the spinal cord to the cerebral cortex for processing
  - Assists with maintaining posture and coordinating movements
  - Disruptions in proprioception are generally caused by either vestibular dysfunction or neuropathy.
- Temperature
  - Maintaining body temperature is crucial to sustain life and depends on balancing heat production, heat loss, and conservation of body heat.
  - A healthy range for body temperature is 36.2° to 37.7° C (97.2° to 99.9° F).
  - The hypothalamus is the location of temperature regulation in the brain.
    - Body heat is produced by two main processes.
      - Nonshivering thermogenesis
      - Metabolism via chemical reactions
    - Conservation of body heat occurs by
      - Increased muscle tone
      - Shivering
      - Constriction of blood vessels
    - Heat loss occurs by
      - Evaporation
      - Convection
      - Radiation
      - Conduction
      - Vasodilation
      - Muscle relaxation
  - Disruptions in temperature control
    - Hyperthermia
      - Temperature less than 99.9° F
      - Severe hyperthermia may lead to seizures, damage to neural tissue, and eventual death.
      - Types of hyperthermia include
        - Heat cramps
          - Excessive loss of sodium and fluid
          - Cramping in trunk and extremities
          - Vital signs may reflect tachycardia and hypertension.

- ○ Heat exhaustion
  - ○ Excessive dilation of blood vessels and sweating
  - ○ Individual may be weak and confused.
  - ○ Vital signs reflect hypotension and tachycardia.
- ○ Heat stroke
  - ○ Regulatory center in the brain fails and body cannot compensate
  - ○ Individual's core temperature is elevated but unable to perspire to decrease temperature.
  - ○ May lead to coma and death
- Hypothermia
  - Temperature less than 95° F
  - Types of hypothermia
    - Accidental hypothermia
      - Unplanned exposure to cold water or ambient temperature leading to a decrease in core body temperature
    - Therapeutic hypothermia
      - Medically induced hypothermia
      - The goal is to reduce metabolic demands and preserve tissue after trauma or surgery.

APPLICATION AND REVIEW

20. What is considered a healthy range of body temperature?
1. 96.8° to 98.9° F
2. 97.2° to 99.9° F
3. 98.0° to 100.0° F
4. 98.8° to 100.2° F

See Answer on page 187–189.

ANSWER KEY: REVIEW QUESTIONS

1. **4 Pain is an unpleasant but protective mechanism of defense for the human body that provides a warning that the body may be experiencing damage.**

   1 Although providing clients with an opportunity express their concerns is appropriate, it does not provide information. **2** Although discussing pain management/coping strategies is appropriate, it does not provide information. **3** Arranging for additional pain medication, which is possibly appropriate, it does not provide information.

   Client Need: Physiological Adaptation; **Cognitive Level:** Analysis; **Nursing Process:** Implementation

2. **4 Pain can occur for a variety of reasons including trauma such as stretching of tissue.**

   1 This is an appropriate assessment question, but it does not address the cause or the pain trigger. **2** This is an appropriate assessment question, but it does not address the cause or the pain trigger. **3** This is an appropriate assessment question, but it does not address the cause or the pain trigger.

   Client Need: Physiological Adaptation; **Cognitive Level:** Analysis; **Nursing Process:** Assessment

3. **Answers: 1, 3, 5.**

   1 A delta fiber nociceptor is covered by a myelin sheath. **3** A delta fiber nociceptor transmits pain sensations quickly. **5** A delta fiber nociceptor sensations may be described as sharp and/or sudden.

   2 C fiber nociceptors lack a myelin sheath. **4** C fiber nociceptors transmit sensations that are dull or diffuse.

   Client Need: Physiological Adaptation; **Cognitive Level:** Understanding; **Integrated Process:** Teaching and Learning

4. **1 Nociception occurs in four stages. The first stage, transduction, includes the triggering of nociceptors in the body's periphery.**

    2 Stimulated message moves from the source of injury up the spinal cord during the transmission stage. **3** The meaning of pain is processed in the cerebral cortex during the perception stage. **4** During the modulation stage, inhibitory neurotransmitters, such as GABA, may be released.

    Client Need: Physiological Adaptation; **Cognitive Level:** Understand; **Integrated Process:** Teaching and Learning

5. **Answers: 1, 2, 3.**

    1 Nonverbal pain cues include an increase in pulse and blood pressure. **2** Nonverbal pain cues include guarding a part of the body that would result in a reluctance to move about. **3** Nonverbal pain cues include restlessness and even agitation.

    4 Nonverbal pain cues include pallor not a red hue to the skin. **5** Diaphoresis not shivering is a characteristic of pain.

    Client Need: Physiological Adaptation; **Cognitive Level:** Applying; **Nursing Process:** Assessment

6. **Answers: 1, 2, 5.**

    1 Acute pain is characterized by a sudden onset. **2** Acute pain usually lasts less than 3 to 6 months. **5** Acute pain is often associated with an increase in pulse and blood pressure.

    3 Chronic pain is often more difficult to treat than acute pain. **4** Chronic pain may be a trigger for depression.

    Client Need: Physiological Adaptation; **Cognitive Level:** Analysis; **Nursing Process:** Assessment

7. **3 Phantom pain would be the term that accurately describes pain a patient continues to feel despite the loss of an amputated limb.**

    1 Hyperalgesia refers to excessive sensitivity to a stimulus. **2** Allodynia is pain caused by a trigger that does not usually induce pain. **4** Referred pain arises in one area, but the pain sensation is felt in a different area.

    Client Need: Physiological Adaptation; **Cognitive Level:** Knowledge; **Integrated Process:** Teaching and Learning

8. **2 Retinal damage caused by the increased intraocular pressure of glaucoma is progressive and permanent if the disease is not controlled.**

    1 Early treatment may prevent blindness. **3** One eye may be affected, and there is no restriction on the use of either eye. **4** Surgery can improve drainage and permanently reduce pressure.

    Client Need: Physiological Adaptation; **Cognitive Level:** Applying; **Nursing Process:** Planning

9. **3 Cranial nerves III, IV, and VI control the movement of the eye.**

    1 Photophobia, sensitivity to light, is not associated with cranial nerve III damage. **2** Color blindness is associated with improper functions of the cones located in the retina. **4** Intraocular pressure is associated with the production and drainage of fluid in the eye (aqueous humor).

    Client Need: Physiological Adaptation; **Cognitive Level:** Application; **Nursing Process:** Assessment

10. **Answers: 2, 3, 5.**

    2 Myopia causes images to be focused too far in front of the retina and can be treated with corrective lens. **3** Hyperopia causes images to be focused behind the retina and can be treated with corrective lens. **5** Astigmatism results in an abnormal curve of the cornea or lens and can be treated with corrective lens.

    1 Ptosis is associated with the paralysis of the upper eyelid. **4** Nystagmus is a neurologic disorder that results in abnormal, jerky eye movements.

    Client Need: Physiological Adaptation; **Cognitive Level:** Applying; **Nursing Process:** Planning

11. **1 Conjunctivitis can be spread by contamination from hands and other objects. Frequent handwashing will help minimize the risk of cross-contamination between family members.**

    2 Conjunctivitis can be a result of bacterial or viral infections, but the statement does not address managing cross-contamination effectively. **3** Although pink eye is another term used to describe conjunctivitis, the knowledge that medical treatment is necessary for this disorder does not effectively address managing cross-contamination. **4** Although vitamin C has some effect on minimizing the risk of developing some infections, using it does not address managing cross-contamination effectively.

    Client Need: Physiological Adaptation; **Cognitive Level:** Applying; **Nursing Process:** Evaluation

12. **1 Trachoma is a bacterial infection that can be transmitted by flies carrying the bacteria into the eyes.**
    2 Trachoma presents with an irritated, scratchy sensation in the affected eye, but there is no associated drainage.
    3 Trachoma is not transmitted via contaminated water. **4** Trachoma is not transmitted via bites or scratches.
    Client Need: Physiological Adaptation; **Cognitive Level:** Applying; **Nursing Process:** Assessment

13. **4 Glaucoma is a result of the increased production of aqueous humor that increases intraocular pressure. Normal intraocular pressure is between 12 and 20 mm Hg.**
    1 The diagnosis of a specific type of glaucoma is not dependent on an increase of intraocular pressure alone but rather the cause of the increase. **2** A reading of 14 mm Hg is within the normal intraocular pressure range. **3** The results are not inconclusive; making this statement incorrect.
    Client Need: Physiological Adaptation; **Cognitive Level:** Analysis; **Nursing Process:** Analysis

14. **1 Glaucoma and the associated uncontrolled increase in intraocular pressure can result in eye pain, loss of peripheral vision, and ultimately blindness.**
    2 Specks or floaters are not associated with glaucoma. **3** Peripheral, not central, vision loss is associated with glaucoma. **4** Watery eyes are not associated with glaucoma.
    Client Need: Physiological Adaptation; **Cognitive Level:** Analysis; **Nursing Process:** Evaluation

15. **4 Secondary glaucoma results from another existing condition, such as a tumor, that obstructs the flow of aqueous humor.**
    1 Closed-angle glaucoma (or narrow-angle glaucoma) occurs when the iris blocks the drainage angle in the eye. **2** Acute angle glaucoma is characterized by a sudden increase in intraocular pressure. **3** Congenital glaucoma is present from birth and results in malformations of certain eye structures.
    Client Need: Physiological Adaptation; **Cognitive Level:** Understanding; **Integrated Process:** Teaching and Learning

16. **4 Cataracts are a clouding of the lens resulting from nutrient and metabolic changes. Risk factors for cataract development include age and metabolic disorders such as diabetes. The client with both factors has an increased risk for developing cataracts.**
    1 The client has one risk factor—age. A closed head injury is not a risk factor for the development of cataracts. **2** The client has one risk factor—age. Hyperopia (farsightedness) is not a risk factor for the development of cataracts. **3** The client has one risk factor—age. Ptosis (upper eyelid paralysis) is not a risk factor for the development of cataracts.
    Client Need: Physiological Adaptation; **Cognitive Level:** Analysis; **Nursing Process:** Analysis

17. **2 Macular degeneration is associated with pathophysiology involving the retina. A risk factor for this disorder includes smoking.**
    1 A risk factor for this disorder includes hypertension, not normal blood pressure. **3** Cataracts are not a risk factor of this disorder. **4** Antihistamine therapy is not a risk factor for this disorder.
    Client Need: Physiological Adaptation; **Cognitive Level:** Applying; **Nursing Process:** Assessment

18. **1 Treatment for dry/atrophic macular degeneration includes nutritional therapy that ensures adequate amounts of antioxidants and zinc.**
    2 Although a good eye health practice, sunglasses are not a part of treatment for this eye disorder. **3** Although bending from the waist increases intraocular pressure, avoiding such movement would not positively affect treatment of macular degeneration. **4** Photodynamic therapy is a treatment for wet/exudative macular degeneration.
    Client Need: Physiological Adaptation; **Cognitive Level:** Applying; **Nursing Process:** Implementation.

19. **3 The semicircular canal, located in the inner ear, contains the receptors for maintaining equilibrium.**
    1 The cochlea holds the organ of Corti, which contains hearing receptors. It has no role in dizziness (equilibrium). **2** The Eustachian tube serves to equalize pressures on both sides of the tympanic membrane. It has no role in dizziness (equilibrium). **4** The tympanic membrane vibrates, causing the bones of the middle ear to vibrate. It has no role in dizziness (equilibrium).
    Client Need: Physiological Adaptation; **Cognitive Level:** Understanding; **Integrated Process:** Teaching and Learning

20. **2 A healthy range for body temperature is 36.2° to 37.7° C (97.2° to 99.9° F).**
    1 This range is too low. **3** This range is too high. **4** This range is too high.
    Client Need: Physiological Adaptation; **Cognitive Level:** Remembering; **Integrated Process:** Teaching and Learning

10 Musculoskeletal System Disorders

MUSCULOSKELETAL SYSTEM OVERVIEW

Musculoskeletal System

- The musculoskeletal system gives the body form and stability; it allows for movement and interaction with objects in the environment.
- The musculoskeletal system is composed of two systems that work together to provide an individual with mobility.
  - Skeleton (bones and joints)
  - Soft tissue (muscle, tendons, and ligaments)

Structure and Function of Bones

- Bone is classified as a unique connective tissue of intercellular matrix and bones.
- Matrix has microscopic structural units named haversian systems or osteons.
  - Lamellae are rings of matrix that surround a haversian canal with blood vessels.
    - Composed of collage fibers and calcium phosphate salts
    - Provide the strong structure of bone
  - Lacunae, the spaces between the rings of matrix, contain osteocytes or mature bone cells.
  - Canaliculi are small passages that provide routes for communication between the lacunae and haversian canals.

Embryonic Bone Development

- There are two primary mechanisms for normal bone development.
- Endochondral ossification uses a cartilage template.
  - Mesenchymal stem cells differentiate into preosteblast or chondrocytes.
  - Produces a mineralized cartilage platform
  - Permits formation of osteoblast
  - Results in formation of long bones and bone elements
- Intramembranous ossification occurs during fetal development.
  - Does not involve cartilage framework
  - Mesenchymal stem cells develop into preosteoblast and then osteoblast.
  - Produces skull and flat bones

New Bone Formation

- A balance is maintained between osteoblasts that produce new bone, and osteoclasts that reabsorb bone.
- Hemostasis of the bone is maintained by the
  - Osteoblast
  - Osteoclast
- Hormone levels and stress imposed on the bone material guide
  - Bone formation
  - Resorption activity

- Osteoblast function is to secrete the matrix of the bone.
  - Osteoprogenitor cells originate from mesenchymal cells.
    - Develop into osteoblast
  - Active on outer surface of bone
    - Form a single layer of cells
    - Responsive to parathyroid hormone
    - Produce osteocalcin, a protein when stimulated by 1,25-dihydroxy-vitamin D_3
    - Through synthesis of osteoid (nonmineralized bone matrix) new bone is formed.
    - Final differentiation stage for osteoblast is transforming to osteocytes.
      - Minerals that enter ossification harden the osteoblast.
      - Osteocytes are the most prevalent cells in bone.
- Osteoclast function is the dissolution and reabsorption of bone.
  - Macrophage progenitor cells produce the osteoclast.
  - Bone is reabsorbed through secretion of substances to digest collagen.
    - Hydrochloric acid
    - Acid proteases (cathepsin K)
    - Matrix matalloproteinases
  - Osteoclast binds to bone surfaces through podosomes.
    - Podosomes contain proteins, enzymes, and receptors.
    - Calcitonin binds to receptor areas of osteoclast to loosen the osteoclast from the cell surface.
    - After reabsorption, osteoclast resumes an inactive or resting state.
- Osteoblast and osteoclast are dependent on hormones to regulate their activity.
  - Calcitonin stimulates osteoblast.
  - Parathyroid hormone stimulates osteoclast.
- Bone cells have a cyclic function to produce and repair bone tissue.
  - New bone tissue is produced.
  - Old bone tissue is reabsorbed.
- Collagen is the fiber that gives bones strength.
- Additional factors impacting bone formation and remodeling
  - Transforming group factor-beta (TGF-β) superfamily
    - Responsible for initiating, differentiating, and providing the precursor cells into osteoblast
  - Bone morphogenetic protein is a member of TGF-β.
    - Regulates at the molecular level different functions in the skeletal system
  - Wnt genes
    - Protein-signaling factors
    - Necessary for development of bone, remodeling, and bone healing
    - Signaling regulates production and differentiation of osteoblast and osteoclast.
    - Affects bone density and mass, formation of joints, bone remodeling, and repair
    - Wnt genes can affect some bone disorders.

Types of Bone

There are two types of bone tissue depending on the density.
- Compact bone
  - Derived from packed tightly haversian systems
  - Produces a strong and rigid structure
  - Forms the outermost covering of bone

- Cancellous or spongy bone
  - Less dense and lacks haversian systems
  - Composed of plates and bars of bone adjacent to cavities that contain bone marrow
  - Bone marrow is a source of mesenchymal (nonhematopoietic) stem cells
    - Generate bone cells
    - Generate cartilage cells
    - Generate fat cells
    - Assist in the development of blood cells and connective tissue
  - The second function of bone marrow cavities within bones is to store cells.
    - For hematopoietic stem cells that develop into blood and immune cells
- Skeletal system functions
  - Provides the body with support
  - Protects internal organs
  - Produces blood cells
  - Works with other structures to provide movement
- Bones provide
  - Support and shape
  - Protection for internal organs
  - Serve a metabolic function
    - Formation of red blood cells in the bone marrow (hematopoiesis)
    - Metabolism and storage of calcium
- Skeletal divisions
  - Axial: bones that forms the vertical and central axis of the body
    - Composed of 80 bones
    - Skull
    - Vertebral column
    - Ribs
    - Sternum
  - Appendicular: the bones of the upper and lower extremities
    - Composed of 126 bones
    - Pelvic girdle
    - Clavicle
    - Scapula

APPLICATION AND REVIEW

1. What client actions would be markedly impaired by a musculoskeletal disorder? **Select all that apply.**
   1. Knitting a scarf
   2. Standing upright
   3. Cutting with scissors
   4. Hearing the telephone ring
   5. Ambulating to the bathroom
2. A genetic disorder that affects fetal bone formation will have an impact on the development of what bones?
   1. Skull bones
   2. Femur bones
   3. Humerus bones
   4. Vertebral bones

3. What process must be in hemostasis to maintain stable new bone replacement?
   1. A balance between the function of both healthy osteoblasts and healthy osteoclasts
   2. Parathyroid production sufficient to stimulate effective osteoclast activity
   3. Sufficient collagen to produce fiber in quantities needed for bone strength
   4. Sufficient production of calcitonin to stimulate osteoblast activity
4. A bone disorder affecting bone density and mass would likely be triggered by what genetic dysfunction?
   1. Overproduction of osteoclasts
   2. Insufficient production of osteoblasts
   3. Dysfunctional wnt gene production
   4. Ineffective TGF-β superfamilies
5. A client with dysfunctional bone marrow cavities will be at risk for what health-related issue?
   1. Myocardial infarction (MI)
   2. Frequent infections
   3. Jaundice
   4. Asthma
6. A client diagnosed with a disease process that affected the function of the skeletal system would require what nursing intervention?
   1. Frequent hematologic monitoring
   2. Education on dietary potassium sources
   3. Instructions of the importance of avoiding sun exposure
   4. Instituting effective stress management practices into daily practice
7. Which sports-related activity places the client at greatest risk for an axial skeletal injury?
   1. Skiing
   2. Football
   3. Catching a ball
   4. Kicking a soccer ball

See Answers on pages 215–217.

Classification of Bones

Bones are classified according to their shape.
- Long bones
  - Consist of thin shaft (diaphysis) with two bulbous ends (epiphyses)
  - Diaphysis is compact bone enclosed in a medullary cavity with marrow.
    - Diaphysis can accommodate bending force in bone.
    - Contains yellow marrow
      - Composed of primarily fatty tissue
      - Promotes red bone marrow in hematopoiesis during stress
  - Epiphyses is spongy bone formed where the shaft broadens at the metaphysis.
  - Hyaline cartilage or articular cartilage
    - Covers the epiphysis to facilities free movement between two bones
  - Epiphyseal cartilage (growth plate)
    - Area where longitudinal bone growth occurs in response to growth and sex hormones
  - Bone growth stops when epiphyseal plate ossifies during adolescence or early adulthood.
  - Epiphyseal plate is referred to as epiphyseal line after long bone closure.
    - Femur
    - Humerus
- Short (cuboidal) bones
  - Provide stability and movement

- Spongy bone has a thin cover of compact bone.
- Square in shape
  - Wrist
  - Ankle bones
- Flat bones
  - For ribs and scapular, the two plates of bone are almost parallel to each other.
  - A spongy bone lies between the compact plates.
  - Thin and curved
  - Ribs
  - Scapular
- Irregular bones
  - Several projections and a variety of shapes
    - Vertebrae
    - Mandible
    - Facial bones
  - Thin portion is composed of two plates of compact bone.
    - Spongy bone between plates
  - Thick portion is composed of spongy bone enclosed by compact bone.
- Sesamoid bones
  - Round
    - Found in tendons
    - Patella bone

APPLICATION AND REVIEW

8. What is the purpose of the diaphysis of a bone?
   1. Provide minimal friction at union points
   2. Give a degree of bendability
   3. Produce a spongy quality
   4. Develop the growth plate
9. Which client is at greatest risk for impaired bone growth?
   1. Preschool child diagnosed with a deficiency in sex hormones
   2. A young adult who was born with a congenital facial anomaly
   3. An adolescent who experienced a severe femur fracture
   4. An older adult diagnosed with osteoporosis
10. A client has been diagnosed as having fractured an irregular bone. What nursing intervention should the nurse consider for inclusion in the client's plan of care?
    1. Medicate for wrist pain as needed
    2. Provide a straw for the intake of liquids
    3. Demonstrate how to support the chest for coughing
    4. Monitor color and temperature of the foot every 4 hours

Bone Layers/Components

- Periosteum
  - Covers the bone
  - Composed of fibrous connective tissue
  - Contains osteoblast, nerves, blood vessels, and lymphatics

- Bone marrow
  - Produced through hematopoiesis
  - Red marrow is found in ribs, cranium, vertebrae, sternum, and ilia.
  - Bone cells: the homeostatis of bone is maintained by the dynamic equilibrium of the production and reabsorption of bone.
    - Osteoblasts are responsible for producing new bone.
    - Osteoclasts are responsible for reabsorption of bone.
    - Osteocytes lie in lacunae spaces and are mature bone cells.

Bone Remodeling

- Process where old bone is removed (by osteoclast)
- New bone is produced (by osteoblast).
- Maintains equilibrium by a continuous renewal of the skeletal system
- Remodeling allows adaption to challenges from the environment to regulate mineral metabolism.
- Three phases of bone remodeling
  - Phase 1 is activation.
    - Stimulus (physical stress, drugs, vitamins, hormones) activates cell death (apoptosis)
    - Apoptosis provides osteoclast information where to begin bone reabsorption.
  - Phase 2 is resorption.
    - Osteoclast attaches to bone matrix through multiple proteins that form podosomes (foot-like structures).
    - Once attached, osteoclast produces lysosomal enzymes that digest the bone.
    - Bone and degraded by-products are released into the vascular system.
  - Phase 3 is formation of new bone.
    - Osteoblast expresses osteoid and alkaline phosphatase into the walls of the resorption cavity.
      - Forming sites for calcium and phosphorus deposits
    - Osteoid mineralizes and forms new bone.
    - Additional layers of new bone are formed until the resorption cavity is a narrowed haversian canal surrounded by a blood vessel.
    - As new haversian systems are formed, the new trabeculae form spongy bone.
    - Process takes 4 to 6 months in a healthy human
  - Remodeling repairs small, microscopic bone injuries.
- Hormones
  - Calcitonin stimulates osteoblast that secretes the matrix of bone.
  - Parathyroid hormone stimulates osteoclast that reabsorbs bone.
  - Bone density can change because of the effect of three hormones.
    - Growth
    - Parathyroid
    - Cortisol
  - Bone growth
    - Appositional: increase in bone diameter
    - Endochondral: increase in length of bone

Structure and Function of Joints

- The major function of joints is to aid with mobility and stability of the skeleton.
  - The location and structure of the joint determines its function.

- Joint (articulation) is the area where two or more bones meet.
- Joints are classified by degree of movement or connecting tissue.
  - Movement
    - Synarthrosis
      - Immovable joint
    - Amphiarthrosis
      - Slightly movable joint
  - Diarthrosis
    - Freely movable joint
- Fibrous joints
  - Fibrous connective tissues connect the joint to the bone.
    - Usually synarthrosis (or immovable) joint
    - Fibrous joints do allow for movement.
    - Degree of the joint movement depends on
      - Distance between bones
      - Flexibility of fibrous connective tissue
- Subdivision of fibrous joints
  - Suture
    - Flat bones in skull of infants and young children are interlocked.
    - Thin layer of dense fibrous tissue
    - Sutures are locked together and allow no movement.
    - In adulthood, bone replaces the fibrous connective tissue.
  - Syndesmosis
    - Ligament or membrane joins two bony surfaces.
    - Limited motion
    - Ligament fibers have flexibility.
    - Examples are bone pairs such as the radius and ulna of the arm.
    - Other examples are the tibia and fibula of the leg.
  - Gomphoses
    - Fibrous joint that has a unique conical projection
    - Held by ligament in a complementary socket
    - Examples are teeth in the mandible or maxillary bone.
  - Cartilaginous joints
    - Both symphysis and synchondrosis
    - Symphysis cartilaginous joints are joined by a disk or pad of fibrocartilage.
      - Two articulating bones covered by hyaline cartilage
      - Broad pad of fibrocartilage acts as a buffer and stabilizer.
      - Examples are intervertebral disks and pubic bones.
    - Synchondrosis cartilaginous joints joined by hyaline cartilage
      - Hyaline cartilage is referred to as costal cartilage.
      - Allows some movement between ribs and sternum for breathing
      - Between rib and sternum
  - Synovial joints (diarthrosis)
    - Most complex and movable joint
    - Articular capsule
      - Fibrous joint capsule
      - Interlocking layers of white fibrous tissue
      - Attaches capsule to the periosteum, ligaments, and tendons

- Covers ends of bones where they meet the joint
  - Blood supply and lymphatic system is robust.
  - Nerves are responsive to compression, tension, vibration, pain, and tempo and direction of motion.
- Synovial membrane
  - Lines inner surface of joint capsule
  - Two layers: subintima and intima
  - Subintima is vascular layer.
    - Composed of fibers, fat cells, fibroblast, macrophages, mast cells, and loose fibrous connective tissue
  - Intima is a cellular layer.
    - Synovial cells encapsulated in a fiber-free intercellular matrix
    - Synovial cells type A
      - Ingest bacteria and particles of debris
    - Synovial cells type B
      - Secrete hyaluronate
      - ~~g~~ ~~g~~ ~~gives viscosity to synovial fluid.~~
- Joint cavity (synovial cavity)
  - ~~Fluid space is located~~ between the articulating surfaces of bones.
  - Allows two bones to move in opposition
  - Encircled by a synovial membrane and contains synovial fluid
- Synovial fluid
  - Synovial fluid is a lubricant for the joint cavity.
  - Well-filtered plasma originating from synovial membrane
  - Loss of synovial fluid leads to a rapid decay of articular cartilage.
- Articular cartilage
  - Covers the end of each joint with a layer of hyaline cartilage
  - Is a pad for joining bony surfaces
  - Collagen fibers reduce friction and disperse forces of weight bearing.
  - Composed of chondrocytes or cartilage cells
  - Chrondrocytes produce the intercellular matrix.
  - Three layers of cartilage
    - Collagen fibers at surface are parallel to the joint surface and are compact and dense.
    - Middle layer (proliferative zone) fibers are tangential to the surface to allow then to absorb forces, such as weight bearing.
    - Bottom layer (hypertrophic zone) fibers are perpendicular allowing resistance to forces. In a calcified layer of cartilage the collagen fibers are anchored by the tidemark.
  - The cartilage matrix is 60% dry weight collagen fibers.
    - Cartilage is secured to underlying bone.
    - Tight framework for cartilage
    - Controls any fluid loss from the cartilage
    - Prevents protein polysaccharides (or proteoglycans) from escaping
  - Usually articular cartilage has no nerves or blood and lymph vessels, therefore repair is slow and it is insensitive to pain after an injury.
  - Healing and regeneration usually occur at the location where the synovial membrane converges with the articular cartilage.

- Advances in cartilage regeneration
  - Mesenchymal stem cell therapy to restore articulate cartilage
  - Mesenchymal stem cells secrete restorative factors in the injured area of the articular cartilage.
    - Promotes repair through tropic effects
  - Gene therapy can target a variety of genes involved at the cellular level (inflammatory, anabolic pathways). TGF-β and other growth factors are described as assisting in cartilage regenerations.

Structure and Function of Skeletal Muscle

- The four functions of skeletal muscle
  - Muscle contraction aids body movement.
  - Muscle tone enhances body position.
  - Stabilizes joints by minimizing excessive movement
  - Maintains body temperature by heat generated through muscle contraction
  - Primarily skeletal muscles are under voluntary control, but there are exceptions.
    - Respiratory movement
    - Pupillary reflexes
    - Blinking
    - Shivering
    - Reflexes
- Multiple signaling factors control formation of skeletal muscle.
- Muscle derives from mesodermal progenitor cells; the largest amount are somites.
- Myogenesis is embryonic muscle formation.
  - Protein kinase is an enzyme that adds phosphate groups to substrate proteins.
  - These factors guide the formation of myoblast.
  - Myoblast fuse with each other to form myotubes that eventually become muscle fibers.
  - Final muscle type is determined by transcription factors in pre- and post-natal muscle development.
- Voluntary muscles
  - Begin as mesodermal layer as an embryo
  - Skeletal muscle differentiation is directed by transcription factors, in particular myoblast determination protein.
  - Myoblast (satellite cells when dormant) guides muscle regeneration and growth.
  - Satellite cells are activated during a muscle injury and increase the number of transcriptional factors to form myoblast needed for repair.
- Skeletal muscles are composed of millions of individual fibers that are needed for movement by contraction or relaxation.
- Muscle constitutes 40% of an adult and 50% of a child's body weight.
- Muscle is made of 75% water, 20% protein, and 5% organic/inorganic compounds.
- Of all protein for energy and metabolism, 32% is stored in muscle.

APPLICATION AND REVIEW

11. Which client would be at risk for impaired red bone marrow storage?
    1. A client who has a fractured mandible
    2. A client who has a fractured femur
    3. A client who has a fractured sternum
    4. A client who has a fractured tibia

12. What factor triggers the process of apoptosis?
    1. Physical stress to the bone
    2. Increased production of osteoblasts
    3. A decrease in circulating sex hormones
    4. A marked lack of forming sites for calcium and phosphorus
13. Which hormones influence bone density? **Select all that apply**.
    1. Sex
    2. Growth
    3. Calcitonin
    4. Thyroxine
    5. Parathyroid
14. Where are suture joints located?
    1. Skull of an infant
    2. Pelvis of an adolescent
    3. Cervical spine of an adult
    4. Rib cage and sternum of an older adult
15. What composes the subintima layer of a synovial membrane? **Select all that apply**.
    1. Fat cells
    2. Mast cells
    3. Fibroblasts
    4. Synovial cells type A
    5. Synovial cells type B
16. What statement by the nurse demonstrates an understanding of the result of a prolonged loss of synovial fluid in a client's knee?
    1. "A surgical procedure will be necessary to replace the fluid."
    2. "The articular cartilage in the knee has decayed significantly."
    3. "The joint between the patella and the fibula will need to be rebuilt."
    4. "The patella will dislocate frequently, requiring manual manipulation."
17. What processes involving skeletal muscles are under involuntary control? **Select all that apply**.
    1. Shivering
    2. Blinking
    3. Respirations
    4. Pupil reflexes
    5. Joint stabilization

See Answers on pages 215–217.

Whole Muscle

- There are more than 350 muscles in the body that are usually paired to provide movement; the length and shape vary according to function.
  - Fusiform muscles extend from one joint to another and are elongated in shape.
  - Pennate muscles are broad and flat and extend obliquely to a muscle's long axis.
- Fascia is a three-part connective tissue frame that encircles each skeletal muscle.
  - Muscle fibers are protected by connective tissue.
  - Attach muscle to bone
  - Network for blood vessels, nerve fibers, and lymphatic channels
- Outer layer of muscle is the epimysium.
  - Located on the muscle surface and tapers at each end to form a tendon
  - Tendons permit a short muscle to exert power on a distal joint.
- Second layer is the perimysium.
  - Connective tissue surrounding muscle fibers
  - Bundles also referred to as fascicles
- Third layer is the endomysium.
  - Surrounds the muscle fascicles

- Connective tissue is composed of the ligaments, tendons, and fascia, and acts as a safeguard to protect limbs from sudden changes in speed or strains.

Skeletal Muscle

- Voluntary muscles controlled by the central nervous system
- Striated denotes a striped pattern of muscle organized into contractile units referred to as sarcomeres.
- Extrafusal muscle fibers differ from other contractile fibers.
- Motor and sensory nerve fibers supply the nerve function to provide the electrical impulses needed for motor function.

Motor Unit

- Originating anterior horn cell of spinal cord
- Axons of motor nerve branch to specialized muscle fibers.
- Motor units consist of the anterior horn cell and its axon and muscle fibers.
- Motor units, which extend to skeletal muscle, are made of lower motor neurons.
- Functional unit refers to the motor unit and it contracts with an electrical impulse.

Sensory Receptors

- Muscles contain sensory receptors.
- Sensory receptors send different signals to the central nervous system.
- Spindles lie parallel to muscle fibers and they respond to stretching.
- Golgi tendon organs, which are near the neuromuscular junction, are dendrites that branch to tendons.
- Motor and sensory neurons secrete neuroregulin.
  - Increase the number of acetylcholine receptors
  - Aid in formation of muscle spindle fiber
  - System of afferent signals responsible for muscle tone and stretch response

Muscle Fibers

- A single muscle cell composes a muscle fiber.
  - Long, cylindric cell is surrounded by a membrane with the ability to provide excitement and impulse.
- Muscle fiber is composed of bundles of myofibrils.
  - Muscle fibers develop from myoblast at birth.
  - Voluntary muscles originate from the mesodermal layer of the embryo.
  - Peripheral nerves impact the motor unit and muscle fiber.
    - Type II fibers (white fast-motor) are dependent on short-term anaerobic glycolytic systems for fast transfer of energy.
      - Ocular muscles contain more type II muscle fibers.
    - Type I fibers are postural muscles; they are highly resistant to fatigue.
- Quantity of muscle fibers depends on location and diameter.

Components of Muscle Fiber

- Muscle membrane
  - Two-part membrane
    - Sarcolemma contains the plasma membrane and basement membrane.
      - Composed of lipid molecule and protein systems

  - Transports nutrients and protein synthesis
  - Sodium-potassium pump and cell's cholinergic receptor
- Basement membrane contains proteins and polysaccharides.
  - Cells microskeleton to maintain muscle shape
  - Diffusion of electrolytes
- Myofibrils
  - Most abundant subcellular muscle
  - Functional units of muscle contraction
  - Contains sarcomeres, composed of proteins
    - Actin
    - Myosin
    - Titin
    - Nebulin
  - Conversion of chemical energy into movement
- Sarcotubular system
  - Similar to endoplasmic reticulum in other cells
  - Sarcoplasmic reticulum part of calcium transportation
  - Contraction of muscle at sarcomere, a portion of myofibril
- Sarcoplasm
  - Cytoplasm of the muscle cell
  - Contains intracellular components
  - Aqueous substance with a matrix to encapsulate the myofibrils
  - Provides enzymes and proteins for the cell's energy, protein synthesis, and storage of oxygen.
    - Mitochondria house enzymes for energy production.
    - Regulate citric acid cycle and adenosine triphosphate (ATP) formation
    - Also contains
      - Ribosomes (RNA)
      - Cell nucleus
      - Satellite cells
      - Glycogen granules
      - Lipid droplets suspended in sarcoplasmic matrix
      - Blood vessels, nerve endings
      - Muscle spindles and Golgi tendon organs
      - Mitochondria

Muscle Function

Goal of muscle function is to accomplish work, or amount of energy released or force exerted over a distance (work = force × distance).
- Muscles contract while at work.
- Muscle contraction at molecular level results in observable movement.

Four Steps of Muscle Contraction

- Excitation
  - Muscle fiber action potential is the electrical impulse in the muscle fiber membrane.
  - Action potential advances along the sarcolemmal membrane.
  - Trigger voltage-sensitive receptors in T-tubule wall
  - Release calcium from sarcoplasmic reticulum

- Coupling
  - After depolarization of T-tubules, coupling occurs.
  - Migration of calcium ions to the myofilaments
  - Calcium affects troponin and tropomyosin, muscle protein.
  - Proteins are attracted to calcium ions in the presence of calcium.
- Contraction
  - Starts as the calcium ions combine with troponin
  - Actin slides toward the thick filament myosin.
  - Ends of myofibril shorten after contraction.
  - Myosin heads attach to the actin module.
- Relaxation
  - Begins with sarcoplasmic reticulum absorbing calcium molecules
  - No interaction with troponin
  - Calcium is replaced into sarcoplasmic reticulum by means of active transport.
  - Cross-bridges detach and sarcomere lengthens.

APPLICATION AND REVIEW

18. What event triggers the contraction of a muscle?
  1. Calcium ions combine with troponin.
  2. Release of calcium from sarcoplasmic reticulum.
  3. Migration of calcium ions to the myofilaments.
  4. The sarcoplasmic reticulum absorbs calcium molecules.
See Answer on page 215–217.

Muscle Metabolism

- Skeletal muscles require fuel for the process of muscle contraction, ATP, and phosphocreatine.
- Muscle contraction involves dynamic cross-bridges of actin and myosin together.
- Transportation of calcium from sarcoplasmic reticulum to myofibril
- Protein synthesis requires ATP to replenish constituents of muscle and growth and repair.
  - Rate of synthesis related to hormone levels (insulin, amino acid)
  - During activity the need for ATP increases dramatically.
  - Short-term stored glycogen and blood glucose are converted anaerobically to maintain brief activity.
  - During intense activity the levels of lactic acid increase, causing the breakdown of glycogen, and a corresponding shift in pH.
  - When more oxygen is required (anaerobic threshold reached)
    - Increase in lactic acid
    - Increase in oxygen consumption
    - Increase in heart rate, respiratory rate, and muscle blood flow
  - Strenuous exercise requires oxygen and promotes aerobic glycogen pathway for ATP formation.
  - Oxygen debt is the amount of oxygen needed to convert accumulated lactic acid and replenish ATP and phosphocreatine reserves.
  - Indirect measure of energy expenditure is timed activity, and heart and respiratory rate.
  - Direct measure of energy expenditure is based on heat production because heat is released with work.

Mechanics of Muscles

- Many factors determine whole muscle contraction.
- Twitch is a motor unit that responds to a single nerve stimulus.
- Phasic contraction occurs; this is termed a twitch.
  - Contraction generated will be a maximum contraction.
- The central nervous system varies the discharge frequency of each active motor unit and adds other motor units.
- Repetitive discharge is the adding of motor units within a muscle.
- Tetanus occurs when the summation of contractions reaches a critical frequency.
- Contraction
  - Static or holding is when the muscle has constant length as tension increases.
    - Example: push against an immovable object.
- Motor unit refers to the muscle fibers stimulated by the spinal cord.
    - Neuromuscular junction is the synapse between the motor nerve and receptor in muscle.
      - Chemical transmitter acetycholine is produced.
      - After muscle contraction, Ach is inactivated by enzyme acetylcholinesterases.
      - Drugs that block Ach relax skeletal muscles.
      - Drugs that interfere with cholinesterase may enhance muscle activity.
- Muscle contractions
  - Begin at the neuromuscular junction
  - End with contraction of the muscle fibers
    - Motor neuron relays action potential to presynaptic terminal.
    - Depolarization of the presynaptic terminal
    - Calcium influx causes exocytosis of neurotransmitter (Ach) into synaptic cleft.
    - Diffusion of the neurotransmitter results in muscle action potential.
    - Muscle action potential goes from t-tubules to another messenger activation.
    - Release of calcium from sarcoplasmic reticulum causes contraction of muscle fiber.
    - Relaxation and contraction of muscle utilizes cellular energy (ATP).
- During exertion, blood supply to the muscle is increased, resulting in an
  - Increased supply of oxygen and nutrients (fatty acids and glucose)
    - Provide energy to muscle and remove waste products
  - Myoglobin is an oxygen-binding protein located in the muscles that can store a small amount oxygen.
- Glycogen is glucose stored in muscle.
- Aerobic respiration to produce ATP occurs in muscle fibers dependent upon adequate oxygen from
  - Myoglobin
  - Circulation blood
  - Anaerobic respiration starts if oxygen supply to muscle decreases.
    - Primary energy source is glucose.
    - Oxygen debt results.
    - Produces lactic acid and small amounts ATP
    - Produces a state of acidosis and an increase in respiration to compensate by decreasing carbon dioxide levels in blood

- Lactic acid can result in local muscle pain and cramps (muscle contraction) owing to irritation of metabolic waste.
- During strenuous activity, anaerobic metabolism results in excessive lactic acid in blood, which results in metabolic acidosis.

Bone Abnormalities

- Curvature of the spine disorders can be caused by common conditions such as arthritis or osteoporosis.
- Kyphosis: abnormal rounding of upper back (commonly called hunchback)
  - Other causes
    - Poor posture
    - Spina bifida
    - Scheuermann disease
    - Spinal tumors
    - Spinal infections
- Lordosis: abnormal curvature inward at the lower back (commonly called sway back)
  - Other causes
    - Obesity
    - Discitis (inflammation in spinal disc)
    - Achondroplasia
    - Vertebrae slip forward
- Scoliosis: abnormal C or S shape sideways curvature of the spine
  - Other causes
    - Genetic
    - Disease
    - Trauma

Trauma

- Fractures
  - Incidence depends on
    - Bone involved
    - Age
    - Gender
- Classification of fractures
  - Complete
    - Broken into two sections
  - Incomplete
    - Damaged but intact in one section
- Fractures are further subdivided into
  - Closed fracture (formerly referred to as a simple fracture)
    - No break in skin near fracture
  - Open fracture (formerly referred to as a compound fracture)
    - Break in skin near fracture
- Fractures classified by the direction of the fracture line (Fig. 10.1)
  - Linear: the break is parallel to the long axis of the bone.
  - Transverse: the break occurs across the bone.
  - Oblique: the break is slanted to the long axis of the bone.
  - Spiral: the break circles around the bone.

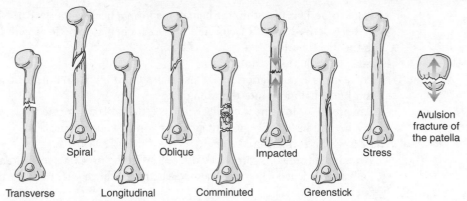

FIG. 10.1 Types of fractures. (From Banasik, J. L., & Copstead, L. E. C. [2019]. *Pathophysiology* [6th ed.]. St. Louis: Elsevier.)

- Comminuted: the bone breaks into more than two fragments.
- Greenstick: the bone bends and cracks.
  - Common incomplete fracture in children
- Compression: bone collapses, such as vertebrae.
- Types of fractures
  - Impacted
    - End of bone telescoped into another bone
  - Pathologic
    - Fracture caused by weakness in bone
    - Caused by a condition such as osteoporosis or tumors
  - Stress fracture
    - Owing to summative effect of repeated activity
  - Fatigue fracture
    - Stress fracture owing to abnormal stress on the normal bone
  - Insufficiency fracture
    - Stress fracture owing to normal stress on the abnormal bone
  - Depressed
    - Occurs in the skull when a section of bone is broken
    - Compresses the brain
- Diagnosis
  - X-rays to confirm the presence of a fracture
- Fracture healing
  - Healing time depends on age.
  - Average time needed for healing is
    - One month in children
    - Two months for adults
    - Longer fracture healing time for geriatric clients

Five Phases of Healing

- For gross injuries, such as fractures or surgical wounds (osteotomies), healing is the same as soft tissue injuries. The bone remodeling process can only repair minor (microscopic) bone injuries.
  - Phase 1: Hematoma
    - Hemorrhage occurs when blood vessels are damaged.

- Platelets and fibrin within the hematoma form a healing meshwork.
- Platelet-derived growth factor and TGF-β are hematopoietic growth factors that assist in the initial healing.
  - Phase 2: Procallus formation
    - Procallus is a granulation tissue that is produced by fibroblasts, osteoblasts, and capillary buds that move into the wound.
    - The precursor to bone is cartilage (types I, II, and II are formed).
    - Insulin and insulin-like growth factors aid in this healing process.
  - Phase 3: Callus formation
    - Wove bone (callus) is formed by osteoblasts in the procallus membranous.
    - Callus is hardened when enzymes increase phosphate content and permit it to join with calcium.
  - Phase 4: Replacement
    - Callus consisting of the multicellular units is replaced by trabecular or lamellar bone.
  - Phase 5: Remodeling
    - Endosteal and periosteal surfaces of the bone are remodeled to the size and shape of the bone prior to injury.
- Factors that influence healing time
  - Local soft tissue
  - Bone damage
  - Extensive damage to the periosteum (fibrous membrane covering the bone)
  - Blood vessels can hinder healing.
  - The ends of the bone are approximated closer
    - Faster healing and immobility of the healing bones
    - Critical to prevent damaging the fragile bridge of new tissue
  - Infection can delay healing.
  - Foreign body can delay healing.
  - Comorbidity
    - Diabetes
    - Circulatory issues
    - Anemia
    - Nutritional deficiencies
    - Administration of medications (e.g., glucocorticoids)
- Complications
  - Muscle spasm
  - Infection
  - Ischemia
  - Compartment syndrome (necrosis of the muscle)
  - Fat emboli
  - Nerve damage
  - Long-term increased incidence of
    - Osteoarthritis as an adult
    - Stunted growth in children

Sprains and Strains

- Strains
  - Tear in tendon

- Avulsion
  - Ligament or tendon separated from bone
  - Signs and symptoms
    - Pain
    - Tenderness
    - Swelling
    - Discoloration
- Diagnosis
  - X-rays
- Healing
  - Granulation tissue at the site
  - Collagen fibers form
  - Fibrous tissue joins tendon/ligament to the bone.

Dislocation

- Caused by trauma, such as a fall
- Can be associate with a fracture or owing to disease or other damage (torn ligament)
- Soft tissue damage occurs to
  - Ligaments
  - Nerves
  - Blood vessels
- Bone is separated from the joint.
  - Subluxation occurs when bone is partially displaced.
- Signs and symptoms
  - Pain
  - Swelling
  - Tenderness
  - Inflammation
  - Bleeding
  - Deformity and limited movement
- Diagnosis
  - Confirmed by x-ray

Muscle Tears

- Tears along a muscle or where it attaches to bone
- Result of trauma or overuse
- Three degrees of muscle tear
  - First-degree tear affects a small percentage of muscle and causes mild pain and minimal loss of strength or range of motion.
  - Second-degree tear is when a larger area of muscle is affected, but a complete tear does not appear. Pain is more severe and substantial loss of strength and range of motion occur.
  - Third-degree tear is across the width of the muscle. Muscle cannot contract and large amount of internal bleeding occurs.
    - May require surgery to heal
  - Third-degree tear may require surgery, and scar tissue can permanently reduce flexibility and muscle strength.
  - Repeated injuries can result in fibrous scar tissue.
    - Decreased mobility

- Permanent joint damage
- Development of osteoarthritis

Repetitive Strain Injury

A disorder affecting muscles, nerves, and tendons that occurs over time
- Repetitive movements decrease circulation to the area.
- Over time soft tissue damage results.
- Primarily affects adults aged 30 to 50 years
- Signs and symptoms
  - Pain
  - Weakness
  - Numbness
  - Sleep disturbance
- Diagnosis
  - History
  - X-ray
  - Arthroscopic examination

BONE DISORDERS

Osteoporosis

- Metabolic disorder
- Decrease in bone density and mass
- Loss of bone mineralization
- Loss of bone matrix
- Higher incidence in women
- Primary osteoporosis
  - Age-related (senile)
  - Postmenopause
  - Idiopathic (unknown cause)
- Secondary osteoporosis
  - Related to disease
  - Hyperparathyroidism
  - Cushing syndrome
  - Medication (e.g., glucocorticoid)
  - Sedentary lifestyle
- Pathophysiology
  - Bone resorption exceeds bone formation.
  - Bones are thin and fragile.
  - Cancellous bone is more often affected.
  - Bone mass peaks in young adults.
    - Bone mass decreases with age.
    - Calcium intake as a child and young adult is important to bone mass maintenance in later life.
- Predisposing factors
  - Aging
    - Older individuals
    - Postmenopausal women with estrogen deficiency

- Sedentary lifestyle
    - Muscle activity puts stress on bone required for osteoblastic activity.
    - Prolonged bedrest
    - Inactivity owing to aging or chronic conditions
- Hormonal factors
    - Hyperparathyroidism
    - Cushing syndrome
    - Use of prednisone or glucocorticoids
- Vitamin or mineral deficits
    - Related to diet deficient in calcium, vitamin D, or protein
    - Childhood malabsorption disorder
- Cigarette smoking
- Light, small bone structure
- Excessive caffeine ingestion
- Signs and symptoms
    - Early stages are asymptomatic
    - Compression fractures of the vertebrae resulting in abnormal curvature of the spine
        - Kyphosis
        - Scoliosis
    - Loss of height
    - Nerve compression

Rickets and Osteomalacia

- Deficit of vitamin D and phosphates necessary for bone mineralization
- Caused by deficiency in diet
- Malabsorption
- Lack of sun
- Medication (prolong use of phenobarbital)
- Signs and symptoms
    - Soft bone
    - Weak or deformed bones owing to calcification of cartilage at the epiphyseal plate
    - Characteristic bowed legs referred to as "rickets"
    - In children, height is below normal
    - In adults, kidney disease referred to as "renal rickets"

Osteomyelitis

- Infection in bone
- Causes
    - Usually caused by bacteria or less frequently fungi
    - Organism enters blood through infection in the body and the organism(s) spreads to the bone.
    - Can be associated with surgery, such as a pin or structural insert
- Signs and symptoms
    - Local and systemic
    - Localized to area
        - Inflammation
        - Bone pain
    - Systemic
        - Fever

- Chills
- Excessive sweating
- Overall malaise
- Diagnosis
  - Symptoms and examination
  - O Blood test
  - Biopsy

Paget Disease (Osteitis Deformans)

- Progressive bone disorder that occurs in adults aged 40 or older
- Cause
  - Unknown etiology
  - Related to childhood infection with a virus
  - Possible genetic factor involved
- Signs and symptoms
  - Bone destruction
  - Healthy bone replaced with fibrous tissue and abnormal bone
  - Can be asymptomatic
  - Pathologic fractures likely
  - Vertebrae involvement could lead to compression fractures and kyphosis.
  - Skull involvement could lead to increased pressure and compression of cranial nerves.
  - Can result in heart failure and cardiovascular disease
- Diagnosis
  - X-ray demonstrates structural abnormalities
  - Thickening and enlargement of
    - Long bones
    - Vertebrae
    - Pelvis
    - Skull

Bone Tumors

- Most primary bone tumors are malignant.
- Common site for secondary tumors related to metastatic bone cancer
  - Malignant tumors that originate in breast, lung, or prostate often spread to bone.
- Cause
  - Osteosarcoma (osteogenic sarcoma)
    - Primary malignant neoplasm
    - Originates in femur, tibia, or fibula (children, young adults)
  - Ewing sarcoma
    - Malignant neoplasm
    - Occurs in long bones, often in adolescents
  - Chondrosarcomas
    - Originate in cartilage cells
    - Occur commonly in adults aged over 30 years
    - Develop in pelvic bone or shoulder girdle
    - Metastasize to the lung

- Signs and symptoms
  - Tumors grow quickly and metastasize to lungs.
  - Pathological fracture
  - Bone pain is common; constant with rest, increases in severity, and occurs at night
  - Bone pain develops late with chondrosarcoma.
- Diagnosis
  - Biopsy
- Survival rate depends on stage of cancer and the histologic aspects of the tumor.

JOINT DISORDERS

Osteoarthritis

- Injury to join owing to "tear and wear"
- Damaged cartilage results in a loss of alignment.
- Loss of smooth working of the articular cartilage
- Causes
  - Sports injuries
  - Repetition in the workplace
  - Congenital predisposition
- Signs and symptoms
  - Large weight-bearing joints often affected
  - Hips
  - Knees
  - Pain is initially mild but increases as the degenerative process progresses.
  - Limitation of the joints
  - Enlarged joint hardens
  - Development of osteophytes (bone spurs)
  - Crepitus
  - Not a systemic disorder
- Diagnosis
  - Radiology review
  - Rule out systemic disorders with laboratory testing

Rheumatoid Arthritis (Fig. 10.2)

- Autoimmune disorder resulting in joint deformity
- Higher incidence in women and the elderly
- Major cause of disability
- Cause
  - Abnormal immune response
- Signs and symptoms
  - Begins with smaller joints (fingers)
  - Progresses to other larger joints (elbows, wrist, knee, hips)
  - Results in the inflammation of synovial membrane
  - Vasodilation
    - Red, painful joints

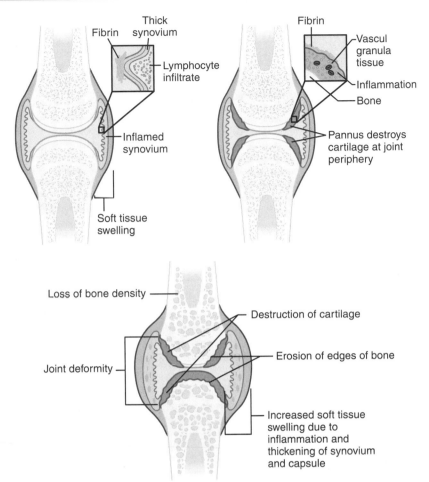

FIG. 10.2 Schematic presentation of the pathologic changes in rheumatoid arthritis. The inflammation (synovitis) leads to pannus formation, obliteration of the articular space, and, finally, ankylosis. The periarticular bone shows disuse atrophy in the form of osteoporosis. (From Banasik, J. L., & Copstead, L. E. C. [2019]. *Pathophysiology* [6th ed.]. St. Louis: Elsevier.)

- Rheumatoid factor (RF) is an antibody that can be present in synovial fluid.
- Over time, the inflammation results in a growth of granulation tissue (pannus).
  - Destroys the cartilage
- Cartilage erodes and fibrosis occurs.
  - Leaving the joint fixed and deformed (ankylosis)
- Inflammation can lead to
  - Muscle atrophy
  - Stretching of adjoining tendons and ligaments
  - Muscle spasm
  - Bone misalignment
- Systemic signs and symptoms include
  - Limited joint function
  - Impairment of activities of daily living

- Fatigue
- Mild temperature elevation
- Anorexia
- Lymphadenopathy
- Generalized malaise
- Diagnosis
  - Presence of RF or other markers in synovial fluid
  - RF is not required for diagnosis.

Juvenile Rheumatoid Arthritis

- Several different types of juvenile rheumatoid arthritis (JRA)
- Signs and symptoms
  - Onset more acute than adult rheumatoid arthritis
  - Large joints often affected
  - Systemic form referred to as Still disease
  - Rash
  - Fever
  - Lymphadenopathy
  - Hepatomegaly
  - Joint involvement
  - Second form of JRA causes polyarticular inflammation.
  - Third form of JRA called uveitis involves four or fewer joints, and inflammation of the iris, ciliary body, and choroid in the eye.
- Diagnosis
  - RF usually not present
  - Abnormal antibodies such as antinuclear antibodies

Infectious (Septic) Arthritis

- Usually develops in a single joint
- Cause
  - Often a history of trauma, surgery, or spread from a nearby infection
- Signs and symptoms
  - Joint is red, swollen, and painful.
- Diagnosis
  - Analysis of synovial fluid aspirated from joint
  - Culture and sensitivity confirms diagnosis, which is usually gonococcus or staphylococcus, but can be anaerobic bacteria.

Gout Arthritis

- Results from abnormal deposits of uric acid and uric acid crystals in the joint
- Causes an inflammatory process
- Uric acid is a byproduct of purine metabolism.
  - Normally excreted through the kidneys
- Hyperuricemia develops if the kidney excretion is inadequate.
  - Genetic factor (deficiency of an enzyme uricase)
  - Results in elevated uric acid levels
- Signs and symptoms
  - A single joint is affected (usually the big toe).

- Inflammation is the result of deposits of uric acid.
- A large, hard nodule can be present, which is called a tophus.
- Signs and symptoms are transient.
- Joint swells and severe pain occurs.
- Diagnosis
  - Confirmed by blood test
  - Analysis of synovial fluid

Ankylosing Spondylitis

- Chronic and progressive inflammatory condition
- Cause
  - Thought to be an autoimmune disease
  - Genetic basis
  - Presence of HLS-B27 in blood serum analysis
- Signs and symptoms
  - Affects the sacroiliac joints, intervertebral spaces, and costovertebral joints
  - Women have greater chance of peripheral joint involvement.
  - Most common in men
  - Onset age 20 to 30 years
  - Cyclic remission and exacerbations
  - Vertebral joints become inflamed.
  - Fusion, calcification, and fibrosis of joints
    - Ankylosis or fixation of joint
    - Loss of mobility with joint
  - Inflammation progress from sacroiliac joint to spine.
    - Described as "poker back," stiff back
    - Kyphosis develops from rigidity and loss of normal spine curvature.
    - Osteoporosis can contribute to kyphosis owing to compression of vertebrae.
  - Lung expansion is diminished owing to calcification of costovertebral joints.
    - Flexion, extension, and rotation of spine
  - Some individuals develop systemic symptoms.
    - Fever
    - Fatigue
    - Weight loss
  - Uveitis (iris), eye inflammation

DISORDERS OF MUSCLE, TENDONS, AND LIGAMENTS

Muscular Dystrophy

- Group of inherited disorders
  - Degeneration of skeletal muscle
  - Differences exist between disorders based on
    - Affected area
    - Age of onset
    - Rate of progression
  - Result is the progressive weakness of skeletal muscle
  - Duchenne or pseudohypertrophic muscular dystrophy is the most common.
    - Associated with X gene, it occurs in young males

- A deficit of dystrophin (muscle cell membrane protein)
- Results in degeneration and necrosis of the cell
- Muscle function is lost.
- Fat and fibrous tissues replace normal connective tissues in the muscle.
- Signs and symptoms
  - Early signs occur in preschool-age children as weakness and regression in motor function.
  - Difficulty standing up or climbing stairs
  - Disease progresses with mental retardation.
  - Cardiac abnormalities
- Diagnosis
  - Genetic abnormalities
  - Elevated creatine levels
  - Electromyography
  - Muscle biopsy
  - Presence of defective serum dystrophin in female carriers of the defective gene
  - Chorionic villus testing can be performed at 12 weeks' gestation.
  - Prognosis is poor.
  - Death results in early adulthood owing to respiratory or cardiac failure.

Primary Fibromyalgia Syndrome

- Group of disorders that affects the muscles, tendons, and surrounding soft tissues
  - Presents with pain and stiffness
- Etiology unknown
  - Alterations in neurotransmissions promote soft tissue sensitivity to substance P.
    - Neurotransmitter that deals with the sensation of pain
- Incidence in women aged 20 to 50 years
  - Normally a history of trauma or osteoarthritis
  - Other factors include stress
    - Sleep deprivation
    - Fatigue
- Signs and symptoms
  - General malaise
  - Aching pain
  - Depression
  - Sleep disturbance
  - Occasionally irritable bowel or urinary symptoms

ANSWER KEY: REVIEW QUESTIONS

1. **Answers: 1, 2, 3, 5.**
   1 The musculoskeletal system gives the body form and stability, and allows for movement and interaction with objects in the environment. Impairment would possibly interfere with hand movement needed for knitting. **2** The musculoskeletal system gives the body form and stability needed for standing upright. **3** The musculoskeletal system gives the body form and stability, and allows for movement and interaction with objects in the environment such as scissors during the act of cutting. **5** The musculoskeletal system gives the body form and stability, and allows for movement needed for walking.
   4 Hearing is a sensory function not markedly reliant on the musculoskeletal system.
   Client Need: Physiological Adaptation; **Cognitive Level:** Analysis; **Nursing Process:** Assessment

2. **1 Intramembranous ossification occurs during fetal development and produces skull bones.**

    2, 3 Endochondral ossification uses a cartilage template and results in long bones such as femur and humerus bones **4** Irregular bones such as the vertebra are not formed by the intramembranous ossification process.
    Client Need: Physiological Adaptation; **Cognitive Level:** Analysis; **Nursing Process:** Analysis

3. **1 A balance must be maintained between osteoblasts that produce new bone, and osteoclasts that reabsorb bone.**

    2 Parathyroid stimulates osteoclast function, one part of the necessary balance. **3** Collagen is the fiber that gives bones strength; a component of healthy, new bone. **4** Calcitonin stimulates osteoblast, one part of the necessary balance.
    Client Need: Physiological Adaptation; **Cognitive Level:** Understanding; **Integrated Process:** Teaching and Learning

4. **3 Wnt genes are protein-signaling factors that affect bone density and mass.**

    1 An overproduction of osteoclasts would affect the reabsorption of bone. **2** Insufficient production of osteoblasts would affect new bone production. **4** Ineffective factor-beta (TGF-β) superfamilies would affect initiating, differentiating, and providing of the precursor cells into osteoblast.
    Client Need: Physiological Adaptation; **Cognitive Level:** Understanding; **Integrated Process:** Teaching and Learning

5. **2 A function of bone marrow cavities within bones is to store hematopoietic stem cells that develop into blood and immune cells. This dysfunction increases the risk for infections.**

    1, 3, 4 Bone marrow cavities do not play a significant role in disorders such as MI, jaundice, or asthma.
    Client Need: Physiological Adaptation; **Cognitive Level:** Applying; **Nursing Process:** Assessment

6. **1 An impaired skeletal system function increases the risk for dysfunctional blood cell production which would require frequent monitoring.**

    2 Dietary intake is not directly associated with ineffective skeleton system function. **3** Sun exposure is not directly associated with ineffective skeleton system function. **4** Stress production is not directly associated with ineffective skeleton system function.
    Client Need: Physiological Adaptation; **Cognitive Level:** Appling; **Nursing Process:** Planning

7. **2 The skull, which is considered a part of the axial skeletal system, is often at risk for fracturing while playing football.**

    1 Leg bones are considered a part of the appendicular skeletal system and are at risk for facture when skiing. **3** The hands are considered a part of the appendicular skeletal system and are at risk for facture when attempting to catch a ball. **4** The foot is considered a part of the appendicular skeletal system and is at risk for facture when kicking objects as in soccer.
    Client Need: Physiological Adaptation; **Cognitive Level:** Analysis; **Nursing Process:** Assessment

8. **2 Diaphysis is compact bone that can accommodate bending force in bone.**

    1 Hyaline cartilage or articular cartilage covers the epiphysis to facilitate free movement between two bones. **3** Epiphyses is spongy bone formed where the shaft broadens at the metaphysis. **4** Epiphyseal cartilage (growth plate) is an area where longitudinal bone growth occurs
    Client Need: Physiological Adaptation; **Cognitive Level:** Understanding; **Integrated Process:** Teaching and Learning

9. **1 Bone growth occurs at sites of epiphyseal cartilage (growth plate). These areas are where longitudinal bone growth occurs in response to growth and sex hormones. A lack of such hormones would result in impaired bone growth.**

    2 Bone growth stops when the epiphyseal plate ossifies during adolescence or early adulthood regardless of existing anomalies. **3** A fractured femur would not necessarily interfere with bone growth unless the fracture occurred at the site of the growth plates. **4** Osteoporosis affects bone strength. Bone growth stops when the epiphyseal plate ossifies during adolescence or early adulthood.
    Client Need: Physiological Adaptation; **Cognitive Level:** Analysis; **Nursing Process:** Assessment

10. **2 The mandible is an example of an irregular bone. Using a straw may be an appropriate intervention for such a fracture.**

    1, 4 The wrist and ankle bones are classified as short or cuboidal bones. **3** Fractured ribs produce pain when coughing, so clients are provided with methods to help minimize the discomfort and encourage coughing to manage secretions.

    Client Need: Physiological Adaptation; **Cognitive Level:** Applying; **Nursing Process:** Planning

11. **3 Bone marrow is produced through hematopoiesis. Red marrow is found in ribs, cranium, vertebrae, sternum, and ilia.**

    1, 2, 4 Neither the femur, the mandible, nor the tibia is a storage location for red bone marrow.

    Client Need: Physiological Adaptation; **Cognitive Level:** Analysis; **Nursing Process:** Assessment/Analysis

12. **1 Stimulus, including physical stress, drugs, vitamins, and hormones, activate cell death (apoptosis).**

    2 Osteoblast production affects the formation of new bone. **3** Sex hormones affect bone growth prior to young adulthood. **4** Forming sites for calcium and phosphorus affect new bone growth.

    Client Need: Physiological Adaptation; **Cognitive Level:** Understanding; **Integrated Process:** Teaching and Learning

13. **Answers: 2, 3, 5.**

    2, 3, 5 Bone density can change because of three hormones; growth, parathyroid, cortisol.

    1 Sex hormone affects bone growth. **4** Thyroxine's principal function is to stimulate the consumption of oxygen and thus the metabolism of all cells and tissues in the body.

    Client Need: Physiological Adaptation; **Cognitive Level:** Understand; **Integrated Process:** Teaching and Learning

14. **1 Suture joints are locked together, allowing no movement; they are found between the flat bones in the skull of infants and young children.**

    2 The pelvis contains symphysis cartilaginous joints. **3** Symphysis cartilaginous joints are found between two bones, such as between cervical vertebrae. **4** The rib cage-sternum joint is a synchondrosis cartilaginous joint.

    Client Need: Physiological Adaptation; **Cognitive Level:** Understanding; **Integrated Process:** Teaching and Learning

15. **Answers: 1, 2, 3.**

    1, 2, 3 The subintima is a vascular layer composed of fibers, fat cells, fibroblast, macrophages, mast cells, and loose fibrous connective tissue.

    4, 5 The membrane's intima is a cellular layer that contains both synovial cells type A and B.

    Client Need: Physiological Adaptation; **Cognitive Level:** Understanding; **Integrated Process:** Teaching and Learning

16. **2 Synovial fluid is a lubricant; loss of the fluid leads to a rapid loss of the affected articular cartilage.**

    1 Synovial fluid cannot be surgically replaced. **3** The loss of synovial fluid cannot be corrected by rebuilding the patella-fibula joint. **4** The loss of synovial fluid will not result in dislocation of the patella.

    Client Need: Physiological Adaptation; **Cognitive Level:** Analysis; **Nursing Process:** Evaluation

17. **Answers: 1, 2, 3, 4.**

    1, 2, 3, 4 Primarily skeletal muscles are under voluntary control, but there are exceptions that include respiratory movement, pupillary reflexes, blinking, and shivering.

    5 Joint stabilization is a result of voluntary control.

    Client Need: Physiological Adaptation; **Cognitive Level:** Understanding; **Integrated Process:** Teaching and Learning

18. **1 Actual contraction starts as the calcium ions combine with troponin.**

    2 The release of calcium from sarcoplasmic reticulum begins the excitation step of the muscle contraction process. **3** The migration of calcium ions to the myofilaments occurs in the coupling step of the muscle contraction process. **4** The relaxation of the muscle contraction occurs when the sarcoplasmic reticulum absorbs calcium molecules.

    Client Need: Physiological Adaptation; **Cognitive Level:** Understanding; **Integrated Process:** Teaching and Learning

11 Integumentary System Disorders

SKIN OVERVIEW

Skin Functions

- The skin is the largest body organ.
- The skin makes up 20% of the body's weight.
  - Primary functions of the skin
    - Protects the underlying tissues and organs of the body
      - Provides a covering to protect the internal organs and skeletal system
      - Acts as a barrier to the external environment
        - Different cells within the epidermal layers have specialized jobs to help protect, fight, and aid the immune system.
        - These specialized cells protect against viruses, bacteria, ultraviolet radiation, foreign objects, environmental damage, and mechanical stress.
    - Secretion
      - Sebum from sebaceous glands lubricates the surface of the skin.
      - Sweat produced by sweat glands also lubricates the skin.
    - Provides sensory perception for environmental stimuli
      - Nerve endings and receptors in the skin relay information to the brain.
      - Relayed information includes pain, pressure, vibration, touch, cold, and heat.
    - Temperature regulation
      - Occurs two different ways
        - Vasoconstriction or vasodilation
          - Blood vessels are controlled by expansion and contraction to maintain ideal body temperature.
        - Excretion
          - Perspiration: 600 to 900 mL water lost daily
    - Vitamin D synthesis
      - Dependent on sun exposure (ultraviolet [UV] B [UVB] radiation)

Skin Layers

- Epidermis
  - Outer layer of the skin
  - The epidermis is 0.3 to 1.5 mm thick.
  - Consists of five layers
    - Stratum germinativum
      - Also called stratum basale
      - Base layer
      - Deepest layer
      - Formation of new epithelial cells occurs in this layer.
      - Keratinocytes are formed in this layer and move up.
        - Keratinocytes produce keratin.

- ○ Keratin is a protein that protects the epithelial cells from stress and damage.
- ○ Melanocytes are located in this layer.
- ○ Melanocytes produce melanin, which determines skin color and protects against harmful UV radiation.
  - ▪ Stratum spinosum
    - ▪ Spiny layer
    - ▪ Located above stratum germinativum
    - ▪ Langerhans cells are located in this layer.
      - ○ Langerhans cells aid the immune system by protecting the skin from bacteria and viruses.
    - ▪ Keratinization begins in this layer.
      - ○ Keratin is the main component in hair, nail, and skin cells.
  - ▪ Stratum granulosum
    - ▪ Granular layer
      - ○ The keratinocytes from the stratum spinosum become granular cells in this layer.
    - ▪ Granular cells bind keratin filaments together.
    - ▪ Waterproofing layer prevents fluid loss
  - ▪ Stratum lucidum
    - ▪ Clear or transparent layer
    - ▪ This skin is found only on the soles of feet and palms of the hands.
    - ▪ Thicker skin for extra protection
    - ▪ Protects and reduces against force or friction
  - ▪ Stratum corneum
    - ▪ Outermost layer of the epidermis
    - ▪ Protects and provides a waterproof barrier
    - ▪ Contains mostly dead cells that shed
- • The epidermis is renewed about every 30 days.
- • Dermis
  - • Located under the epidermis
  - • The dermis is 1.0 to 4.0 mm in thickness.
  - • Composed of connective tissues that provide support for blood vessels and nerves in the dermis
    - ▪ Collagen
      - ▪ Group of proteins found naturally in the body
      - ▪ Responsible for the strength of the skin
    - ▪ Reticulin
      - ▪ A protein that is similar to collagen
    - ▪ Elastin
      - ▪ A protein that is elastic and allows things in the body to return to their shape after stretching and contracting.
  - • Dermis cells
    - ▪ Fibroblasts are the primary cell type in the dermis.
      - ▪ Fibroblasts produce collagen and elastin
  - • Mast cells
    - ▪ Important in wound healing
    - ▪ Participate in allergic reactions by releasing histamine and cytokines

- Nerves
  - Signals are transmitted to and from the sweat glands, hair muscles, and blood vessels by the nerves in the dermis.
  - Information about temperature change (hot, cold), pain, and pressure are relayed to the brain via the nerves in the skin.
- Blood vessels
  - Blood flow is controlled through the skin.
  - Vasoconstriction
    - When the body is cold, the blood vessels contract to try and keep the internal body temperature.
  - Vasodilation
    - When the body is too hot, the blood vessels expand allowing heat to be released through the skin's surface.
- Hair follicles
  - Originate from the dermis or root
  - Each hair follicle is attached to an arrector pili muscle.
  - The arrector pili muscle connects the root of the hair to the hair follicle thus allowing for contraction when cold.
  - Main function is to act as a touch receptor.
  - Sebaceous glands are associated with each hair follicle; they secrete sebum, an oily substance that provides a waterproof barrier to prevent drying.
- Sebaceous glands
  - Sebum, an oily secretion, is produced by sebaceous glands.
  - Provides a waterproof barrier to the skin and hair to prevent drying
- Sweat glands
  - The two types of sweat glands are
    - Eccrine glands
    - Apocrine glands
- Subcutaneous layer
  - Also called hypodermis
  - Located below the dermis
  - Composed of connective tissue
  - Mainly used for fat storage
    - Adipose cells
      - Provide insulation
  - Macrophages
    - Type of white blood cell that protects and ingests foreign invaders
    - Plays a key role in aiding the immune system
  - Fibroblasts
    - Produce collagen and elastin
  - Blood vessels
  - Nerves
  - Serves as an appendage base
    - Hair follicles, sebaceous and sweat glands

APPLICATION AND REVIEW

1. A nurse teaches a nursing student about the functions of the skin. Which statements, if made by the student, indicate that teaching was successful? **Select all that apply**.
   1. "The skin provides protection for the kidneys."
   2. "The skin helps regulate magnesium levels."
   3. "The skin is important in temperature regulation."
   4. "The skin serves as a barrier to bacteria."
   5. "The skin has nerve endings that relay pain signals."
2. What is the deepest layer/stratum of the epidermis?
   1. Granular
   2. Corneum
   3. Spinosum
   4. Germinativum
3. What layer/stratum of the epidermis is found only on the soles of the feet and the palms of the hands?
   1. Corneum
   2. Spinosum
   3. Lucidum
   4. Granulosum
4. What statement concerning the epidermis is correct?
   1. It consists of four layers
   2. It is renewed every 30 days
   3. It is between 1 and 4 mm thick
   4. It supports blood vessels in the dermis
5. Which type of cells support the immune system?
   1. Keratinocytes
   2. Melanocytes
   3. Langerhans
   4. Sebum
6. What component of the skin is responsible for providing the skin with strength?
   1. Elastin
   2. Collagen
   3. Mast cells
   4. Nerve cells
7. Which process occurs in the skin to conserve body heat?
   1. Vasodilation of blood vessels
   2. Decreased sebaceous secretion
   3. Vasoconstriction of blood vessels
   4. Accelerated perspiration production
8. Damage to which skin layer would impact normal hair growth?
   1. Dermis
   2. Corneum
   3. Epidermis
   4. Germinativum
9. Insufficient amounts of what type of dermis cell would affect the elasticity and strength of the skin?
   1. Mast
   2. Fibroblasts
   3. Macrophages
   4. Melanocytes

See Answers on pages 236–238.

Skin Glands (Fig. 11.1)

- Sebaceous
  - Secretes sebum
    - Consists mainly of lipids
    - Prevents the skin and hair from dryness by providing an oily lubrication
    - Sebum is emptied into the hair follicles.
  - Dependent on sex hormones
    - Sebum production and secretion are predominantly regulated by testosterone levels.
  - Located on most areas of the skin
    - Most abundant on the face, upper chest, and back
    - Not located on the soles of the feet and palms of the hands

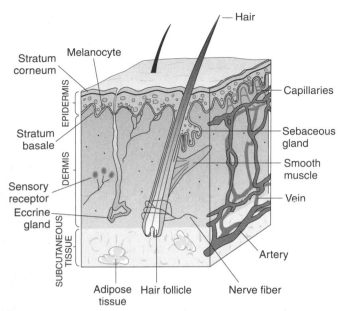

FIG. 11.1 Diagram of the skin. (From Hubert, R. J., & VanMeter, K. C. [2018]. *Gould's pathophysiology for the health professions* [6th ed.]. Philadelphia: Saunders.)

- Sweat
  - Eccrine
    - Widely distributed over the body
    - Most abundant on the forehead, soles of feet, and palms of hands
    - Main functions
      - Decrease body temperature by evaporation
      - Excrete waste products through skin pores
      - Moisturize surface cells
  - Apocrine
    - Main locations include the breast areolae, armpits, genital area, and eyelids
    - These glands contain ducts that have an entrance directly into the hair follicles.
    - Secrete a substance that produces an odor when in contact with bacteria on the skin's surface

Skin Lesions

See Table 11.1 for descriptions of common skin lesions.

Congenital Skin Abnormalities

- Birthmarks
  - Visible mark on the skin at birth or shortly thereafter
  - Can be vascular, pigmented, or nonpigmented
    - Vascular
      - Hemangioma
        - Noncancerous formations or growths of benign tumors from fast growing vascular endothelial cells
        - Occur when an abnormal proliferation of blood vessels develops in one specific area of the body

TABLE 11.1	Description of Some Skin Lesions
Macule	Small, flat, circumscribed lesion of a different color than the normal skin
Papule	Small, firm, elevated lesion
Nodule	Palpable elevated lesion; varies in size
Pustule	Elevated, erythematous lesion, usually containing purulent exudate
Vesicle	Elevated, thin-walled lesion containing clear fluid (blister)
Plaque	Large, slightly elevated lesion with flat surface, often topped by scale
Crust	Dry, rough surface or dried exudate or blood
Lichenification	Thick, dry, rough surface (leatherlike)
Keloid	Raised, irregular, and increasing mass of collagen resulting from excessive scar tissue formation
Fissure	Small, deep, linear crack or tear in skin
Ulcer	Cavity with loss of tissue from the epidermis and dermis, often weeping or bleeding
Erosion	Shallow, moist cavity in epidermis
Comedone	Mass of sebum, keratin, and debris blocking the opening of a hair follicle

From Hubert, R. J., & VanMeter, K. C. (2018). *Gould's pathophysiology for the health professions* (6th ed.). Philadelphia: Saunders.

- ○ Hemangiomas first occur as a red birthmark, which then forms into a bump that extends above the skin's surface.
- ○ Can be on the skin's surface or deeper, such as the liver, brain, kidneys, or colon
- ○ Skin hemangiomas appear as small red bumps.
- ○ Skin hemangiomas on the face are called strawberry hemangiomas.
- ▪ Pigmented
  - ▪ Moles
    - ○ Also called nevi, they are benign lesions on the skin.
    - ○ Appear as small brown spots
    - ○ Pigmented cells (melanocytes) grow in a cluster instead of spreading out.
    - ○ At ages 3 to 5 years, mole formation usually occurs.
    - ○ Moles can appear anywhere on the skin, alone or in groups.
    - ○ Moles may be removed by a surgical excision if necessary.
  - ▪ Nonpigmented (melatonin disorders)
    - ▪ Epidermis contains melanocytes, which produces melanin.
    - ▪ Melanin or dark pigment establishes skin color.
    - ▪ Melanin protects against UV radiation.
    - ▪ Genetics and environmental factors play a role in melanin production.
      - ○ Albinism
        - ○ A disorder that results in a deficiency of melanin production
        - ○ Physical characteristics include
          - White hair
          - White skin
          - Absence of color in the iris of the eye
      - ○ Avoidance of sun exposure is critical.

- Vitiligo
  - Lack of pigment occurs in small areas of the body owing to melanocyte loss.
  - The melanocytes stop producing melanin or die.
  - May be related to autoimmune disorder, stressful trigger, or genetics
  - Appears as patchy loss of skin color
  - Loss of skin color first starts on the face, lips, hands, and feet.
  - Larger areas may become affected over time and can include most of the body.
  - No medications can stop the process of vitiligo.

APPLICATION AND REVIEW

10. Which statements accurately describe the structure and function of apocrine gland secretion? **Select all that apply**.
    1. Located in the armpits
    2. Secreted directly in the hair follicle
    3. Regulate body temperature
    4. Serve to moisturize the surface of the skin
    5. Secretion odor results from contact with bacteria
11. Which statement by the nurse demonstrates an understanding of moles?
    1. "Most moles are formed by age five."   3. "Black is the primary color of moles."
    2. "Moles appear primarily on the torso."   4. "It is difficult to remove a mole surgically."

See Answers on pages 236–238.

Inflammatory Integumentary Disorders

- Contact dermatitis
  - Allergic contact dermatitis
    - Inflammation of the skin from an irritant.
    - Irritant exposure to
      - Chemicals, soaps, metals, drugs, latex, or poison ivy
  - Type IV cell-mediated hypersensitivity
    - First exposure sensitization occurs.
    - Second exposure to an irritant produces dermatitis symptoms.
    - T cells are a major player in allergic contact dermatitis.
  - Signs and symptoms
    - Itching at site
    - Reddened area
    - Inflamed area
    - Rash
    - Lesions at site of irritant
- Irritant contact dermatitis
  - Chemical irritants cause an inflammatory dermatitis.
  - Direct contact with a substance that damages the epidermis
  - Signs and symptoms
    - Swollen area
    - Reddened area
    - Pain can occur
    - Itching can occur

- Atopic dermatitis
  - Also known as atopic eczema
  - More prevalent in infants and children
  - Cause not fully known, but genetics along with an immune system dysfunction is involved
  - Many people with atopic dermatitis develop asthma and allergies later in life.
  - Signs and symptoms
    - Extreme itching
    - Swelling
    - Scaly and red appearance to skin
    - Dry and cracked skin
    - Rash
- Urticaria
  - Also known as hives
  - Type I hypersensitivity reaction occurs.
    - An allergic reaction occurs as a result of re-exposure to a specific type of irritant or allergen.
    - Can be caused by shellfish, heat, cold, stress, sunlight, specific fruits, perfumes, detergents, lotions, latex, nickel, or drugs
  - Signs and symptoms
    - Lesions occur that are red, swollen, raised, and circular in appearance
    - Edema of the lips, tongue, or throat can occur.
    - Extremely itchy lesions anywhere on the skin
- Psoriasis
  - Autoimmune disease
  - There are five different types of psoriasis.
  - Categorized as a chronic inflammatory skin disorder
  - T-cell mediated
  - Involves the skin, scalp, and nails
  - Genetic mechanisms involved
  - Disease can range from mild to severe
  - Exacerbations and remissions occur as part of the disorder.
  - Signs and symptoms
    - Red patches of skin covered with gray-like scales
    - Dry, cracked skin
    - Itching
    - Burning
    - Swollen and stiff joints
- Plaque psoriasis
  - Most common type of psoriasis
  - 80% to 90% of people with psoriasis are affected by this type.
  - Lesions are mainly on the face, torso, knees, elbows, and head.
  - Lesions are concentrated, rough, and red in appearance.
  - Lesions have normal-looking skin surrounding the outer perimeter.
    - Inverse psoriasis
      - Rare type of psoriasis
      - Lesions form in the creases of body parts such as genital, underarm, and stomach areas.
      - Lesions are flat, dry, and red in color.
      - Often mistaken for fungal infections

- Guttate psoriasis
  - Prevalent in children
  - May appear after a streptococcal infection in the lungs
  - Appear as small pimple-like bumps
  - Usually emerges unexpectedly on the torso, arms, or legs
- Pustular psoriasis
  - Present as cysts with draining pus that evolve over plaque psoriasis
- Erythrodermic psoriasis
  - Also called exfoliative psoriasis
  - Pruritus and pain are common.
  - Big red lesions that spread over large body areas
  - Lesions are rough in appearance.
  - Fever and chills are often associated with this type of psoriasis.
- Psoriatic arthritis
  - Arthritis associated with the inflammatory response that causes the psoriatic skin lesions
  - Can appear years after primary psoriasis diagnosis
  - Presents as painful, swollen, and stiff joints
  - Any joint can be affected.

Infectious Integumentary Disorders

- Bacterial
  - Common causative agents are *Staphylococcus aureus* and streptococci
    - Folliculitis
      - Hair follicle inflammation
      - Usually caused by *S. aureus*
      - Bacterial enzymes and inflammatory factors cause the inflammation of the follicle.
      - Excessive skin moisture, restrictive clothing, bad hygiene, makeup, and trauma to the skin add to folliculitis development.
      - Signs and symptoms
        - Red rash at site
        - Itchy
        - Bumps develop at site
    - Furuncles
      - Also known as boils
      - Hair follicle inflammation that spreads to the dermis
      - Caused by an untreated folliculitis
      - *S. aureus* is the causative agent.
      - Large cystic bumps or lesions with cellulitis develop.
      - Lesions may contain pus and dead tissue.
    - Impetigo
      - Most commonly occurs in children ages 2 to 5 years
      - Caused by *S. aureus* and streptococcus
      - Highly contagious
      - More prevalent in hot, humid climates
      - Red lesions, crust, and itching occur.
    - Cellulitis
      - Dermis and subcutaneous tissue are affected.
      - Caused by staphylococcus, methicillin-resistant *S. aureus*, or group B streptococci

- Signs and symptoms
  - Reddened area of skin
  - Warm to touch
  - Inflammation present
  - Pain at and around area
- Viral
  - Herpes simplex virus 1 (HSV-1)
    - HSV-1 is spread by saliva that is infected.
    - Contagious
    - Common body areas infected with HSV-1 include oral (cold sores, fever blisters) and the eye (cornea).
    - Herpes virus can live dormant in humans for a lifetime.
    - Virus invades the nervous system.
    - Signs and symptoms
      - HSV-1 presents as itchy, vesicular groupings.
      - Recurrent infections
      - Avoid kissing, touching, or direct contact with other individuals when lesions are open to prevent spread of the virus.
  - Chickenpox
    - Also known as varicella
    - Causative agent is varicella-zoster virus (VZV).
    - Affects people that have never been exposed to VZV before
    - Commonly occurs in children
    - Very contagious
    - Spread by direct contact and airborne droplets
    - Signs and symptoms
      - Fever
      - Itching
      - Small bumps on the torso, face, or head, with spreading to the arms and legs later
      - There can be vesicles ranging in amount from 100 to 300 at one time on an individual's body.
      - Vesicles eventually crust.
      - VZV vaccine has prevented children from acquiring chickenpox since the year 1995.
  - Herpes zoster
    - Also known as shingles
    - Caused by VZV, same virus that causes chickenpox
    - Herpes zoster is contagious to immunosuppressed individuals, people who have not had chickenpox, or individuals who have not been vaccinated against chickenpox.
    - VZV remains dormant until the virus is triggered again by factors such as
      - Major stressful life event
      - Decreased immunity
    - Signs and symptoms
      - Very painful
      - Blisters form along nerve distribution lines through the body.
      - Itching
    - In 2017, a new shingles vaccine called Shingrix was licensed by the US Food and Drug Administration (FDA).

- The Centers for Disease Control and Prevention (CDC) recommends adults over 50 years of age and individuals who have had shingles get vaccinated with Shingrix to prevent shingles and the complications associated with the disease.
- Warts
  - Also known as verrucae
  - Caused by human papillomaviruses (HPV)
  - HPV is categorized by many types that are associated with different diseases.
  - Found anywhere on the body but most common areas are the hands and feet
  - Direct contact can spread warts from person to person.
  - Signs and symptoms
    - Overgrowth of flesh-colored cells on the epidermis
    - Growth is usually a bumpy, elevated lesion that is tender or painful when pushed on.
- Hand, foot, and mouth disease
  - Very contagious viral disease that mainly occurs in babies and children.
  - Causative agents include the coxsackievirus A16 and enterovirus 71.
  - Signs and symptoms
    - Fever
    - Rash-like disease that occurs in the mouth, and on the hands and feet
    - Painful
    - No vaccine is available yet for this disease.
- Fungal
  - Dead keratinized epidermal cells on the skin are used as food for fungi to survive.
    - Tinea capitis
      - Many different types of skin infections (ringworm) are caused by tinea.
      - Scalp infection (ringworm) caused by the organism *Trichophyton tonsurans*
      - Sign and symptoms
        - Red patches
        - Scaly and circular in appearance on scalp
        - Loss of hair at infected area
    - Tinea corporis
      - Ringworm of the body
      - Causative organism is *Microsporus canis*.
      - Affects the areas without hair on the face, torso, arms, and legs of the body
      - Cats and dogs are common causes that serve as modes of transmission of the microorganisms.
      - Signs and symptoms
        - Red, scaly rings on the body
        - Clear center in the middle of the rings
        - Itching may occur.
        - Possible stinging pain can occur.
    - Tinea pedis
      - Also known as athlete's foot
      - Causative organism is *Trichophyton mentagrophytes* or *Trichophyton rubrumis*.
      - Common areas for increased risk of infection include gymnasiums, locker rooms, or swimming pool areas.
      - Signs and symptoms
        - Red areas around skin on toes

- ○ Burning sensation on feet
- ○ Bad smell may also be present.
  - ▪ Tinea unguium
    - ▪ Also called onychomycosis or nail fungus
    - ▪ Occurs as a nail infection
    - ▪ Most commonly affects the toenails
    - ▪ Signs and symptoms
      - ○ Toenail turns white first.
      - ○ Thick nail develops and becomes brittle.
      - ○ Pain
      - ○ Foul odor is present.
  - ▪ Thrush
    - ▪ Causative agent is *Candida albicans*
    - ▪ Can also be caused by long-term antibiotic or steroid therapy
    - ▪ Found mainly inside an infant's oral area
    - ▪ Yeast-like fungus present on mucosa of the mouth
    - ▪ Symptoms
      - ○ Tongue usually has white lesions.
      - ○ Lesions make mouth and tongue sore and painful.
- Parasitic
  - Scabies
    - ▪ Causative agent is a mite.
      - ▪ *Sarcoptes scabiei*
        - ○ Process of infection
          - ○ Female mite invades the epidermal layer and lays eggs.
          - ○ Female mite dies after laying eggs and male mite dies after fertilization occurs.
          - ○ Larvae hatch and move to the skin surface.
          - ○ Larvae invade the skin to look for food.
          - ○ Larvae grow into adults and repeat the cycle.
        - ○ Signs and symptoms
          - ○ Red, itchy lesions are present.
          - ○ Linear burrowing by mites is visible as brown lines on the skin.
          - ○ Swollen areas associated with mite burrowing are also visible on the skin.
- Pediculosis
  - Also known as lice
  - Can be found on the scalp, body, and pubis
  - Female lice lay white eggs (nits) on hair shafts.
  - The white eggs or nits hatch and are called louse.
  - A hatched louse is sustained by human blood.
  - Head lice are spread by direct contact with the hair of someone who is infected.
  - Head lice infestations are not related to cleanliness.
  - Lice cannot fly or hop; they move by crawling.
  - Signs and symptoms
    - ▪ Itchy scalp
    - ▪ Red bumps form

Traumatic Integumentary Disorders

- Burns
  - Burns can cause tissue damage and harm to the body that ranges from mild to severe.
  - Burns are categorized two ways.
    - How deep the burn penetration was, which resulted in damage to the skin layers
    - How much area the burn covered on an individual's body
      - Superficial
        - Burns that affect and cause harm to the outer layer of the skin or epidermis
        - The top part of the dermis may also be affected.
        - Long-term tissue damage is rare.
        - First-degree burn examples include sunburns or quick heat flash burns.
  - Signs and symptoms
    - Redness or pink color present at site of burn
    - Pain that subsides over a few days
    - Dry skin
    - Peeling skin
  - Partial thickness (superficial and deep)
    - Burns that cause harm to all of the epidermis and much of the dermis
    - These burns are also known as second-degree burns.
    - Infection risk is high.
  - Symptoms
    - Redness
    - Very tender
    - Very painful
    - Weeping surface
    - Swelling with fluid-filled vesicles present
- Full-thickness
  - Tissue damage to all the skin layers
  - Referred to as third-degree burns
  - Bone and muscle may be involved.
  - Symptoms
    - Dry and leathery skin
    - May be black and white in color
    - The outer layer tissues become tight, causing stress and tension on the other underlying tissues.
    - Muscles, tendons, or bones may be visible.

Chronic Integumentary Disorders

- Acne vulgaris
  - Most prevalent skin condition that affects over 75% of the population
  - People ranging from 12 to 25 years of age are affected by this skin disease.
  - Acne vulgaris coincides with the beginning of puberty.
  - Acne is found mainly on the face, upper portion of the back, and neck areas.
  - The sebaceous glands and associated hair follicles are involved.
  - Acne develops owing to follicular blockage or inflammation of the sebaceous glands.

- There is noninflammatory acne and inflammatory acne.
  - Noninflammatory acne contains both blackheads (open) and whiteheads (closed).
  - Inflammatory acne or cystic acne produces whiteheads that cause irritation, swelling, and redness in the dermis, which causes pain.
- Many components contribute to acne formation.
  - Hair follicle inflammation
  - Too much sebum is produced.
  - Presence of the *Propionibacterium acnes* bacteria
  - Hyperproliferation of the cells lining the hair follicle
- Signs and symptoms
  - Pain
  - Redness
  - Tenderness

Skin Cancers

- Basal cell carcinoma
  - Nonmelanoma skin cancer that does not develop from melanocytes
  - Most prevalent skin cancer in the world.
  - Develops in sun-exposed areas of the body
  - Basal cells continue to form, which results in a mass.
  - Slow-growing tumor that rarely spreads beyond the skin
  - Several factors contribute to an individual acquiring basal cell carcinoma.
    - Prolonged exposure to UV light
    - Individuals who are older in age
    - Radiation
    - Individuals who have had weakened immune systems for a long period of time
    - Lighter skinned individuals
  - Signs and symptoms
    - Appear mainly on the face, arms, hands, head, and neck areas of the body
    - Borders of mass are white in color and raised.
    - Mild redness
- Squamous cell carcinoma
  - Nonmelanoma skin cancer
  - Develops in the squamous cells of the epidermis
  - Can spread to the dermis and lymph nodes
  - Cigarettes, cigars, and pipe smoking are also responsible for this type of cancer.
  - Other contributing factors include
    - UV exposure
    - Radiation
    - Lighter skinned individuals
    - Individuals with weakened immune systems
    - Genetics
  - Signs and symptoms
    - In the initial stages, lesions are hard, rough, and may have possible discharge.
    - In later stages, lesions form a crust-type layer.
- Malignant melanoma
  - When melanoma originates in the skin, it is called cutaneous melanoma.

- Malignant melanoma is a cancerous tumor that begins in the melanocytes.
- Melanoma is able to metastasize to any organ in the body such as the heart and brain.
- Considered the deadliest skin cancer
- Exact cause is unknown.
- Risk factors that contribute to melanoma include
  - Sun exposure to natural and artificial UV radiation
  - Genetics
  - Lighter skinned individuals
  - Individuals with weakened immune systems
  - A gene alteration (B-RAF)
- Signs and symptoms
  - Can occur on sun-exposed areas such as the head, neck, back, chest, arms, and legs
  - Appear mostly as brown or black in color, but can be red, blue, gray, or white
  - Color is irregular.
  - Surface is irregular.
  - Borders of lesion are irregular.
  - Can be raised or flat
- Cutaneous melanomas
  - Categorized by their patterns of growth
  - Superficial spreading melanoma
    - Most prevalent type of melanoma
    - Most curable type
    - Most commonly found on the upper portion of the back and the legs. These areas of the body usually have the most sun exposure.
  - Lentigo maligna melanoma
    - Occurs in the elderly and are found on the face
    - Appear first as brown patches that later turn into cancer.
  - Acral lentiginous melanoma
    - Appears on the palms of hands, mucous membranes, soles of feet, and ends of fingers
    - More prevalent in dark skinned individuals and people of Asian descent.
  - Nodular melanoma
    - Can occur anywhere on the body
    - More commonly found in males
    - Looks very similar to a blood blister and is therefore often incorrectly diagnosed
    - Threatening type of melanoma that can evolve and penetrate very quickly

ABCDE Rule for Skin Cancer Assessment

- Rule or guide used to assess suspicious lesions on the body
- A is for Asymmetry.
  - Each half of a mole or birthmark does not match the other half.
- B is for Border.
  - The border is irregular, jagged, or not clear.
- C is for Color.
  - The color of the lesion has variation. The lesion may be brown or black and may also have shades of blue, white, red, or pink.
- D is for Diameter.
  - If the diameter of the lesion is bigger than 6 mm across, then it needs to be checked.

- E is for Evolving or Elevation.
  - Determine if the lesion is elevated in any way, such as a raised appearance.
  - Determine if the lesion is changing in size, shape, and color.
- Merkel cell carcinoma
  - A very intrusive and uncommon carcinoma
  - Mainly occurs on the head and neck areas
  - Factors that contribute to this type of cancer include
    - UV exposure
    - Individuals with weakened immune systems
    - An infection in the Merkel cells
    - Males
    - Individuals older than 50 years of age
  - Signs and symptoms
    - Present as purple or flesh-colored lesions
- Kaposi sarcoma
  - Forms cells from the cells surrounding the blood vessels
  - Kaposi sarcoma can be differentiated into four different categories.
    - Classic
    - Immunocompromised
    - Epidemic
    - AIDS-related and most common form
      - Endemic (African)
  - Signs and symptoms
    - Reddish, purple bumps on skin
    - Lesions occur on the legs at first.
    - In HIV-infected individuals, the lesions are usually on the upper part of the body, such as the face and mouth areas.
    - Lesions are painful and itchy.

APPLICATION AND REVIEW

12. Which statement made by the nurse demonstrates knowledge related to the ethnic risks associated with skin cancer?
    1. "A specific form of melanoma is seen more often in people of Asian descent."
    2. "Arab ancestry is a risk factor for developing cutaneous melanomas."
    3. "Regular skin screenings are important for those of Jewish descent."
    4. "People of African ancestry have a very low risk for skin cancers."
13. What lifestyle factors puts a client at a higher risk for developing a squamous cell carcinoma?
    1. Pipe smoking
    2. Having several tattoos
    3. Use of perfumed lotions
    4. Treatment with beta blockers
14. What assessment findings are characteristic of a second-degree burn? **Select all that apply**.
    1. Skin is taut
    2. Skin is white in color
    3. Skin is leathery looking
    4. Reports pain at a 6 of 10
    5. Blisters are noted over burn area

See Answers on pages 236–238.

Disorders of the Hair

- Alopecia
  - Hair loss that occurs on the body or the head
  - Occurs owing to hair follicle growth interruption
  - Hair loss can happen owing to numerous factors.
    - Deficiency in iron levels in the body
    - Chemotherapy
    - Poor nutrition
    - Hair pulling
    - Chemicals used on the hair
    - Hormone changes
- Androcentric alopecia
  - Also known as male-pattern baldness in males
  - Involves the androgen receptor (AR) gene
  - A deviation in the AR gene
  - Affects more males than females with alopecia
  - Hair loss occurs in a pattern which starts on the sides above the temples and progresses over the top of the head.
- Female-pattern alopecia
  - Mostly affects women ages 20 to 40 years and women older than 70 years of age
  - Hair loss mainly occurs on the crown of the head as well as the areas behind the ears.
  - Genetics plays a role.
  - Adrenal androgen dehydroepiandrosterone sulfate is found to be increased in women who are afflicted with female-pattern alopecia.

Integumentary Changes Associated With Aging

- Skin changes that occur with aging include many factors.
  - Genetics
  - Gravity
  - Environmental influences
    - Sun exposure (UV radiation) to natural and artificial light
      - UV radiation is harmful and known to cause wrinkles and skin cancer.
  - Diet
    - A diet high in sugars, fats, and dairy can lead to inflammation and can affect the skin's appearance.
  - Smoking history
    - Tobacco smoke can lead to wrinkles, deprives the body of necessary oxygen, and causes much damage to an individual's skin integrity over prolonged periods of time.
  - Alcohol consumption history
    - Chronic alcohol consumption is harmful not only to the body but also can lead to changes in the skin's integrity over time.
  - Weight
    - An underweight individual has insufficient natural fat which can cause the skin to sag, making wrinkles more prominent.
    - Being overweight can lead to health problems causing integumentary issues to develop, which can add to the aging process.

- Poor nutrition leads to aging skin when there is a decreased intake of fats, calories, proteins, and vitamins.
  - Hydration
    - Individuals need a significant amount of water or healthy fluids for the skin to maintain a healthy appearance.
    - The skin is an organ made up of cells that need water to properly function.
    - Without proper hydration, the skin is dry, which leads to the skin having less elasticity.
  - Chronic exposure to a cold environment
    - A constant cold environment can have a negative impact on the skin's integrity and cause wrinkles and thinning of the skin.
  - Chemical exposure history
    - Medications that an individual takes on a daily basis, in oral form or applied to the skin, can cause harmful effects to the skin thus adding to the aging process.
- Structural changes that occur with age
  - Melanocytes and melanin decrease.
    - With age, melanocyte loss occurs, which results in reduced UV protection.
    - Melanocyte loss also causes hair to turn gray in color.
      - Langerhans cells decrease.
        - With age, these cells decline, resulting in decreased immunity in the skin's response to fight off harmful bacteria and viruses.
      - Skin loses elasticity.
        - The dermis becomes thinner with an elastic fiber deficit giving the skin a clear-like and paper consistency.
        - Collagen fibers and fibroblasts disintegrate, which results in increased wrinkling and sagging of skin.
        - Loss of elastin results in wrinkles.
  - Adipose tissue volume loss
    - Usually occurs in the face, which leads to a thin facial appearance
    - Decreased subcutaneous fat can increase the risk of trauma to the skin, skin tearing, and hypothermia.
  - Oil production decrease
    - Dry, rough, flaky skin
    - Coarse hair and scalp
  - Sebaceous and sweat gland deterioration
    - Decreased activity of the apocrine and sebaceous glands results in dry skin with minimal perspiration.
  - Capillary frailty
    - Capillaries become increasingly fragile and weak, which leads to increased bruising.
  - Decreased blood supply
    - Skin gets cold easily.
  - Nerve endings
    - Reduction occurs with age
  - Receptors associated with touch and pressure
    - The number of receptors diminishes with age, which results in decreased attention to pain, temperature, and touch.

APPLICATION AND REVIEW

15. What assessment data support that an older adult client is experiencing expected age-related integumentary system changes? **Select all that apply**.
    1. Skin on face presents with an increase in sagging
    2. Several skin tears noted on both lower arms
    3. Claims bruised area, "only hurts a little."
    4. Being treated for acne vulgaris
    5. Several moles noted on torso
16. Which statement demonstrates the nurse's understanding of the effect of smoking on the skin?
    1. "Facial wrinkling is often the result of long-term smoking."
    2. "Poor hydration of the skin has been attributed to chronic smoking."
    3. "Smoking deposits nicotine on the skin, which contributes to tissue loss."
    4. "Smoking damages the melanocytes leading to a loss of ultraviolet protection."
17. What risks to the function of the skin are incurred when the diet is dramatically low in dietary fat? **Select all that apply**.
    1. Increases risk of poor skin hydration
    2. Accelerates the normal skin aging process
    3. Accelerates secretion of sweat production
    4. Increases sensitivity to changes in temperature
18. The nurse is caring for an elderly client. Which statement, if made by the client, would the nurse attribute to the loss of adipose tissue related to the normal aging process?
    1. "Oily hair and skin were never a problem when I was younger."
    2. "I sweat so much I have to bathe at least twice a day."
    3. "My face is so much thinner than it used to be."
    4. "My skin feels warm most of the time."
19. Which assessment findings support a probable diagnosis of female-pattern alopecia? **Select all that apply**.
    1. Age: 34 years
    2. Hair color: Light auburn
    3. Menarche: Started at age 14
    4. Hair loss is noted behind both ears
    5. Family history of premature hair loss

See Answers on pages 236–238.

ANSWER KEY: REVIEW QUESTIONS

1. **Answers: 1, 3, 4, 5.**
   1 A primary function of the skin involves protection of internal organs. **3** A primary function of the skin involves temperature regulation. **4** A primary function of the skin is to protect against bacteria. **5** A primary function of the skin involves sensory perception of pain.
   2 Magnesium balance is not regulated by the integumentary system (skin).
   Client Need: Physiological Adaptation; **Cognitive Level:** Applying; **Nursing Process:** Planning
2. **4 Stratum germinativum is the deepest layer of the epidermis.**
   1 Stratum granular is above the germinativum. **2** Stratum corneum is the outer most layer of the epidermis. **3** Stratum spinosum is located above the germinative layer
   Client Need: Physiological Adaptation; **Cognitive Level:** Understanding; **Integrated Process:** Teaching and Learning

3. **3 The stratum lucidum is thicker skin found on the soles of the feet and the palm of the hands to protect those surfaces from friction damage.**

   1 The stratum corneum is a waterproofing layer that contains mostly dead skin cells. **2** The stratum spinosum is where keratin, the main component of hair, nails, and skin cells is created. **4** The stratum granulosum is the waterproofing layer found on most body surfaces.

   Client Need: Physiological Adaptation; **Cognitive Level:** Understanding; **Integrated Process:** Teaching and Learning

4. **2 The epidermis is renewed about every 30 days.**

   1 The epidermis consists of five layers. **3** The epidermis is between 0.3 and 1.5 mm thick. **4** The dermis supports the blood vessels found in the epidermis.

   Client Need: Physiological Adaptation; **Cognitive Level:** Understanding; **Integrated Process:** Teaching and Learning

5. **3 Langerhans cells aid the immune system by protecting the skin from bacteria and viruses.**

   1 Keratinocytes produce keratin. **2** Melanocytes produce melanin, which determines skin color. **4** Sebum from sebaceous glands lubricates the surface of the skin.

   Client Need: Physiological Adaptation; **Cognitive Level:** Understanding; **Integrated Process:** Teaching and Learning

6. **2 Collagen, a group of proteins found naturally in the body, is responsible for the strength of the skin.**

   1 Elastin is a protein that provides the skin with the ability to return to its original shape after stretching. **3** Mast cells are important in wound healing. **4** Nerve cells transmit sensory information to the brain.

   Client Need: Physiological Adaptation; **Cognitive Level:** Understanding; **Integrated Process:** Teaching and Learning

7. **3 When the body is cold, the blood vessels contract to increase the internal body temperature.**

   1 When the body is too hot, the blood vessels expand allowing heat to be released through the skin's surface. **2** Sebaceous glands are associated with each hair follicle; they secrete sebum, an oily substance that provides a waterproof barrier to prevent drying, not heat, regulation. **4** Perspiration increases when the body needs to release not conserve heat.

   Client Need: Physiological Adaptation; **Cognitive Level:** Understanding; **Integrated Process:** Teaching and Learning

8. **1 Hair follicles originate in the dermis.**

   2, 3, 4 The corneum and the germinativum are layers that comprise the epidermis.

   Client Need: Physiological Adaptation; **Cognitive Level:** Understanding; **Integrated Process:** Teaching and Learning

9. **2 Fibroblasts produce both collagen and elastin, which are responsible for providing the skin with strength and elasticity.**

   1 Wound healing is affected by the presence of mast cells. **3** A macrophage is a type of white blood cell that protects and ingests foreign invaders. **4** Melanocytes produce melanin, which determines skin color and protects against harmful UV radiation.

   Client Need: Physiological Adaptation; **Cognitive Level:** Understanding; **Integrated Process:** Teaching and Learning

10. **Answers: 1, 2, 5.**

    1 An apocrine gland secretion site is in the armpits. **2** Apocrine glands contain ducts that have an entrance directly into the hair follicles. **5** Apocrine secretions are odorless until exposed to skin bacteria. **3** Eccrine gland secretions are used to help decrease body temperature. **4** Eccrine gland secretions are used to help moisturize the cells on the surface of the skin.

    Client Need: Physiological Adaptation; **Cognitive Level:** Understanding; **Integrated Process:** Teaching and Learning

11. **1 At ages 3 to 5 years, mole formation usually occurs.**

    2 Moles can appear anywhere on the skin, alone or in groups. **3** Moles appear as small brown spots. **4** Moles may be removed by surgical excision if necessary.

    Client Need: Physiological Adaptation; **Cognitive Level:** Understanding; **Nursing Process:** Evaluation

12. **1 Acral lentiginous melanoma appears on the palms of hands, mucous membranes, soles of feet, and ends of fingers, and it is more prevalent in dark skinned individuals and people of Asian descent.**

    2 Although the risk is higher among light skinned persons, dark skinned individuals also have a risk for the development of skin cancers. **3** People of all cultures at risk for skin cancer should be screened. **4** Africans are not at higher risk for skin cancer than other populations.

    Client Need: Physiological Adaptation; **Cognitive Level:** Analysis; **Nursing Process:** Analysis

13. **1 Cigarettes, cigars, and pipe smoking increase the risk for developing a squamous cell carcinoma.**

    2 Although traumatizing for the skin, there is no known link between tattoos and squamous cell carcinoma. **3** There is no known link between perfumed lotions and squamous cell carcinoma. **4** There is no known link between beta blocker therapy and squamous cell carcinoma.

    Client Need: Physiological Adaptation; **Cognitive Level:** Applying; **Nursing Process:** Assessment

14. **Answers: 4, 5.**

    4 Signs and symptoms of a second-degree burn include moderate to severe pain. **5** Signs and symptoms of a second-degree burn include the presence of fluid-filled vesicles.

    1, 2, 3 Signs and symptoms of a third-degree burn include skin that is taut, dry, and leathery, which appears white or even black in color.

    Client Need: Physiological Adaptation; **Cognitive Level:** Applying; **Nursing Process:** Assessment

15. **Answers: 1, 2, 3.**

    1 Aging causes decreased subcutaneous fat, which can increase the risk of sagging skin. **2** Aging causes decreased subcutaneous fat, which can increase the risk of trauma to the skin such as skin tears. **3** The number of receptors diminishes with age, resulting in decreased attention to pain, temperature, and touch.

    4 Acne vulgaris, although prevalent, is not a result of aging. **5** Moles are not a result of aging, but can be either benign or cancerous and require monitoring.

    Client Need: Physiological Adaptation; **Cognitive Level:** Analysis; **Nursing Process:** Analysis

16. **1 Tobacco smoke can lead to wrinkles and causes much damage to an individual's skin integrity over prolonged periods of time.**

    2 Skin hydration is not generally affected by smoking. **3** Nicotine is deposited in the lungs not necessarily on the skin. **4** Aging, not smoking, significantly affects melanocyte production.

    Client Need: Physiological Adaptation; **Cognitive Level:** Analysis; **Nursing Process:** Evaluation

17. **2 Poor nutrition leads to aging skin when there is a decreased intake of fats, calories, proteins, and vitamins.**

    1 Hydration is not directly affected by fat consumption. **3** Skin secretion is not directly affected by fat consumption, but rather by aging. **4** Decreased sensitivity to temperature changes is a result of aging.

    Client Need: Physiological Adaptation; **Cognitive Level:** Analysis; **Nursing Process:** Analysis

18. **3 Adipose tissue volume loss usually occurs in the face, which leads to a thin facial appearance.**

    1 Oil production decreases, which results in dry, rough, flaky skin and coarse hair and scalp. **2** Decreased activity of the apocrine and sebaceous glands results in dry skin with minimal perspiration. **4** A decreased blood supply causes the skin to get cold easily.

    Client Need: Physiological Adaptation; **Cognitive Level:** Analysis; **Nursing Process:** Analysis

19. **Answers: 1, 4, 5.**

    1 Female-pattern alopecia mostly affects women aged 20 to 40 years and women older than 70 years of age. **4** Female-pattern alopecia commonly presents with hair loss behind both ears. **5** Genetics play a role in female-pattern alopecia.

    2 Hair color is not a risk factor for female-pattern alopecia. **3** Onset of menarche does not appear to be a risk factor for female-pattern alopecia.

    Client Need: Physiological Adaptation; **Cognitive Level:** Analysis; **Nursing Process:** Analysis

Hematologic System Disorders 12

OVERVIEW

- The various systems that compose the human body are distinct but are also interrelated.
- One universal standard for all systems within the body is a method to provide oxygen to the tissues and additional nutrients for cellular metabolism, and for the timely removal of waste by-products.
- The distribution of blood through the body by vessels is critical in the body's function of transporting blood to the heart.
- Blood and lymph are vital body fluids that are carried via a complex system of tubes (blood vessels) throughout the body and by the pumping action of the heart.
- Blood plays a critical role in the immune system.
  - Helps defend the body
  - Removes cell waste
    - Transports oxygen to tissue with nutrients to aid in cellular metabolism
- Blood, a component that all systems depend on
  - To transport essential oxygen
  - Is required for cellular metabolism

Blood Vessels

- A closed system, consisting of
  - Veins
  - Capillaries
  - Arteries
- Veins, capillaries, and arteries distribute blood throughout the body.
  - Two circulations
    - Pulmonary circulation: allows for oxygen and carbon dioxide in the lungs to be exchanged.
    - Systemic circulation: throughout the body nutrients and wastes are exchanged between the blood and cells.
  - Blood is transferred away from the heart by the arteries through the body tissues and lungs.
  - Small branches of the arteries, called arterioles, control the portion of blood that flows through capillaries to certain areas by the contraction of smooth muscle (vasoconstriction or dilation) in the vessel walls.
  - Very small vessels, also known as capillaries, are categorized into copious networks that make up the microcirculation.
    - Precapillary sphincters determine how much blood flows from the arterioles to the individual capillaries.
      - Blood flows slowly into capillaries.
      - Blood flow depends on the metabolic needs of the tissues.
  - Blood from the capillary beds flows through small venules conducting blood toward the heart.

- Veins are called capacitance vessels because approximately 70% of blood is located in the veins at one time.
  - Venules drain blood into the larger veins.
  - Skeletal muscle action affects blood flow into the veins through gravity and respiratory movements.
  - Respiratory movements support the movement of blood through the trunk.
  - The valves have an important role in the larger veins by keeping blood flowing to the heart.
- Three layers of walls of arteries and veins are
  - The inner layer, also known as the endothelial layer, or tunica intima
  - The middle layer
    - Controls the diameter and lumen diameter of the blood vessel
    - A layer of smooth muscle, the tunica media
    - The outer connective tissue layer
    - Contains collagen and elastic fibers
- Vasa vasorum
  - Made up of tiny blood vessels that supply blood to the tissues of the wall of large blood vessels
- During the cardiac cycle bigger arteries are highly elastic and adjust to blood volume changes that occur.
  - Systolic pressure can rise too high if the aorta does not expand during systole.
  - To maintain adequate diastolic pressure the walls must recoil.
  - Arteries, unlike veins, have larger walls and more smooth muscle.
- Autoregulation is a reflex adjustment in a tiny area of an organ or tissue.
  - It can vary depending on the needs of the cells within the area.
  - It also controls localized vasodilation or vasoconstriction in arterioles.
  - Histamine, a release of chemical mediators, can increase temperature at a specific area and cause vasodilation.
  - If pH decreases and carbon dioxide increases, a decrease in oxygen can cause local vasodilation.
  - Systemic blood pressure is not affected by local changes.
- Epinephrine and norepinephrine
  - Stimulate the $alpha_1$-adrenergic receptors located in the walls of the arterioles
  - Another potent vasoconstrictor is angiotensin.
  - Continued circulation of blood is distributed throughout the body by partial vasoconstriction.
  - The sympathetic nervous system maintains constant blood flow even at times of rest, through the vasomotor center.
- Capillary walls consist of a single endothelial layer and through this layer flows
  - Fluid
  - Carbon dioxide
  - Oxygen
  - Glucose
  - Electrolytes
  - Other nutrients and wastes

Blood

- Oxygen and glucose, which are carried from the blood, provide essential nutrients, cell wastes, and electrolytes.
  - Serves as the body's defense by transporting
    - Antibodies

- White blood cells (WBCs)
  - Antibodies and WBCs rapidly expunge all foreign material.
- Body temperature is regulated by distributing core heat throughout peripheral tissue, promoting homeostasis.
  - Hormones measure and adjust various controls such as
    - Blood pressure
    - Body fluid levels, where blood is the medium
- Hemostasis occurs through clotting factors continually circulating in the blood.
  - Aids in clotting to help stop the bleeding process
  - Keeps blood within a damaged blood vessel
- The blood maintains a stable pH of 7.35 to 7.45 because of buffer systems in place.

APPLICATION AND REVIEW

1. What are functions of the blood? **Select all that apply**.
   1. Defends the body against infection
   2. Removes cellular waste produces
   3. Transports oxygen to the tissues
   4. Supports cellular metabolism
   5. Balances body fluids
2. What blood vessel is considered a part of the body's microcirculation?
   1. Arteriole
   2. Venule
   3. Capillary
   4. Vein
3. Which client diagnosis is associated with impaired pulmonary circulation?
   1. Chronic malnutrition
   2. Acute kidney failure
   3. Deep vein thrombosis
   4. Left-sided heart failure
4. What is the primary factor that controls the amount of blood flow to the capillary system?
   1. Precapillary sphincters in the venule system
   2. Precapillary sphincters in the arteriole system
   3. The smooth muscle layer of the associated vessel
   4. The amount of blood in the microcirculation at any time
5. What is the primary concern related to the ineffective expansion and contraction of the aorta during the cardiac cycle?
   1. The resulting poor circulation to the brain
   2. Ineffective management of diastolic blood pressure
   3. Increased risk for the development of arteriosclerosis
   4. Dangerous rise in systolic blood pressure during systole
6. What is the role of histamine in the reflexive process of autoregulation associated with blood vessels?
   1. It stimulates the muscle layer of the vessel causing vasoconstriction
   2. It increases the temperature at a specific site causing vasodilation
   3. It stimulates the sympathetic nervous system to trigger vasodilation
   4. It stimulates the $alpha_1$-adrenergic receptors located in the walls of the arteriolar
7. What events are examples of the various functions of blood? **Select all that apply**.
   1. Delivering white blood cells (WBCs) to the site of a skin wound
   2. Clotting a blood vessel that has been cut
   3. Stabilizing pH through a buffer system
   4. Draining interstitial fluid from tissues
   5. Supporting the process of sweating

See Answers on pages 263–265.

Composition of Blood

- The average adult body is composed of approximately 5 liters of blood.
  - 55% of the blood volume is composed of water and dissolved solutes.
  - 45% the remaining percentage of blood is composed of
    - Erythrocytes
    - Formed liquid elements or cells
    - Thrombocytes
    - Platelets
    - Leukocytes
    - Hematocrit
  - Suggests the viscosity of blood, erythrocytes, proportion of cells
    - Males have a higher hematocrit, which averages 42% to 52%.
    - Females' hematocrit ordinarily falls within 37% to 47%.
  - Elevated hematocrit indicative of
    - Dehydration (loss of body fluids)
    - Excess number of red blood cells (RBCs)
  - Lower hematocrit indicative of
    - Anemia
    - Blood loss
- Plasma
  - Remaining clear yellowish fluid after the cells have been detached
- Serum
  - After cells and fibrinogen have been removed from the plasma the fluid or solutes that remain; serum contains
    - Plasma proteins include albumin, which is essential for preserving osmotic pressure in the blood.
      - Globulins
      - Antibodies
      - Fibrinogen (essential for the formation of blood clots)

Blood Cells and Hematopoiesis

- Red bone marrow is where all blood cells are derived.
- Red bone marrow is found in the following bones of adults
  - Pelvis
  - Sternum
  - Vertebrae
  - Ribs
  - Irregular and flat bones
- When a biopsy is performed the iliac crest is a common site for removing bone marrow.
- Hematopoiesis is also known as hematopoiesis.
  - Various blood cells developing from a single stem cell (pluripotential hematopoietic stem cell)
  - Committed stem cells for each type of blood cell are formed from the basic cell differentiation process (Fig. 12.1).
  - Matured and proliferated cells provide the particular functional cells needed by the body.
- Dyscrasia
  - Disorders involving cellular components of the blood
  - Pathologic condition

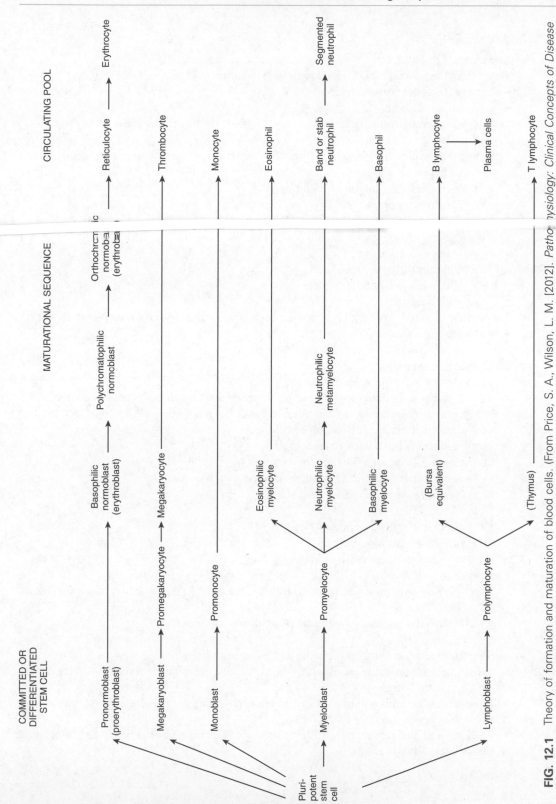

FIG. 12.1 Theory of formation and maturation of blood cells. (From Price, S. A., Wilson, L. M. [2012]. *Pathophysiology: Clinical Concepts of Disease Processes* [6th ed.]. St. Louis, Mosby.)

Red Blood Cells

- Erythrocytes or RBCs
  - Erythrocytes, or red blood cells, Are flexible discs (biconcave).
  - Mature RBCs are non-nucleated.
  - Contain hemoglobin
  - RBC size and structure are crucial to easy transport to the smaller capillaries.
- Erythropoietin
  - A hormone, which encourages erythrocyte production in the red bone marrow in response to tissue hypoxia, emerges from the kidney.
    - RBC comprise the largest cell volume in blood.
    - RBC values range from 4.2 to 6.2 million/mm^3.
    - For RBCs to produce and mature, they require the following raw materials, such as
      - Amino acids
      - Iron
      - Vitamin B_{12}
      - Vitamin B_6
      - Folic acid
- Hemoglobin is a red protein that is in charge of transporting oxygen in the blood.
  - Hemoglobin is made up of
    - Globin portion
    - Four heme groups
    - Two pairs of amino acid chains
  - Each is composed of a ferrous iron atom to which the oxygen molecule can adhere.
  - When hemoglobin becomes fully saturated with oxygen in the lungs, the oxygen binding sites are approximately 98% occupied.
  - Heme causes the red color in hemoglobin.
  - Oxyhemoglobin is formed in the combination of
    - Hemoglobin by combining oxygen in oxygenated blood
    - It is responsible for the bright red color.
  - Deoxyhemoglobin
    - Hemoglobin is not bound with oxygen.
    - Found in venous blood
    - Results in a dark or bluish red color
- Carbon dioxide
  - Hemoglobin (carbaminohemoglobin) transports a miniscule proportion of carbon dioxide in the blood.
    - The biocarbonate ion transports carbon dioxide in blood.
    - Buffer pair
- Carbon monoxide can easily replace the oxygen in the hemoglobin.
  - When carbon monoxide binds with iron in the hemoglobin, the result is a severe oxygen deficit or lethal hypoxia.
  - Pulse oximetry levels will overestimate the arterial oxygenation of the blood with carbon monoxide poisoning.
  - Early detection of carbon monoxide poisoning can be noted by the bright red color in the lips or face of the victim.

- Life span of RBCs
  - Every 120 days RBCs start a new life span.
  - As the RBCs become old, stiff, and fragile they submit to phagocytosis.
    - The spleen or liver breaks down the RBC into two components.
      - Globin
      - Heme
        - Amino acids break down globin, which becomes reused in the amino acid pool.
        - Iron is returned to the bone marrow and liver to be used in the synthesis of more hemoglobin.
        - Excessive iron is stored as ferritin or hemosiderin in the
          - Blood
          - Liver
  - Other body tissues
    - Hemochromatosis is a genetic disorder, caused by iron overload.
      - Is caused by copious amounts of hemosiderin assembled in the liver, heart, and other organs
      - Can cause organ damage
    - Bilirubin is the remainder of the converted heme component.
      - Bilirubin moves through the blood to the liver.
      - Combines or conjugates with glucuronide to make it more dissolvable then discharged in the bile
- Hemolysis is the elimination of excess RBCs.
  - May result in increased levels of serum bilirubin levels, which can lead to jaundice, when the sclera of the eyes and skin become yellow in color

Leukocytes

- Leukocytes or WBCs comprise only 1% of the blood volume and numbers 5000 to 10,000 cells/mm^3.
- Can grow and change from the original stem cell in bone marrow
  - Are subdivided into three types of granulocytes and two types of agranulocytes
- Leukopoiesis is the creation of WBCs.
  - Stimulated by colony-stimulating factors (CSF) produced by different cells such as macrophages and T lymphocytes
    - For example, production of granulocyte CSF or multi-CSF (interleukin-3) is increased to produce additional types of WBCs to respond to an inflammatory process.
  - Diapedesis or ameboid action (movement through an intact capillary wall) allows WBCs to escape through the capillaries and enter the tissues, to defend the system.
- Five types of leukocytes
  - Lymphocytes are small leukocytes that make up 30% to 40% of the WBCs.
    - Two main types: B and T lymphocytes
  - Neutrophils are the most common leukocyte, making up 50% to 60% of WBCs, living only 4 days.
    - First responders to tissue damage and commence phagocytosis
  - Basophils can enter tissue that has migrated from the blood and become mast cells that release histamine and heparin.
    - Can be fixed or wandering

- Eosinophils can fight the effects of histamine.
  - Response heightened by allergic reactions and parasitic infections
- Monocytes can become macrophages.
  - After entering the tissue acting as phagocytes when tissue damage has occurred
- Differential count is used when making a diagnosis.
  - It represents the different types of WBCs in the blood.
  - With allergic reactions or parasitic infections there is an increase in eosinophil count, a bacterial infection or inflammatory condition increases neutrophils.
- Platelets, also called thrombocytes, assist in blood-clotting or hemostasis.
  - Although not cells, thrombocytes are small sporadic pieces from larger megakaryocytes.
  - A platelet plug, formed from platelets sticking to damaged tissue
    - Adheres to small breaks in blood vessels with rough surfaces and foreign material
    - Initiated the coagulation process
    - Aspirin can lead to an increase in bleeding by reducing the formation of adhesions.
- Hemostasis is the procedure that stops bleeding; consisting of three steps.
- Vasoconstriction or vascular spasm is the first response to blood vessel damage.
  - A platelet plug may form in small blood vessels because of a reduction of blood flow.
  - At the site of injury thrombocytes stick to underlying tissue.
  - With smaller blood vessels a platelet plug will develop.
    - Coagulation mechanism is needed for larger blood vessels and the inactive forms of clotting factors are activated in a particular sequence.
  - Cascade of reactions is the method for coagulation.

Blood Clotting

- Clot formation (coagulation) requires an arrangement or avalanche of events.
  - The production of prothrombin activator occurs after the injured tissue and platelets produce factors that begin a sequence of reactions.
  - The inactive prothrombin or factor II converts into thrombin.
    - Thrombin serves as both an anticoagulant and a procoagulant.
  - Fibrinogen (factor I) through the action of thrombin fibrin is converted.
  - Fibrin mesh by collecting cells form a solid clot and halts the flow of blood.
  - The clot gradually diminishes and drags the edges of injured tissue closer together and secures the site.
- The liver produces the circulation clotting factors.
  - With the help of fat-soluble vitamins, such as vitamin K, which is required for the production of most clotting factors
  - Calcium ions are essential for many steps in the clotting process.
- Other methods can be used to aid in the clotting process, such as
  - Applying pressure
  - Applying cold with pressure to the site
  - Thrombin solution to the area that needs blood flow reduced will aid in clotting.
- Fibrinolysis
  - The body regulates the need to clot to prevent excessive blood loss with the potential for infarctions can be caused by unnecessary clotting.
  - Although some individuals are able to form clots easily, others are susceptible to excessive bleeding.
    - Antithrombin III is a coagulation inhibitor in the bloodstream that prevents thrombus from forming.

- A prostaglandin is discharged to prohibit platelets from sticking to nearby undamaged tissue, through thrombin.
- Thrombomodulin, an endothelial cell receptor protein, attached to thrombin, triggers a sequence of reactions that lead to fibrinolysis.
- Heparin is an anticoagulant, blocks thrombin, is discharged from basophils or mast cells in the tissues, and can be administered intravenously to individuals at risk for thrombus formation.
- Heparin does not get rid of clots, but does prevent growth of the thrombus.
- Fibrinolysis is a natural process that allows for freshly formed clots to be broken down.
  - Inactive plasminogen is circulated through the blood.
  - After an injury inactive plasminogen can become converted by tissue plasminogen activator and streptokinase into plasmin.
  - The final stage, or product plasmin, di~~~~~~~~~~
- Fibrinolysis is localized and plasmin is quickly deactivated by the plasmin inhibitor.
- The body maintains a balance with clotting in the regulation of defense mechanisms.
- An example of these mechanisms are a group of "clot busting" medications, such as streptokinase.
  - Frequently used to help reduce blood clots that can form with heart attacks and strokes
  - Reducing the incidence of blood clots can reduce the risk of tissue damage.
  - Careful monitoring of clotting times and administration methods is needed to reduce the potential for unwanted bleeding and hematoma formation.
  - The most reliable technique to ensure the patient is properly healing is to monitor to prevent excessive bleeding or hematoma formation.
  - New studies and procedures are being developed in the United States that will further allow for increased safety and better recovery for patients.

Antigenic Blood Types

- An individual's blood type, which is uniquely formed, is determined by antigens found on the cell membranes of the individual's erythrocytes.
- Based on the presence of type A or B antigens or agglutinogens allow ABO groups to acquire characteristics.
  - After birth the antibodies of the mother in the fetal circulation can react with antigens in the blood of the newborn infant.
  - Similar antigen-antibody reactions can also occur with a blood transfusion with incompatible blood types.
  - Agglutination is the clumping and hemolysis of the recipient's RBCs and is a sign of incompatible blood transfusion, an antigen-antibody reaction.
- Matching blood types before transfusion is essential; therefore, individuals are carefully checked, including red cell antigen typing.
  - Individuals who are blood type O are considered universal donors because they lack A and B antigens.
  - Individuals with AB blood type are universal recipients.
  - Signs and symptoms of a transfusion reaction
    - Decreased blood pressure
    - Rapid pulse
    - Pain in the chest and abdomen
    - Headache
    - Fever and chills

- ▪ Flushing in the face
- ▪ Feeling of warmth in the vein receiving the transfusion
- Rh factor is an inherited protein located on the surface of RBCs.
  - Blood incompatibility can result in the mother is Rh negative and the fetus is Rh positive.
  - Erythroblastosis fetalis is a condition where the blood is incompatible between an Rh-negative mother and an Rh-positive fetus.
- Diagnostic tests
  - Complete blood count includes a count of the total number of
    - ▪ RBCs
    - ▪ WBCs
    - ▪ Platelet count
    - ▪ Cell morphology (shape and size)
    - ▪ WBC differential count
    - ▪ Hemoglobin (amount and concentration)
    - ▪ Hematocrit
- Screening tools have many diagnostic uses
  - Leukocytosis (an increase WBC) is frequently associated with inflammation and infection.
    - ▪ Leukopenia is a decrease in leukocytes; it can be caused by radiation, chemotherapy, or a viral infection.
    - ▪ An allergic reaction can be associated with an increase in eosinophils.
  - Individual cells can be observed for
    - ▪ Size
    - ▪ Shape
    - ▪ Maturity
    - ▪ Hemoglobin amounts
    - ▪ Uniformity
  - Observation of cells can help distinguish different types of anemia by size and shape, and presence of a nucleus in the RBC.
    - ▪ Hematocrit displays the percentage of blood volume made up of RBCs.
      - ▪ Illustrates fluid and cell contents
      - ▪ Anemia can be indicated by low RBC levels.
  - The mean corpuscular hemoglobin is an indication of the amount of hemoglobin per cell.
    - ▪ Indicates the oxygen-carrying capacity of the blood
  - Checking reticulocyte (immature non-nucleated RBC) counts is a way to assess bone marrow function.
  - Serum levels of the different components are determined by chemical analysis of the blood and certain components, such as vitamin B_{12}, iron, folic acid, urea, cholesterol, and bilirubin, can indicate metabolic disorders.
  - Blood clotting disorders can be differentiated by different tests.
    - ▪ Bleeding time is a measure of platelet functioning.
    - ▪ International normalized ratio (INR) and prothrombin time are measurements of the extrinsic pathways.
      - ▪ Used to evaluate anticoagulation therapy with warfarin
    - ▪ Partial thromboplastin time (PTT) is a measurement of the intrinsic pathway and the activity of various factors that comprise the coagulation process.
      - ▪ Also used to evaluate anticoagulation therapy with heparin

APPLICATION AND REVIEW

8. A blood transfusion is started after a client has had emergency surgery. What signs and symptoms would suggest that the client is experiencing a transfusion reaction? **Select all that apply.**
1. Temperature of 101.2° F (38.4° C)
2. Facial flushing
3. Reports of chest pain
4. Blood pressure of 160/110 mmHg
5. Moderate headache

See Answer on pages 263–265.

Blood Therapies

- Anemia or thrombocytopenia is treated by platelets and packed RBCs
- When stabilizing hydrostatic pressures and balancing osmotic, colloidal volume-expanding solutions or plasma can be infused without the risk of a reaction because they contain no antibodies and antigens.
- A variety of man-made blood products are available; however, none can perform all the intricate functions of normal human whole blood.
  - Artificial or substitute blood products are compatible with all blood types.
    - Although there are studies being conducted and various drugs that are being tested, none of the artificial blood products have been approved by the US Food and Drug Administration (FDA).
  - Multiple blood transfusions increase the risk of infection, but the use of epoetin alfa (Procrit), a type of erythropoietin, delivered by injection can stimulate RBC production before certain procedures.
- Stem cell or bone marrow transplants can be used to treat specific cancers, severe blood cell disease, and immune deficiencies.
  - Bone marrow is extracted from a donor's pelvic bone and instilled into the recipient's veins.
  - Within several weeks the new normal cells should develop.
  - With some cancers, the treatment involving chemotherapy or radiation may kill the tumor cells prior to the transplant.
- For patients with abnormal clotting conditions, drugs are available to assist with the clotting process. Some drugs have been approved for use by the FDA.
  - Romiplostim activates the production of platelets by the bone marrow.
  - Coagulation factor VIIa recombinant is used to treat hemophiliacs, but it also has been utilized in the treatment of combat trauma.
  - Some complications have arisen by use of these clotting agents, such as unintended clotting.

BLOOD DYSCRASIAS

Anemia

- Anemia is a reduction in hemoglobin content that impairs the transportation of oxygen in the blood.
- A number of factors can account for a low hemoglobin count
  - A decline in protein production
  - A decline in the number of erythrocytes
  - A combination of these and other factors

- Anemias are categorized by different attributes, such as cell shape (morphology), etiology, or size.
  - Loss of oxygen can cause the following events to occur
    - A loss of energy by cells, reduction in cell metabolism, and slowing of reproduction
    - Peripheral vasoconstriction and tachycardia are compensation mechanisms that occur to enhance oxygen.
    - General signs and symptoms of anemia
      - Pallor (pale color; most evident on face and palms)
      - Tachycardia (rapid heart rate)
      - Dyspnea (difficulty breathing)
      - Fatigue (extremely tired)
    - Reduced regeneration of epithelial cells can cause the digestive tract to become irritated, inflamed, and ulcerated, resulting in
      - Stomatitis or ulcers in the oral mucosa
      - Irritated and cracked lips
      - Dysphagia or difficulty swallowing
      - Changes in the skin and hair
    - Chronic anemia can be attribute to
      - Angina or chest pain (if during stress, the supply of oxygen to the heart is insufficient)
      - Severe cases of chronic anemia can result in congestive heart failure.
- Anemia(s) can be a result of one of the following factors
  - Lack of a required nutrients
  - Impaired bone marrow function
  - Blood loss
  - Excessive destruction of erythrocytes

Iron Deficiency Anemia

- Common type of anemia
- Pathophysiology
  - Lack of iron inhibits the production of hemoglobin, therefore lowering the amount of oxygen delivered in the circulatory system.
  - Erythrocyte appearance changes owing to the lower amount of hemoglobin in each cell
    - Microcytic or smaller erythrocytes
    - Hypochromic or erythrocytes with less color
    - Low iron is very common in all age groups and can range from mild/moderate to severe.
  - Estimated 20% of women are affected with some degree of anemia, and a higher percentage for pregnant women.
  - Source of the underlying problem needs to be identified.
    - Reduced iron stores can be associated with a lower
      - Serum ferritin
      - Hemosiderin
      - Histiocytic with less iron in the bone marrow
- Etiology
  - Some of the main causes of iron deficiency anemia include
    - Consumption of iron as part of the diet is insufficient to meet the daily standards. The need for iron-containing foods, such as vegetables and meats, is particularly high during adolescence, pregnancy, and while breastfeeding.
      - On average 5% to 10% of ingested iron is absorbed, but this can increase to 20% during periods when there is a demand for more iron absorption.

- Chronic and excessive blood loss, which can be caused by menstrual bleeding, cancer, hemorrhoids, and bleeding ulcers, leads to a shortage of iron and reduced hemoglobin levels.
  - Even small but steady losses in blood can have an impact on iron levels because there is less iron in the circulatory system to support an adequate production of hemoglobin.
- Malabsorption syndromes can reduce the absorption of iron in the duodenum, such as
  - Regional ileitis
  - Achlorhydria (deficiency in hydrochloric acid in the stomach)
- Chronic and extensive liver disease can decrease the absorption and storage of iron.
  - A lack of protein can further inhibit hemoglobin synthesis.
- Iron deficiency anemia can occur with some cancers and infections.
  - There are high iron stores but low hemoglobin levels because the iron available is not being utilized correctly.
- Signs and symptoms
  - The body can compensate for mild anemias, but with a continual drop in hemoglobin, the common signs and symptoms of anemia are
    - Pale skin and mucus membranes caused by cutaneous vasoconstriction
    - Feelings of weakness, fatigue, and susceptibility to cold temperatures caused by cell metabolism diminishing
    - Irritability owing to hypoxia and associated central nervous system changes
    - Frail hair and ridged or concave (spoon shaped) nails
    - Glossitis and stomatitis, irritation of the tongue and oral mucosa
    - Irregular menstrual cycles
    - Impaired wound healing
    - With untreated and severe anemia, signs and symptoms become more pronounced owing to the lack of circulating hemoglobin and oxygen
      - Tachycardia
      - Heart palpitations
      - Dyspnea (difficulty breathing)
      - Syncope (fainting)
- Diagnostic tests
  - Laboratory tests will indicate the decreased level of
    - Hemoglobin and hematocrit
    - Mean corpuscular volume and hemoglobin
    - Serum ferritin and iron
    - Transferrin saturation
  - Microscopic evaluation will indicate hypochromic and microcytic erythrocytes.

Pernicious Anemia-Vitamin B$_{12}$ Deficiency (Megaloblastic Anemia)

- Characterized by abnormally large but immature nucleated erythrocytes
- Progressively formed by vitamin deficiencies such as vitamin B$_{12}$ or vitamin B$_9$ (folic acid)
- Pregnant women during the first 2 months of pregnancy are most at risk for megaloblastic anemia owing to a lack of folic acid in the diet.
  - Folic acid deficiency can increase the risk of spina bifida or other spinal abnormalities in the fetus.
  - Folic acid deficits are usually related to dietary intake.
  - Folic acid supplements are recommended for females in childbearing years.
- Pernicious anemia, a type of megaloblastic anemia, is discussed below.

- Pathophysiology
  - Most common type of megaloblastic anemia is caused by reduced absorption of vitamin B_{12}, owing to a lack of intrinsic factor produced by the gastric mucosa glands.
    - Intrinsic factor has to bind with B_{12} in order to be absorbed by the lower ileum.
    - The gastric mucosa parietal cells atrophy and stop producing hydrochloric acid, therefore the amount of acid in the gastric secretions is severely reduced (or missing), which is referred to as achlorhydria.
    - Achlorhydria interrupts the early digestion of protein in the stomach and the absorption of iron.
      - May be associated with iron deficiency anemia
  - Megaloblasts or macrocytes contain nuclei and have extremely large RBCs that die prematurely and this can cause anemia (low erythrocyte count).
    - However, the hemoglobin in the cell is normal, so oxygen transportation is not interrupted.
    - The development of granulocytes is impaired, causing the production of abnormally large hypersegmented neutrophils.
      - Thrombocyte levels may be reduced.
    - A reduction in vitamin B_{12} can cause demyelination of the peripheral nerves and subsequently the spinal cord.
    - Reduction of the myelin sheath can interrupt nerve conduction, and damage may be permanent.
      - Sensory fibers are the first to be affected, followed by motor fibers.
- Etiology
  - Rarely owing to B_{12} deficiency in the diet because small amounts are required
    - Vegans and vegetarians are usually the only group vulnerable to vitamin B_{12} deficiency, owing to a lack of animal foods, therefore they must include other sources of vitamin B_{12} in their diet.
  - Issues with absorption of vitamin B_{12} are most often the cause, and can be a result of
    - Autoimmune reaction, particularly in the elderly
    - Chronic gastritis can lead to atrophy of the gastric mucosa, which is common in alcoholics.
    - Inflammatory processes such as regional ileitis
    - Gastrectomy can also be an underlying cause of deficiency owing to the removal of a portion of the stomach (loss of parietal cells) or resection of the ileum, area of absorption.
- Signs and symptoms
  - In addition to previous signs and symptoms discussed, the signs and symptoms characteristic of pernicious anemia are
    - Neurologic symptoms, such as paresthesia (burning or tingling sensation), in the extremities, decrease in coordination or muscle control (ataxia)
    - Expanded size of tongue, tender, red, and shiny
    - Low levels of gastric acid increases irritation in the digestive tract and is usually accompanied by diarrhea and nausea.
- Diagnostic tests
  - Diminished erythrocytes in peripheral blood appear megaloblastic or macrocytic and nucleated under a microscope.
  - Hyperactive bone marrow with an increase in megaloblast
    - Granulocyte numbers are lower and are hypersegmented.
  - Serum B_{12} level is below the normal range.
  - Shilling test is used to measure absorption by administering a dose of radioactive B_{12}.
  - Gastric atrophy is confirmed by the presence of hypochlorhydria or achlorhydria.

Aplastic Anemia

- Rare, but serious, aplastic anemia results from a syndrome where the bone marrow fails.
- Pathophysiology
  - Bone marrow dysfunction or failure that causes a loss of stem cells and accompanying pancytopenia (loss of erythrocytes, platelets, and leukocytes)
  - Bone marrow has a decrease in cell components and an increase in fatty tissue.
- Etiology
  - The source of the condition, aplastic anemia, determines if it is temporary or permanent.
    - Idiopathic cases or middle-aged individuals represent roughly half of the cases.
    - Myelotoxins (radiation, industrial chemicals (e.g., benzene) and drugs (e.g., chloramphenicol, gold salts, antineoplastic drugs) can injure the bone marrow.
      - Early identification and removal of the agent is important to allow the bone marrow time to heal.
      - Because individuals with cancer are at a greater risk, stem cells may be obtained prior to treatment and then transfused at a later date.
    - Hepatitis C or other viruses
    - Autoimmune diseases (systemic lupus erythematosus) can negatively impact bone marrow.
    - Genetic conditions can affect bone marrow function.
      - Myelodysplastic syndrome (MDS)
      - Fanconi anemia
- Signs and symptoms
  - Onset occurs unnoticed at first.
  - The whole bone marrow is affected and signs and symptoms can include
    - Anemia (and related symptoms, dyspnea, weakness, and pallor)
    - Leukopenia (recurrent or multiple infections)
    - Thrombocytopenia with hemorrhages of the skin (petechiae) and a tendency to bleed (especially orally)
- Diagnostic tests
  - Blood counts and bone marrow biopsy are used to determine pancytopenia (deficiency in RBC, WBC, and platelets).
  - Erythrocyte appearance is usually normal.

Hemolytic Anemia

- Disproportionate elimination of RBCs (or hemolysis), causes depressed total hemoglobin and erythrocyte counts.
  - Causes include
    - Genetic defects (affecting structure)
    - Immune reaction
    - Changes to blood chemistry
    - Presence of toxins in the bloodstream
    - Infections (malaria)
    - Transfusion reactions
    - Blood incompatibility in the neonate (erythroblastosis fetalis)

Sickle Cell Anemia

- Representative of a great number of similar hemoglobinopathies

- Pathophysiology
  - Inherited RBC disorder causes the production of abnormal hemoglobin, hemoglobin S (HbS).
    - One amino acid in the two beta-globin chain transforms from normal glutamic acid to valine.
    - Changed hemoglobin becomes deoxygenated, crystallizes, and changes to form a "sickle-" shape versus a disc-shaped RBC.
    - The cell membrane is injured, causing a shorter lifespan, approximately 20 versus 120 days.
    - Initially the sickling may be reversible, but over time the RBC damage is irreversible and results in hemolysis.
    - HbS is able to transport oxygen, but with a low RBC count the hemoglobin level in the blood is decreased.
    - Obstruction of small blood vessels can occur owing to the elongated and rigid RBCs, causing formation of thrombus and infarctions.
    - With repeated infarctions throughout the body, tissue necrosis occurs.
    - A sickling crisis can occur when an individual has a lung infection or dehydration that reduces oxygen levels.
    - Eventually larger vessels are involved, with multiple infarctions throughout the body, in areas such as organs, bones, and the brain.
    - Hemolysis results in basic anemia, hyperbilirubinemia, jaundice, and gallstones.
- Etiology
  - Hbs gene is recessive.
  - Common among descendants from African and the Middle East
  - In homozygotes normal hemoglobin is replaced by HbS, which results in sickle cell anemia.
    - Intensity of the anemia and the number of sickling crises varies among individuals.
  - In heterozygotes, only half of the hemoglobin is affected and only under certain conditions (pneumonia or high altitudes) will the individual develop symptoms; this is sickle cell trait.
  - Incidence: 1 in 12 African Americans carry the trait, and 1 in 500 have sickle cell anemia.
  - In Africa the number of individuals who are carriers is greater because there is a decrease in malaria with individuals with HbS.
- Signs and symptoms (Fig. 12.2)
  - Clinical signs appear usually at age 1 year, when fetal hemoglobin (HbF) is replaced with HbS. Ratio of HbS to erythrocytes indicates the potential severity of the disease.
  - Severe anemia: pallor, fatigue, dyspnea, and tachycardia
  - Hyperbilirubinemia results in jaundice (yellowing of skin and sclera of eyes). High bilirubin levels can concentrate the bile and may result in gallstones.
  - Splenomegaly or expansion of the spleen (most common in younger individuals owing to sickled cells)
  - Intense pain brought on from vascular occlusions and infarctions, resulting in painful crisis and permanent damage to organs and tissue. Damage can result in
    - Ulcers on lower extremities
    - Necrosis in the bones or kidneys
    - Seizures, strokes, or hemiplegia (from cerebral infarctions)
    - Intense pain
  - Lungs can experience occlusions and infections with associated pain and fever, often causing death.
  - Occlusion in the smaller vessels of the extremities can lead to hand-foot syndrome.

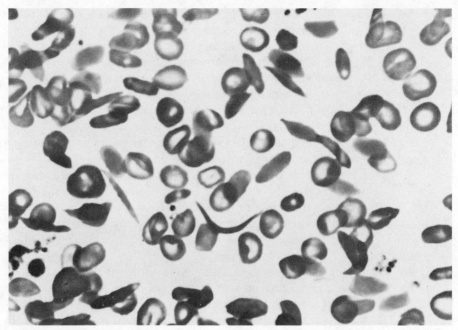

FIG. 12.2 The characteristics of sickle- or crescent-shaped red blood cells are shown in a peripheral smear. (From Price, S. A., & Wilson, L. M. [2012]. *Pathophysiology: Clinical concepts of disease processes* [6th ed.]. St. Louis: Mosby.)

- Delays in growth and development: puberty is delayed, tooth eruption is late, hypoplasia, and intellectual impairment can occur.
- Congestive heart failure owing to increased cardiac load to improve the supply of oxygen, and increased peripheral resistance caused by obstructions.
- Infection is common because of poor healing in underlying conditions, damage to the spleen (cannot filter the blood properly), and pneumonia in children, and is frequently a cause of death. Infections lead to more sickling and a perpetual cycle recurs.
- Diagnostic tests
  - Blood tests determine if individuals are carriers of the gene (hemoglobin electrophoresis).
  - Early identification of the sickle cell trait; individuals with sickle cell trait should avoid hypoxia and sickling episodes (e.g., high altitudes, anemia).
  - Genetic counseling
  - Prenatal diagnosis by reviewing DNA analysis in the fetal blood
  - Older children (over age 1 year); confirm diagnosis by the presence of HbS cells in peripheral blood.
    - Bone marrow is hyperplastic.
    - More reticulocytes (immature RBCs)

Thalassemia

- Anemia results from a genetic defect.
- Pathophysiology
  - Missing one or more genes for hemoglobin. Case is moderate to severe if two genes are involved.

- Interferes with globin chain production and results in a decrease in hemoglobin synthesized, and RBC numbers are lower
  - Hemoglobin is composed of four globin chains, and two alpha and two beta chains.
  - Thalassemia alpha is a reduction or absence of alpha chains.
  - Thalassemia beta is a reduction or absence of beta chains.
  - Results in less normal hemoglobin being produced
  - Even though some chains are missing, other chains accumulate and RBCs are damaged, for example
    - Missing beta chain: the extra alpha chains gather in the RBCs and damage the cell membrane, resulting in hemolysis and anemia.
    - Homozygotes have thalassemia major (Cooley anemia), a severe form of anemia.
    - Heterozygotes have thalassemia minor and exhibit mild signs of anemia.
    - With severe cases, the increase in the hemolysis of RBCs can intensify the anemia and result in splenomegaly, hepatomegaly, and hyperbilirubinemia.
    - Bone marrow is extremely active in an effort to compensate.
- Etiology
  - The most prevalent genetic disorder in the world is thalassemia.
  - Thalassemia beta occurs often in individuals from Mediterranean countries (Greece or Italy).
    - The most common form of thalassemia
  - Thalassemia beta occurs often in individuals from Indian, Chinese, or Southeast Asian descent.
  - If more than one gene is involved, a variety of gene mutations occurs with different effects on hemoglobin synthesis and the severity of anemia.
- Signs and symptoms
  - Usual signs and symptoms of anemia previously discussed
  - Lethargy and slowed development in children caused by hypoxia and possibly by fatigue and inactivity
  - With hyperactivity in the bone marrow, invasion of the bone, and impaired skeletal development
  - Heart failure occurs from compensation that increases the cardiac workload.
- Diagnostic tests
  - RBCs vary in size, are hypochromic (low hemoglobin) and microcytic.
  - An overload of iron can occur.
  - Fetal diagnosis can be done at 12 weeks with chorionic villus assay or at 16 weeks by amniocentesis.

BLOOD-CLOTTING DISORDERS

- Sudden or extensive bleeding after an injury may be indicative of a blood-clotting disorder.
- Other signs and symptoms may be owing to additional factors, such as injured or vulnerable blood vessels and infections.
  - Warning signs
    - Frequent bruising (ecchymosis) and purpura
    - Prolonged bleeding beyond what would be expected by the injury
    - Nosebleeds and periodontal bleeding (from gums or teeth)
    - Petechial rash (similar to a rash on skin that can come from capillary or tiny arteriole hemorrhage)
    - Blood entering a joint (hemarthroses); joint will be swollen, red, painful

- Hemoptysis or hematemesis, coughing or vomiting blood
- Blood in stool, frequently black or bright red
- Anemia
- Hypotension, tachycardia
- Feeling tense and weak
- Causes for excessive bleeding
  - Viral infection in children can cause thrombocytopenia that often resolves in 6 months.
  - Autoimmune reactions in adults, such as chronic idiopathic thrombocytopenic purpura; the chronic form usually has an impact on adults, especially young females, when thrombocytes are destroyed by antibodies.
    - Other causes of thrombocytopenia are human immunodeficiency virus infection, hepatomegaly, splenomegaly, and some medications.
  - Cancers (e.g., leukemia), chemotherapy, and radiation can also reduce platelet counts and result in excessive bleeding.
  - Abnormal platelet responses owing to chronic conditions, such as
    - Uremia with end-stage kidney disease
    - Aspirin therapy or drugs combined with aspirin
    - Nonsteroidal anti-inflammatory drugs should be avoided or used with caution because they interfere with platelet function.
  - Vitamin K may reduce prothrombin and fibrinogen levels.
    - Vitamin K is fat-soluble; it is present in certain foods and supplied by the intestinal bacteria.
    - Vitamin K deficiencies occur with liver disease (and associated decrease in bile secretion) and with malabsorption syndromes.
  - Patients with liver disease have less available vitamin K and select proteins; this has an impact on the production of clotting factors in the liver.
  - Genetic defects can cause bleeding disorders because of a lack of one or more clotting factors. Specific test and factor analysis can be a useful diagnostic tool.
    - Measure prothrombin time (PT) for extrinsic pathway
    - Measure activated partial thromboplastin time (APTT) for intrinsic pathway
    - Thrombin time for last stage (fibrinogen to fibrin)
  - Ebola virus is a hemorrhagic fever virus that can result in bleeding, acute illness, and can have multiple impacts on internal organs.
  - Anticoagulant drugs (e.g., warfarin) are a long-term medication and require close monitoring for excessive bleeding. Therapeutic and toxic drug levels are narrow, and bleeding can occur.
    - Other drugs, herbs, and foods can alter the effect of anticoagulant drugs and can create a serious situation.
- Patients with bleeding disorders are at a great risk of hemorrhage with any invasive procedure. Therefore, precautions should be taken prior to surgical interventions, such as
  - Pre-surgery laboratory test to validate current blood clotting status and the administration of appropriate prophylactic medications
  - Prepare for emergency response to manage excessive bleeding with the application of pressure; have absorbable hemostatic packing materials (absorbabal gelatin powder and styptics) and cold packs available.

Hemophilia A

- Hemophilia A is an X-linked recessive trait that is a common inherited clotting disorder.
- Pathophysiology
  - Lacking in, or abnormal, clotting factor VIII

- Type A results from an X-linked recessive trait (carried by females, but is manifested in males); 90% of hemophiliacs have this type of disorder.
  - A female who is a carrier or a male who is affected can produce a female child who inherits the gene (from both parents).
- Hemophilia B (Christmas disease) is a lack of factor IX.
- Hemophilia C (Rosenthal hemophilia) is a lack of factor XI.
- Even without a family history of a genetic mutation, hemophilia can occur and cause the disease.
- There are 18,000 to 20,000 known cases of hemophilia in the United States.
- Signs and symptoms
  - Extensive hemorrhage materializes after a minor tissue trauma.
  - Hematomas and prolonged oozing of blood occur after a minor trauma.
  - Spontaneous hemarthrosis (bleeding into joints) can lead to deformities as a result of chronic inflammation.
  - Hematuria (blood in urine or feces) as a result of kidney or digestive tract bleeding
- Diagnostic tests for hemophilia A
  - PT will be normal, but PTT and APTT will be prolonged.
  - Decreased blood levels of factor VIII
  - Thromboplastin generation time can help distinguish between lack, or deficits, of factors VIII and IX.

von Willebrand Disease

- Most prevalent genetic blood clotting or bleeding disorder
- Pathophysiology
  - Lack of the von Willebrand factor, which assists platelets in collecting and sticking to the internal lining of blood vessels in the area of injury
  - Three major types of this disease are similar to the signs and symptoms of hemophilia, but to a much lesser degree.
- Signs and symptoms
  - Rashes on the skin
  - Nosebleeds
  - Bruises on the skin
  - Gums bleeding
  - Abnormal menstrual bleeding
- Diagnostic tests
  - Can be difficult to diagnose owing to the vague symptoms
  - Laboratory tests for diagnosis include
    - Bleeding time
    - Blood typing
    - Factor VIII levels
    - Platelet count and aggregation
    - Ristocetin cofactor test
    - von Willebrand factor test

Disseminated Intravascular Coagulation

- Life-threatening condition resulting from excessive bleeding and clotting.
- Pathophysiology
  - Results as a complication owing to numerous primary issues that activate the clotting process throughout the body

- Clotting thought to be caused by the release of tissue thromboplastin or injury to the endothelial cells causing platelets to attach
- Results in multiple infarctions and thrombosis that expend all the clotting factors available and encourage the fibrinolytic process
- Eventually the exhaustion of fibrinolysis and clotting factors results in severe hemorrhage and ultimately shock.
- Chronic disseminated intravascular coagulation (DIC) is a milder form that can be difficult to identify because blood counts may be normal or abnormal.
  - Cause is usually chronic infections; thromboembolism is the prevalent symptom.
- Etiology
  - Examples of disorders that can cause DIC include
    - Amniotic fluid embolus
    - Trauma (burns or crushing injuries)
    - Carcinomas (produce substances that trigger coagulation)
    - Infections (especially gram-negative organisms that result in endotoxins that damage the epithelial and stimulate release of thromboplastin)
    - Abruption placentae (thromboplastin released from placenta)
    - Toxemia in pregnancy
- Signs and symptoms
  - Depending on the underlying cause, obstetric patients develop hemorrhages and cancer patients are likely to develop thrombosis.
  - With hemorrhage the following pattern is noted
    - Low plasma fibrinogen level
    - Thrombocytopenia
    - Prolonged bleeding time (PT, APTT, and thrombin time)
    - Lowered blood pressure; without intervention, ultimately shock
    - Bleeding from multiple sites, mucosal and hematuria
    - Vascular occlusions usually occur in small blood vessels, but can also occur in larger vessels and then cause infarcts in the brain and other organs.
  - Dyspnea and cyanosis
  - Neurologic impairments such as unresponsiveness and seizures
  - Acute renal failure often associated with shock

Thrombophilia

- Collection of inherited or acquired conditions that increases the risk of abnormal clotting in the arteries and veins.
- Can result in pulmonary embolism, deep vein thrombosis, or peripheral vascular disease
  - Inherited case occurs when the genes that regulate the production of coagulation proteins in the blood are mutated.
  - Acquired case occurs during an event (e.g., surgery, injury) that allows for an elevation of the amount of blood clotting factors or an accumulation of antibodies.
- Signs and symptoms
  - Abnormal clotting event can impact any organ to which a clot can travel and obstruct the blood supply.
  - If obstruction occurs in the heart or lung, a myocardial infarction or stroke can occur.
- Diagnosis
  - Blood test for clotting factors and antibody levels

Myelodysplastic Syndrome

- MDS is a classification of diseases that involve inadequate production of cells by the bone marrow.
  - Does not include aplastic anemia and deficiency dyscrasia
  - Can occur after chemotherapy or radiation therapy, or idiopathically
- Diagnosis
  - Patient history
  - Blood test to determine anemia (hemoglobin and hematocrit)
  - Bone marrow biopsy

NEOPLASTIC BLOOD DISORDERS

Polycythemia

- Primary polycythemia is an increased production of erythrocytes or other cells in the bone marrow.
- Serum erythropoietin levels are reduced.
- Secondary polycythemia (erythrocytosis) and an increase in RBCs as a result of hypoxia and accelerated erythropoietin secretion
- In secondary polycythemia the level of RBC is not as high and greater number of reticulocytes are noted in the blood.
- Polycythemia vera: a large increase in RBCs and granulocytes and thrombocytes, resulting in a larger blood volume and increased viscosity
- Etiology
  - Primary polycythemia: unknown origin that develops usually in adults aged 40 to 60 years.
  - Secondary polycythemia may be the body's way of responding to low oxygen levels owing to chronic lung or heart disease, or high altitudes.
- Signs and symptoms
  - Because of engorged blood vessels, patient will appear dusky red or bluish (skin and mucosa).
  - An enlarged liver and spleen
  - Pruritus (itching of skin)
  - Dyspnea, visual disturbances, and headaches
  - Thrombosis and infarctions may develop (systemic).
  - Congestive heart failure owing to increased cardiac load
  - High uric acid level and accompanying joint pain
- Diagnostic tests
  - Increased cell counts (hematocrit and hemoglobin)
  - Polycythemia vera; the erythrocyte is abnormal
  - Bone marrow is hypercellular.
  - Hyperuricemia owing to high cell destruction rate

Leukemia

- Neoplastic disorder involving the WBCs
  - Of the 31,000 new cases each year, approximately 2500 are children.
- Pathophysiology
  - Undifferentiated, immature, and nonfunctional cells

- Cells multiply uncontrollably in the bone marrow.
  - Large number released into the blood circulation
- Leukemic cells invade the lymph nodes, spleen, liver, and other organs.
- Acute leukemia has a large number of immature and nonfunctional (blast) cells.
  - Noted in the bone marrow and peripheral circulation
  - Abrupt onset
- Chronic leukemia has a large number of mature cells with reduced function.
  - Subtle onset
  - Mild signs and better prognosis
- Both acute and chronic leukemia can be subtyped according the cell involved.
  - Acute lymphocytic leukemia (ALL)
  - Chronic lymphocytic leukemia
  - Acute myelogenous leukemia (AML)
  - Chronic myelogenous leukemia
- Most cases of ALL involve precursor B lymphocytes
- Myelogenous leukemia effects can impact multiple granulocytes and can involve all blood cells.
- Major groups can be further subdivided
  - Primitive cells: the term "blast" is used in the name of the type of leukemia.
- The great number of leukemic cells in the bone marrow reduces the production of other cells and can cause
  - Anemia
  - Thrombocytopenia
  - Reduction in normal functional leukocytes
  - Hyperuricemia and associated kidney stones or kidney failure
  - Pain results from pressure on bones owing to the expansion of bone marrow.
    - With progression, the leukemic cell causes congestion and enlargement of lymph tissue, lymphadenopathy, splenomegaly, and hepatomegaly.
- Complications, such as hemorrhage or infection, result in death.
- Etiology
- Chronic leukemia is common in older adults.
- Acute leukemia is common in children and younger adults.
  - ALL is the most common childhood cancer (ages 2 to 5 years.)
  - AML is common in adults.
- Factors associated with leukemia in adults
  - Exposure to radiation
  - Chemicals (benzene)
  - Viruses
  - After chemotherapy (especially alkylating agents)
- Signs and symptoms
- Onset of acute leukemia is characterized by
  - Infection that does not respond to treatment
  - Multiple infections (nonfunctional WBCs)
  - Severe hemorrhage (brain or gastrointestinal tract) owing to thrombocytopenia
  - Signs of anemia (decreased RBCs)
  - Bone pain

- Weight loss, fatigue
- Fever
- Enlarged and painful lymph nodes, spleen, and liver
- If leukemic cells enter the central nervous system, early signs of headache, weakness, visual disturbance, and vomiting occur.
  - Chronic leukemia has milder onset and can be diagnosed with a routine blood test.
- Diagnostic test
  - Peripheral blood smears
    - Indicate immature leukocytes and damaged WBCs
    - High percentage of WBCs are immature and appear abnormal.
    - Number of RBCs and platelets is reduced
    - Confirmed diagnosis with bone marrow biopsy

APPLICATION AND REVIEW

9. A client has been diagnosed with acute leukemia. Which assessments would be performed by the nurse that are specific to this disorder? **Select all that apply.**
   1. Assess for enlarged lymph nodes
   2. Take and record oral temperature
   3. Monitor capillary blood glucose levels
   4. Assess client's need for pain medication
   5. Check oxygen saturation levels
10. A client, who has had a peripheral blood smear to assist in the diagnosis of leukemia, asks the nurse what results would point toward a positive diagnosis. Which responses by the nurse are appropriate? **Select all that apply.**
    1. "The number of red blood cells you have would be below normal."
    2. "It would confirm that your white blood cells are abnormally formed."
    3. "A positive bone marrow biopsy result would confirm diagnosis."
    4. "The leukocytes in your blood would be immature."
    5. "Your platelet count would be very high."
11. The nurse teaches a group of nursing students about leukemia. Which statement, if made by a nursing student, indicates that teaching was successful?
    1. "Chronic leukemia has milder signs and symptoms and a better prognosis than acute leukemia."
    2. "Leukemia causes a large number of abnormal cells to develop, which results in a blood disorder called thrombocytosis."
    3. "The onset of signs and symptoms of chronic leukemia will be abrupt. There will be a much more subtle onset of signs and symptoms with acute leukemia."
    4. "Leukemia is caused by an overproduction of well-differentiated, mature cells being produced in the bone marrow."
12. Which client is at greatest risk for developing lymphocytic leukemia?
    1. A 10-year-old client diagnosed with Down syndrome
    2. A 20-year-old client prescribed chemotherapy for a brain tumor
    3. A 30-year-old client prescribed radiation therapy for thyroid cancer
    4. A 40-year-old client who is human immunodeficiency virus positive

13. What response should the nurse provide when asked why a client diagnosed with leukemia has developed anemia?
    1. "The number of leukemic cells reduces the production of red blood cells by the bone marrow."
    2. "The bone marrow shrinks significantly because of the presence of leukemic cells."
    3. "The chemotherapy prescribed has produced abnormal red blood cells."
    4. "Radiation therapy often damages the bone marrow."

14. What characteristic is associated with primary polycythemia?
    1. The serum level of erythropoietin is reduced
    2. RBC production is triggered by hypoxia
    3. The level of reticulocytes in the blood is increased
    4. Blood viscosity is increased

15. Which client statement supports the presence of signs and symptoms associated with polycythemia? **Select all that apply.**
    1. "My liver has definitely gotten larger."
    2. "I seem to have more headaches than before."
    3. "I'm told I may have congestive heart failure."
    4. "I'm concerned about my skin being pale."
    5. "My hematocrit is up but my hemoglobin is down."

16. Which client has the greatest risk for developing disseminated intravascular coagulation?
    1. A client diagnosed with chronic renal failure
    2. A client experiencing idiopathic hypertension
    3. A client with third-degree burns over 10% of the body
    4. An older adult client recovering from hip replacement surgery

17. What characteristics suggest the client may be developing a blood-clotting disorder? **Select all that apply.**
    1. Petechial rash
    2. Nosebleeds
    3. Hemoptysis
    4. Dyspnea
    5. Fever

18. The nurse is caring for a 3-year-old child who has acute leukemia. What clinical manifestations of the disease should the nurse expect when assessing the child? **Select all that apply.**
    1. Weight loss
    2. Fatigue
    3. Fever
    4. Painful lymph nodes
    5. Purplish rash over trunk

See Answers on pages 263–265.

ANSWER KEY: REVIEW QUESTIONS

1. **Answers: 1, 2, 3, 4.**
   1, 2, 3, 4 Blood plays a critical role in the immune system by defending the body against infection, removing cell waste, and transporting oxygen to tissue with nutrients to aid in cellular metabolism.
   5 The kidney is responsible for balancing body fluids.
   Client Need: Physiological Adaptation; **Cognitive Level:** Understanding; **Integrated Process:** Teaching and Learning

2. **3 Very small vessels, known as capillaries, are categorized into copious networks that make up the microcirculation.**
   1, 2, 4 These vessels are too large to be found in the microcirculation.
   Client Need: Physiological Adaptation; **Cognitive Level:** Understanding; **Integrated Process:** Teaching and Learning

3. **4 Pulmonary circulation allows for oxygen and carbon dioxide in the lungs to be exchanged; heart failure would be associated with impaired pulmonary function.**

   1 Systemic circulation is involved throughout the body with nutrients and waste exchange between the blood and cells. **2** Kidney circulation is not associated with pulmonary circulation. **3** Systemic circulation, especially peripheral veins, is associated with deep vein thrombosis.

   Client Need: Physiological Adaptation; **Cognitive Level:** Applying; **Nursing Process:** Analysis

4. **2 Precapillary sphincters determine how much blood flows from the arterioles to the individual capillaries.**

   1 Venule system carries blood away from the capillary system. **3** Small branches of the arteries, arterioles, control the portion of blood that flows through capillaries to certain areas by the contraction of smooth muscle in the vessel walls. **4** Although the amount of blood in the circulatory system is a factor in blood flow, it is not the primary factor related to the capillary system blood flow.

   Client Need: Physiological Adaptation; **Cognitive Level:** Understanding; **Integrated Process:** Teaching and Learning

5. **4 During the cardiac cycle bigger arteries are highly elastic and adjust to blood volume changes that occur. Systolic pressure can rise too high if the aorta does not expand during systole, which increases the risk for aortic rupture.**

   1 Poor organ perfusion is a concern, but the primary concern is associated with the risk for rupture. **2** Diastolic pressure would be affected by ineffective adjustment to blood flow, but the risk for rupture is of primary importance. **3** Arteriosclerosis is not a risk related to the aorta's ineffective expansion and contraction.

   Client Need: Physiological Adaptation; **Cognitive Level:** Analysis; **Integrated Process:** Teaching and Learning

6. **2 Histamine, which triggers a release of chemical mediators, can then increase temperature at a specific area causing vasodilation.**

   1 Histamine is not responsible for the stimulation of muscle layers within the vessels. **3** Histamine is not responsible for the stimulation of the sympathetic nervous system. **4** Epinephrine and norepinephrine stimulate the alpha1-adrenergic receptors located in the walls of the arteriolar.

   Client Need: Physiological Adaptation; **Cognitive Level:** Understanding; **Integrated Process:** Teaching and Learning

7. **Answers: 1, 2, 3, 5.**

   1 Blood serves as the body's defense by transporting white blood cells to the site of infections. **2** Blood serves to support hemostasis by circulating clotting factors to sites of bleeding. **3** The blood maintains a stable pH of 7.35 to 7.45 because of the buffer systems in place. **5** Blood serves to regulate body temperature by distributing core heat throughout peripheral tissue.

   4 The lymph system drains interstitial fluids, which are then introduced into the blood.

   Client Need: Physiological Adaptation; **Cognitive Level:** Understanding; **Integrated Process:** Teaching and Learning

8. **Answers: 1, 2, 3, 5.**

   1, 2, 3, 5 A patient having a transfusion reaction can exhibit symptoms, including fever, facial flushing, chest pain, and headache.

   5 Hypotension is associated with a transfusion reaction.

   Client Need: Physiological Adaptation; **Cognitive Level:** Applying; **Nursing Process:** Assessment

9. **Answers: 1, 2, 4, 5.**

   1 The onset of acute leukemia is characterized by enlarged, painful lymph nodes. **2** The onset of acute leukemia is characterized by a fever. **4** The onset of acute leukemia is characterized by both bone and lymph node pain. **5** The onset of acute leukemia is characterized by signs of anemia, including low oxygenation saturation levels.

   3 Ineffective glucose utilization is not associated with acute leukemia.

   Client Need: Physiological Adaptation; **Cognitive Level:** Applying; **Nursing Process:** Planning

10. **Answers: 1, 2, 3, 4.**

    1 To contribute to a positive diagnosis, the smear would show a decrease in the number of RBCs. **2** To contribute to a positive diagnosis, the smear would show a high percentage of WBCs being immature and abnormally formed. **3** A diagnosis requires a suggestive smear and a bone marrow biopsy that also confirms the smear results. **4** To contribute to a positive diagnosis, the smear would show immature leukocytes.

5 To contribute to a positive diagnosis, the smear would show a low platelet count.
Client Need: Physiological Adaptation; **Cognitive Level:** Applying; **Integrated Process:** Teaching and Learning

11. **1 Chronic leukemia has milder signs and symptoms and a better prognosis than acute leukemias.**

    2 Leukemia results in thrombocytopenia, not thrombocytosis. **3** Onset of signs and symptoms of acute leukemia will be abrupt. **4** Onset of chronic leukemia signs and symptoms will be more subtle. Leukemia is caused by over-production of abnormal WBCs.
    Client Need: Physiological Adaptation; **Cognitive Level:** Applying; **Integrated Process:** Teaching and Learning

12. **1 ALL is associated with chromosomal abnormalities (e.g., Down syndrome).**

    2, 3, 4 AML is common in adults especially those exposed to radiation, chemotherapy and viruses.
    Client Need: Physiological Adaptation; **Cognitive Level:** Analysis; **Nursing Process:** Assessment/Analysis

13. **1 The great number of leukemic cells in the bone marrow reduces the production of other cells and can cause anemia.**

    2 Bone marrow expands rather than shrinks. **3** It is not the chemotherapy that causes the development of anemia. **4** It is not the radiation that causes the development of anemia.
    Client Need: Physiological Adaptation; **Cognitive Level:** Analysis; **Integrated Process:** Teaching and Learning

14. **1 Primary polycythemia is an increased production of erythrocytes or other cells in the bone marrow, resulting in a reduction of serum erythropoietin levels.**

    2 Secondary polycythemia is triggered by hypoxia. **3** In secondary polycythemia a greater number of reticulocytes are noted in the blood. **4** Polycythemia vera causes a large increase in RBCs, granulocytes, and thrombocytes, resulting in a larger blood volume and increased viscosity.
    Client Need: Physiological Adaptation; **Cognitive Level:** Understanding; **Integrated Process:** Teaching and Learning

15. Answers: 1, 2, 3.

    1, 2, 3 Signs and symptoms of polycythemia include an enlarged liver, headaches, and congestive heart failure.
    4 Skin would appear dusky red or bluish. **5** There would be increases in both hemoglobin and hematocrit.
    Client Need: Physiological Adaptation; **Cognitive Level:** Analysis; **Nursing Process:** Assessment

16. **3 DIC results as a complication of numerous primary issues that activate the clotting process throughout the body, such as burns.**

    1 Renal failure would not trigger the clotting process. **2** Hypertension would not trigger the clotting process. **4** Surgery would not likely trigger such a massive clotting process sufficient to cause DIC.
    Client Need: Physiological Adaptation; **Cognitive Level:** Analysis; **Nursing Process:** Analysis

17. Answers: 1, 2, 3.

    1, 2, 3 Usual or prolonged bleeding would be the common characteristic of a blood-clotting disorder. Petechial rashes, nosebleeds, and coughing up blood (hemoptysis) are all bleeding-related signs.
    4 Dyspnea, difficulty breathing, is not commonly associated with a blood-clotting disorder. **5** Fever is associated with an infection.
    Client Need: Physiological Adaptation; **Cognitive Level:** Analysis; **Nursing Process:** Analysis

18. Answers: 1, 2, 3, 4.

    1, 2, 3, 4 Onset of acute leukemia is characterized by weight loss, fatigue, fever, and painful lymph nodes.
    5 A purplish rash is not associated with acute leukemia.
    Client Need: Physiological Adaptation; **Cognitive Level:** Understanding; **Nursing Process:** Assessment

13 Lymphatic System Disorders

OVERVIEW (Fig. 13.1)

- Lymphatic vessels
  - Originate as microscopic capillaries
  - Capillaries come in contact with tissue cells and the interstitial fluid surrounding the cells.
  - Capillaries form branches, then trunks, and finally ducts.
  - Ducts empty into the left and right subclavian veins.
  - Lymphatic vessels have thinner walls and more valves than veins.
  - Thinner walls allow an increased degree of permeability.
  - Large molecules can be removed from the interstitial spaces.
  - Proteins that eventually accumulate in the interstitial fluids can only be returned to the blood system through the lymphatic vessels.
  - Afferent lymph vessels carry lymph into the lymph node.
  - Efferent lymph vessels take the fluid out of the lymph node and drain into lymph node chains that empty into lymph vessels, which finally drain into the subclavian veins.
  - Interrupted periodically by lymph nodes, at which point the lymph is filtered and more lymphocytes may enter the lymph
  - The vessels of the upper right quadrant of the body empty into the right lymphatic duct, which returns the lymph into the general circulation via the right subclavian vein.
  - The remainder of the lymphatic vessels drain into the thoracic duct in the upper abdomen and thoracic cavity. This duct drains into the left subclavian vein.
  - Lymphatic capillaries in the intestinal villi absorb and transport most lipids as chylomicrons.
  - Any condition that might affect normal return from lymphatic vessels to the blood vessels could have a dramatic effect on blood protein concentration and osmotic pressure with serious or fatal results.
- Lymph fluid
  - Seeps into lymph vessels across a very thin vessel wall
  - Lymph will travel through many nodes because there are many lymph node chains that drain a region of the body.
  - Clear fluid that resembles plasma that bathes body tissues
  - Full of white blood cells (WBCs)
    - Lymphocytes
    - Macrophages
  - Contains antigens
- Lymphoid tissue
  - Lymph nodes
    - Small oval-shaped structures located along a network of lymph channels
    - Most abundant in the head, neck, axillae, abdomen, pelvis, and groin
    - Help remove and destroy unwanted antigens
    - Each lymph node is enclosed in a capsule made of fibrous tissue.

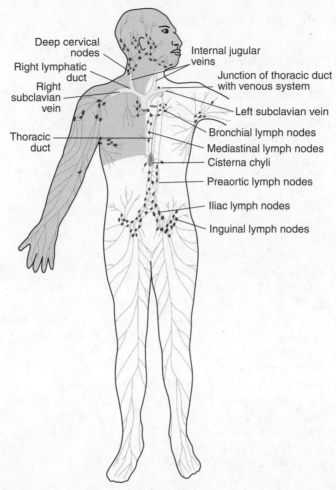

FIG. 13.1 Anatomy of the lymphatic system. (From Monahan, F. D., Sands, J. K., Neighbors, M., Marek, J. F., & Green-Nigro, C. J. [2007]. *Phipps' medical-surgical nursing: health and illness perspectives* [8th ed.]. Philadelphia: Saunders.)

- Node is divided in three parts.
  - Superficial cortex
    - Full of follicles made of B cells
  - Deep cortex
    - Intrafollicular areas that contain mostly T cells
    - Contains phagocytes that attack antigens in the lymph (cleans out the lymph)
  - Medulla
    - Full of plasma cells that secrete immunoglobulins
    - Phagocytic cells that attack antigens in the lymph (cleans out the lymph)
      - When infection is present, the regional lymph nodes are often swollen and tender.

APPLICATION AND REVIEW

1. What characteristic of a lymph vessel has the greatest impact on its ability to absorb fluid?
   1. The thickness of its exterior walls
   2. The number of valves each vessel contains
   3. The sensitivity of its inner filtering system
   4. The vessel drains into the subclavian veins
2. Which statement by a client demonstrates an understanding of the pathophysiology causing lymphatic fluid to accumulate in the abdomen?
   1. "My right lymphatic duct is obstructed."
   2. "The drainage into my left subclavian vein is abnormally large."
   3. "There is an abnormal amount of pressure on my right subclavian vein."
   4. "My thoracic duct is not allowing the lymphatic fluid to flow normally."
3. What would be the outcome of a dysfunction of an afferent lymph vessel node in the right axillary area?
   1. Swelling of the right arm
   2. A back-up of lymph fluid into the right subclavian vein
   3. Poor absorption of lymph fluid by the left subclavian vein
   4. Insufficient reabsorption of protein in the circulation of the right arm
4. What is normally found circulating in lymph fluid? **Select all that apply.**
   1. Antigens
   2. Macrophages
   3. Lymphocytes
   4. Erythrocytes
   5. Platelets
5. Where are T cells found in lymph nodes?
   1. The fibrous capsule
   2. Superficial cortex
   3. Deep cortex
   4. Medulla
6. At what point in the lymphatic system can additional lymphocytes enter the lymph fluid?
   1. At the lymph nodes
   2. Where ducts branch in trunks
   3. By the right or left subclavian veins
   4. Near the origin of the efferent lymph vessels
7. What processes are seriously affected when there is a dysfunction in the return of fluids in the lymphatic vessels and in the blood vessels? **Select all that apply.**
   1. Osmotic pressure
   2. Blood protein concentration
   3. Lymph capillary formation
   4. Diameter of lymph vessel
   5. Impaired lymph fluid production
8. What statement by the nurse demonstrates an understanding of lymph fluid? **Select all that apply.**
   1. "The fluid in the lymph system contains different forms of white blood cells (WBCs)."
   2. "Lymph fluid enters the lymph system by seeping through lymph filters."
   3. "Lymph fluid travels through many nodes before it is reabsorbed."
   4. "Lymph fluid drains different regions of the body."
   5. "Lymph is a cloudy liquid."
9. Where are lymph nodes most densely located? **Select all that apply.**
   1. Head
   2. Axillae
   3. Pelvis
   4. Groin
   5. Extremities

See Answers on pages 274–276.

- Spleen
  - Largest lymph organ
  - Located in the left upper quadrant of the abdomen
  - Size of a fist
  - Dark red, oval structure
  - Splenic pulp
  - White pulp
    - Contains compact masses of lymphocytes surrounding branches of the splenic artery
  - Red pulp
    - Consists of a network of blood-filled sinusoids supported by reticulated fibers and mononuclear phagocytes, lymphocytes, plasma cells, and monocytes
  - Functions of the spleen
    - Phagocytes
    - Break up old red blood cells (RBCs) and hemoglobin is released and then broken down into its components
    - Phagocytes retain and destroy damaged or abnormal RBCs and large amounts of abnormal hemoglobin.
    - Filters and removes bacteria and other foreign substances
    - Substances are promptly removed by splenic phagocytes.
    - Phagocytes interact with lymphocytes to start an immune response.
    - Reservoir for a large amount of blood in the pulp and venous sinuses
    - Can be quickly returned to the circulatory system if needed
    - If the spleen is damaged by trauma, there is chance for splenic rupture, which can be life threatening.
    - If the spleen is removed following trauma or disease, the liver and bone marrow assume its function.
- Thymus gland
  - Two-lobed mass of lymph tissue
  - Found at the base of the heart in the mediastinum
  - Helps form T lymphocytes (T cells)
  - Very active in infancy; after that has no function
  - Shrinks over time
  - Accessory lymphoid organs and tissues
    - Remove foreign debris the way lymph nodes do
    - Located in places where microbes have access to the body
    - Palatine and pharyngeal tonsils
    - When infection is present, the regional lymph nodes are often swollen and tender.
      - Adenoids
      - Appendix
      - Peyer patches (intestines)
  - The lymph nodes and lymphoid tissues act as a defense system, removing foreign or unwanted material.
  - Function of lymphatic system
    - Returns excess interstitial fluid and protein to the blood
    - Filters and destroys unwanted material from body fluids
    - Initiates an immune response

10. The nurse is teaching a group of nursing students about the structure and function of the spleen. What information should be included? **Select all that apply.**
    1. The spleen is normally the size of a human fist.
    2. The spleen is located in the right upper quadrant of the abdomen.
    3. The spleen is the largest organ associated with the lymph system.
    4. The spleen destroys abnormal erythrocytes.
    5. The spleen is a storage location for a large amount of blood.

11. The nurse is caring for a client after a splenectomy (removal of the spleen). What information should the nurse provide to the client?
    1. The role of the spleen will be assumed by the liver.
    2. Blood pressure will become chronically low.
    3. There will be fewer infections.
    4. Red blood cell (RBC) count decreases.

See Answers on pages 274–276.

LYMPHATIC SYSTEM DISORDERS

Lymphomas (Table 13.1)

- Malignant neoplasms with lymphocyte proliferation in the lymph nodes
- Specific causes of lymphomas have not been identified.
- A higher incidence in adults who received radiation treatments during childhood
- Hodgkin lymphoma
  - Epidemiology
    - Incidence has declined in recent years.
    - Onset of the disease occurs in adults 20 to 40 years of age.
    - Equal numbers in males and females.
    - A second peak occurrence is found in those more than 50 years of age, but primarily in males.
    - When caught at an early stage, the prognosis is excellent; many are considered cured with greater than 5-year survival rate.

TABLE 13.1 Clinical Differences in Hodgkin Disease and Non-Hodgkin Lymphoma

Characteristic	Hodgkin Disease	Non-Hodgkin Lymphoma
Pattern of spread	Contiguous spread	Noncontiguous spread
Extranodal disease	Uncommon	More common involvement of gastrointestinal tract, testes, bone marrow
Site of disease	Mediastinal involvement common Bone marrow involvement uncommon Liver involvement uncommon	Mediastinal involvement less common Bone marrow involvement common Liver involvement common
Extent of disease	Often localized	Rarely localized
B symptoms	Common	Uncommon

From Banasik, J. L., & Copstead, L. C. (2019). *Pathophysiology* (6th ed.). St. Louis: Elsevier.

- Pathophysiology
  - Starts in a single lymph node, frequently in the neck
  - The cancer spreads to adjacent nodes and then to organs via the lymph system.
  - T lymphocytes appear to be defective, and the lymphocyte count is decreased.
  - Reed-Sternberg cell in the lymph node is the atypical cell used as a marker for the diagnosis of Hodgkin lymphoma.
  - Extensive testing is required to stage lymphomas accurately.
  - Four subtypes of Hodgkin disease based on biopsy
  - Ann Arbor staging system
    - Stage I cancer affects a single lymph node or region.
    - Stage II affects two or more lymph node regions on the same side of the diaphragm or in a relatively localized area.
    - Stage III involves nodes on both sides of the diaphragm and the spleen.
    - Stage IV represents diffuse involvement outside the lymph system, such as bone, lung, or liver.
- Signs and symptoms
  - The first indicator is usually a lymph node, often cervical, which is large, painless, and nontender.
  - Later splenomegaly and enlarged lymph nodes at other locations may cause pressure effects.
  - Enlarged mediastinal nodes may compress the esophagus.
  - General signs of cancer
    - Weight loss
    - Anemia
    - Low-grade fever
    - Night sweats
    - Fatigue
    - Generalized pruritus is common.
    - Recurrent infection is common because the abnormal lymphocytes interfere with the immune response.
- Non-Hodgkin lymphoma
  - Non-Hodgkin lymphomas are increasing in incidence.
  - Partly owing to the numbers associated with human immunodeficiency virus (HIV) infection
    - In some ways non-Hodgkin lymphomas are similar to Hodgkin lymphoma.
    - 80% of the cases involve B lymphocytes.
    - Non-Hodgkin lymphoma is distinguished by multiple node involvement.
    - Nodes are scattered throughout the body in a nonorganized pattern.
    - Intestinal nodes and organs are frequently involved in the early stage.
      - Widespread metastases at diagnoses
      - The initial manifestation is an enlarged, painless lymph node.
      - The clinical signs, staging, and treatment are similar to Hodgkin lymphoma.
      - It is more difficult to treat when the tumors are not localized.
- Multiple myeloma
  - Onset is usually insidious and the malignancy well advanced before diagnosis.
  - Frequent infections may be the initial sign related to impaired production of antibodies.
  - Proliferation of plasma cells (terminally differentiated B cells)

- Malignant cells overproduce nonfunctional antibodies.
  - Results in immunodeficiency
  - Anemia
  - Abnormal bleeding
    - Elevated serum protein
    - Elevated urine protein
    - Can lead to kidney damage
    - Kidney function is affected because of tubule damage, leading to kidney failure.
    - Occurs most commonly in bones
    - Causes bony destruction
      - Leads to hypercalcemia
      - Bone pain (while at rest)
      - Spinal cord compression
      - Pathologic fractures
- Lymphedema
  - Lymph system absorbs a small amount of protein and interstitial fluid.
  - For lymphatic channels that are surgically removed or become blocked; the protein and fluids leak into the interstitial space, which is called lymph edema.
  - Lymph node tumors or inflammation that obstruct lymphatic flow will lead to lymphedema in the affected area
- Elephantiasis
  - Most common in tropical and subtropical areas
  - Mosquitos become infected with roundworm larvae → mosquitos bite humans → larvae survive in human blood stream and grow → larvae mature and live in the human lymph system for many years damaging the lymph system → causes areas of swelling.
  - Diagnosis is usually late when abnormal swelling is noted.
  - The swelling becomes bulky, lumpy, and eventually the skin becomes stiff and tough.
  - The swollen areas become painful.
  - This condition becomes disabling.
- Castleman disease (CD)
  - Rare disease
  - Estimated 6500 to 7000 new cases each year in the United States
  - Unicentric CD
    - Poorly understood; cause unknown
    - More common in women and younger individuals
    - Affects a single group of lymph nodes often in the chest or abdomen
    - Most common type
    - Signs and symptoms
      - Localized lymphadenopathy and associated compressive symptoms
    - May be asymptomatic
    - Can be cured if the lymph nodes can be removed
  - Multicentric CD (MCD)
    - Affects many lymph nodes
    - Becomes widespread and cannot be surgically removed
    - Signs and Symptoms
      - Flulike symptoms: night sweats that soak the sheets, fatigue, fever, and weight loss
      - Edema, anasarca, ascites, pleural effusion

- Eruptive cherry hemangiomatosis or violaceous papules
- Pneumatosis
- Two types
  - Human herpes virus (HHV)-8 associated MCD
    - Well understood
    - More common in men and individuals with human immunodeficiency virus (HIV)
    - HHV-8 is responsible for all the symptoms of the disease.
    - Signs and symptoms
      - Flu-like symptoms; fever, night sweats that soak the sheets, weight loss, loss of appetite, weakness, and fatigue
      - Shortness of breath
      - Nausea and vomiting
      - Numbness and weakness (neuropathy)
      - Leg edema
      - Skin rashes
      - Hemangioma
      - Pemphigus
      - Kaposi sarcoma
  - HHV-8 negative MCD (iMCD)
    - Poorly understood; cause unknown
    - Slightly more common in men
    - No known risk factors
    - Thought to involve immune dysregulation and a pathway of increased cytokines
    - Other proposed etiologies are autoimmune, autoinflammatory, neoplastic, and infectious mechanisms.
      - POEMS: polyneuropathy, organomegaly, endocrinopathy, monoclonal plasma disorder, and skin changes
        - A paraneoplastic syndrome
        - Caused by cytokine production from monoclonal plasma cells that have undergone mutations or deletions
      - TAFRO: thrombocytopenia, anasarca, myelofibrosis, renal dysfunction, and organomegaly
        - Etiology and pathology completely unknown
      - Not otherwise specified (NOS): thrombocytosis, hypergammaglobulinemia, and plasmacytic features
        - Etiology and pathology completely unknown

APPLICATION AND REVIEW

12. The nurse is caring for a client with multiple myeloma. Which clinical manifestation would the nurse expect the client to report as an early sign or symptom of this disease?
    1. Elevated serum protein from abnormal bleeding
    2. Body pain related to the effects of hypercalcemia
    3. Kidney failure resulting from malfunctioning tubules
    4. Frequent infections because antibody production is severely impaired

13. The nurse is caring for a young adult male with possible non-Hodgkin lymphoma. Which assessment finding would support the diagnosis?
   1. Presence of three enlarged, painless inguinal lymph nodes
   2. A history of two pathologic fractures of long bones
   3. Palpation of an enlarged spleen
   4. Reports of frequent night sweats

14. The nurse is caring for a client with non-Hodgkin lymphoma. Which finding would indicate a good prognosis?
   1. Localization of involved lymph nodes
   2. Initial node involvement noted in the cervical area
   3. The client has tolerated the prescribed drug therapy
   4. The client's treatment includes chemotherapy

15. Which statement by a client demonstrates an understanding of a diagnosis of stage II Hodgkin disease?
   1. "I'm told that my liver is affected."
   2. "I have one affected cervical lymph node."
   3. "Affected lymph nodes have been found on both sides of my diaphragm."
   4. "There are two affected lymph node regions, but all are in a localized area."

16. Which client has an increased risk for the development of lymphomas?
   1. A 17-year-old client who is pregnant
   2. A 72-year-old client who is diagnosed with kidney disease
   3. A 25-year-old client who has abused alcohol for 8 years
   4. A 30-year-old client who underwent radiation treatment as a child

17. What statement by a client undergoing treatment for Hodgkin lymphoma demonstrates an understanding of a basic component of the diagnostic process of this disease?
   1. "The biopsy showed Reed-Sternberg cells in my lymph nodes."
   2. "I'm female and over 50 years old, so my risk is increased."
   3. "Luckily, there is a definitive test to stage lymphomas."
   4. "My lymphocyte count is high and that's a bad sign."

18. Which assessment data support the possible presence of cancer? **Select all that apply**.
   1. An unexplained weight loss of 10 pounds over 6 weeks
   2. Reports of nightly sweats starting 3 months ago
   3. Laboratory results show an increase in the red blood cell count
   4. Low-grade fever for several weeks
   5. Decreased platelet count

See Answers on pages 274–276.

ANSWER KEY: REVIEW QUESTIONS

1. **1 Lymphatic vessels have thin walls that allow for an increased degree of permeability or flow of fluid or fluids from the interstitial space into the vessels.**
   2 The valves contribute to the vessels' ability to move lymphatic fluid along the vessel; they do not affect permeability. **3** The filters and the resulting filtration of the lymphatic fluid are not related to the vessel's permeability. **4** Whereas it is true that the lymphatic system drains the fluid into the subclavian veins, that process does not affect permeability.
   Client Need: Physiological Adaptation; **Cognitive Level:** Analysis; **Integrated Process:** Teaching and Learning

2. **4 The lymphatic vessels drain into the thoracic duct in the upper abdomen and thoracic cavity.**

   1 The vessels of the upper right quadrant of the body empty into the right lymphatic duct. **2** The thoracic duct drains into the left subclavian vein. **3** The vessels of the upper right quadrant of the body empty into the right lymphatic duct, which returns the lymph into the general circulation via the right subclavian vein.

   Client Need: Physiological Adaptation; **Cognitive Level:** Analysis; **Integrated Process:** Teaching and Learning

3. **1 Afferent lymph vessels carry lymph into the lymph node; a disruption of the flow at the node would result in edema prior to the node.**

   2 Flow into the right subclavian vein is a result of malfunction of efferent lymph vessels. **3** Flow into the left subclavian vein is a result of malfunction of efferent lymph vessels managing drainage for the abdomen and thoracic regions. **4** Protein is put back into the blood system by the efferent system of lymph vessels.

   Client Need: Physiological Adaptation; **Cognitive Level:** Analysis; **Integrated Process:** Teaching and Learning

4. **Answers: 1, 2, 3.**

   1, 2, 3 Lymphatic fluid contains white blood cells (lymphocytes and macrophages) and antigens.

   4 Erythrocytes (red blood cells) are not normally found in lymph fluid. **5** Platelets are not normally found in lymph fluid.

   Client Need: Physiological Adaptation; **Cognitive Level:** Understanding; **Integrated Process:** Teaching and Learning

5. **3 The node's deep cortex contains mostly T cells.**

   1 The capsule serves to provide the node with structure; it does not store T cells. **2** The node's superficial cortex is full of follicles made of B cells. **4** The node's medulla contain phagocytic cells.

   Client Need: Physiological Adaptation; **Cognitive Level:** Understanding; **Integrated Process:** Teaching and Learning

6. **1 Lymphatic vessels are interrupted periodically by lymph nodes, at which point the lymph is filtered and more lymphocytes may enter the lymph.**

   2 Lymphocytes may enter the lymph at the nodes not at a branching point. **3** Lymphocytes may enter the lymph at the nodes not at the right or left subclavian veins. **4** Lymphocytes may enter the lymph at the nodes not at the origin of the efferent lymph vessels.

   Client Need: Physiological Adaptation; **Cognitive Level:** Understanding; **Integrated Process:** Teaching and Learning

7. **Answers: 1, 2.**

   1, 2 Any condition that might affect normal return from lymphatic vessels to the blood vessels could have a dramatic effect on blood protein concentration and osmotic pressure with serious or fatal results.

   3 A change in fluid exchange between the lymphatic and blood systems is not directly associated with lymph capillary formation. **4** A change in fluid exchange between the lymphatic and blood systems is not directly associated with lymph vessel diameters. **5** A change in fluid exchange between the lymphatic and blood systems is not directly associated with lymph fluid production, but does affect fluid circulation.

   Client Need: Physiological Adaptation; **Cognitive Level:** Understanding; **Integrated Process:** Teaching and Learning

8. **Answers: 1, 3, 4.**

   1 Lymph fluid is full of WBCs (both lymphocytes and macrophages). **3** Lymph will travel through many nodes because of the many lymph node chains that drain a region of the body. **4** Lymph drains different regions of the body through a system of vessels and node chains.

   2 Lymph fluid seeps into lymph vessels across a very thin vessel wall. **5** Lymph is a clear fluid that resembles blood plasma.

   Client Need: Physiological Adaptation; **Cognitive Level:** Analysis; **Integrated Process:** Teaching and Learning

9. **Answer: 1, 2, 3, 4.**

   1, 2, 3, 4 Lymph nodes are most abundant in the head, neck, axillae, abdomen, pelvis, and groin.

   5 Extremities are not densely populated with lymph nodes.

   Client Need: Physiological Adaptation; **Cognitive Level:** Understanding; **Integrated Process:** Teaching and Learning

10. **Answer: 1, 3, 4, 5.**

    1 The spleen is normally the size of a fist. **3** The spleen is the largest lymph organ. **4** Phagocytes in the spleen retain and destroy damaged or abnormal RBCs (erythrocytes). **5** The spleen is a reservoir for a large amount of blood stored in the pulp and venous sinuses.

2 The spleen is located in the left upper quadrant of the abdomen.
Client Need: Physiological Adaptation; **Cognitive Level:** Understanding; **Integrated Process:** Teaching and Learning

11. **1 If the spleen is removed following trauma or disease, the liver and bone marrow assume its function.**
2 Although the spleen stores about 300 mL of blood, blood pressure will not be affected by its removal. **3** After a splenectomy, there is an increased risk for infections. **4** After a splenectomy, the RBC, WBC and platelet counts will dramatically increase.
Client Need: Physiological Adaptation; **Cognitive Level:** Understanding; **Integrated Process:** Teaching and Learning

12. **4 Frequent infections may be the initial sign related to the impaired production of antibodies.**
1 Although overproduction of nonfunctioning antibodies results in abnormal bleeding, bleeding is not the initial clinical manifestation of multiple myeloma. **2** Although overproduction of nonfunctioning antibodies results in abnormal bleeding, the resulting bone pain is not an initial sign of multiple myeloma. **3** Although overproduction of nonfunctioning antibodies results in abnormal bleeding that can cause damage to the kidney's tubules, kidney failure in not an initial sign of multiple myeloma.
Client Need: Physiological Adaptation; **Cognitive Level:** Evaluation; **Nursing Process:** Evaluation

13. **1 Non-Hodgkin lymphoma is distinguished by multiple node involvement.**
2 Multiple myeloma presents with pathologic fractures. **3** Non-Hodgkin lymphoma presents with splenomegaly in the later stages. **4** Night sweats are a general sign of cancer.
Client Need: Physiological Adaptation; **Cognitive Level:** Application; **Nursing Process:** Assessment

14. **1 Non-Hodgkin's lymphoma is more difficult to treat when the tumors are not localized; prognosis is improved when involved nodes are clustered together.**
2 The location of the initial node involvement is not directly related to prognosis. **3** Drug therapy is commonly prescribed. Although it remains the most successful combination regimen, it is not a factor associated with prognosis. **4** Chemotherapy would be suggested; the decision is not based on prognosis.
Client Need: Physiological Adaptation; **Cognitive Level:** Application; **Nursing Process:** Analysis

15. **4 Stage II affects two or more lymph node regions on the same side of the diaphragm or in a relatively localized area.**
1 Stage IV represents diffuse involvement outside the lymph system, such as bone, lung, or liver. **2** Stage I affects a single lymph node or region. **3** Stage III involves nodes on both sides of the diaphragm and the spleen.
Client Need: Physiological Adaptation; **Cognitive Level:** Evaluation; **Nursing Process:** Evaluating

16. **4 Adults who received radiation treatments during childhood have a higher incidence for the development of lymphomas.**
1 Regardless of age, pregnancy is not considered a risk factor for the development of lymphomas. **2** Kidney disease is not considered a risk factor for the development of lymphomas. **3** Although a known health risk, alcohol abuse is not considered a risk factor for the development of lymphomas.
Client Need: Physiological Adaptation; **Cognitive Level:** Analysis; **Nursing Process:** Analysis

17. **1 Reed-Sternberg cells in the lymph nodes is the atypical cell used as a marker for the diagnosis of Hodgkin lymphoma.**
2 Hodgkin lymphoma is diagnosed in equal numbers in males and females, but a second peak occurrence is found in those more than 50 years of age, but primarily in males. **3** Extensive testing is required to stage lymphomas accurately. **4** Hodgkin lymphoma causes a decreased lymphocyte count.
Client Need: Physiological Adaptation; **Cognitive Level:** Analysis; **Nursing Process:** Evaluation

18. **Answers: 1, 2, 4.**
1 An unexplained, rapid weight loss can be a general sign of cancer. **2** Night sweats can be a general sign of cancer. **4** A persistent low-grade fever can be a general sign of cancer.
3 Anemia with an associated decrease in RBCs can be a general sign of cancer. **5** Platelet count is not generally associated with general cancer signs.
Client Need: Physiological Adaptation; **Cognitive Level:** Understanding; **Integrated Process:** Teaching and Learning

Cardiovascular System Disorders 14

OVERVIEW

- The cardiovascular system is composed of the heart, blood vessels, and about 5 liters of blood circulating through the body.
- The heart is the intricate pump system of the body, pushing blood through the circulatory and pulmonary systems.
- The heart is made of two atria and two ventricles.
- A series of valves within the heart direct blood flow as the heart contracts.
- The heart contracts by activation of its own electrical impulse system.
- Increased age increases the risk for diseases associated with the heart.
- Hypertension is the most common cardiac disease.
- Physical fitness and body weight play a major role in health of the cardiovascular system.
- Certain heart conditions, such as such as severe heart failure and some genetic disorders, are so severe they require heart transplantation to correct.

Functions of the Cardiovascular System

- Branches of the cardiovascular system
  - Circulatory
    - The blood vessels, lymph system, and the heart make up the circulatory system.
    - Transports vital nutrients, oxygen, and cells through the body
    - Transports waste products to the kidney and lungs for removal from the body
    - Managed by the left side of the heart
    - Moves oxygenated blood to body tissues
  - Pulmonary circulation
    - Delivers blood to the lungs for oxygenation
    - Controlled by the right side of the heart
  - Blood vessels
    - Arteries and veins are the vessels of the cardiovascular system.
    - Arteries do not have valves.
    - Valves are present in veins.
    - Arteries have high pressure and carry blood away from the heart.
    - Arterioles are tiny arteries that lead to capillaries, which are microscopic vessels supplying blood to tissues by perfusion.
    - Arteries have smaller lumens and thick walls with a rounded appearance.
    - Veins have low pressure and conduct blood flow toward the heart.
    - Veins appear flat and have large lumens with thin walls.
    - Veins and arteries both have three layers
      - Tunica intima
        - Inner layer of the blood vessel
        - Consists of connective tissue layers and epithelial cells
      - Tunica media
        - Middle layer of the vessel
        - Thicker in arteries

- Tunica externa
  - Outer layer of the vessel
  - Composed of collagenous fibers and elastic fiber bands
  - Help to hold vessels in position

APPLICATION AND REVIEW

1. What is the function of the right side of the heart?
   1. Delivering unoxygenated blood to the lungs
   2. Delivering oxygenated blood to body organs
   3. Delivering oxygenated blood to the lungs
   4. Circulating blood around the body

See Answers on pages 296–298.

- Layers of the heart
  - Pericardium
    - Double-wall sac containing the heart
    - Made of two layers, the parietal and visceral pericardia
    - Normally contains about 20 mL of fluid lubricating the pericardial cavity
    - Protects the heart from infection
    - Stabilizes the structure of the heart when the body moves
    - Contains receptors that play a role in blood pressure and heart rate
  - Myocardium
    - Thickest layer of the heart
    - Consists of muscle
    - Attached to the heart's fibrous skeleton
  - Endocardium
    - Lining inside the heart chambers
    - Membrane from which valves of the heart are formed
  - Epicardium
    - Outer layer of heart
    - Allows the heart to relax and contract
    - Prevents friction with heart contractions
- Blood flow through the heart
  - With each heartbeat unoxygenated blood enters the right atrium through the superior and inferior venae cava and the coronary sinus.
  - Blood flows from the right atrium into the right ventricle through the open tricuspid valve.
  - As the right ventricle fills, 70% of flow is passive through the relaxed right atrium.
  - When the right atrium contracts, it completes ventricular filling by pushing in the last 30%.
  - The right ventricle contracts and the tricuspid valve closes preventing backflow of blood into the right atrium.
  - Increased pressure from contraction causes blood inside the ventricle to rise until the pulmonary semilunar valve is forced open.
  - Blood is pushed into the pulmonary trunk and toward the alveoli of the lungs, where oxygen is picked up and carbon dioxide is discarded for elimination by the lungs.
  - The pumping of the right ventricle forces oxygenated blood in the capillaries of the pulmonary circulation toward the left side of the heart within the pulmonary veins. These veins empty into the left atrium.

- From the left atrium, blood flows into the left ventricle through the open bicuspid valve. As on the right side of the heart, 70% of the blood flow into the left ventricle occurs while the left atrium is relaxed with atrial contraction pushing the remaining 30%.
  - The left ventricle contracts and the bicuspid valve closes, preventing backflow into the left atrium.
  - As the contraction continues, ventricular pressure rises until the aortic semilunar valve is forced open, and blood rushes into the systemic circuit.
  - After traveling to tissue capillaries, blood will return to the right atrium and begin a new cycle.
- Heart conduction pathway
  - The sinoatrial node (SA node), located in the upper wall of the right atrium, is the pacemaker of the heart. It generates nerve impulses that travel through the walls of the heart. These impulses cause the atria to contract.
  - The atrioventricular node (AV node) is located on the right side, near the bottom of the heart wall dividing the atria. Impulses received by the AV node from the SA node are delayed about one-tenth of a second to allow the atria to contract and empty blood into the ventricles prior to ventricular contraction.
  - The electric impulses then move to the atrioventricular bundle, which branch off into two bundles, and are carried down to the center of the heart and both ventricles.
  - The atrioventricular bundles divide further at the base of the heart into Purkinje fibers. When electrical impulses reach the Purkinje fibers, muscle fibers in the ventricles are triggered to contract.
  - The right ventricle sends blood through the pulmonary artery and to the lungs. The left ventricle supplies blood to the aorta.
- Electrical activity
  - Depolarization
    - Change in the charge of the heart cells from negative to positive initiated by the SA node
  - Repolarization
    - Increased positive charge in the heart cells causing potassium channels to open and the occurrence of heart contraction
- Evaluation of cardiovascular function
  - Assessment of risk factor for cardiovascular disease, such as family history, increased age, obesity, hypertension, and lung disease.
  - Chest x-ray
    - Examines size of heart and surrounding structures
  - Computed tomography (CT)
    - Used to visualize structures of the heart and surrounding area
    - Provides information about the presence and degree of calcification in heart valves and vessels
  - Electrocardiogram (ECG)
    - Evaluates the heat rate and rhythm in regard to the electrical conduction system of the heart
    - Provides baseline data about electrical function of the heart
    - Used to detect myocardial infarction and cardiac dysrhythmias
    - Holter monitoring is a wearable device that can detect changes in electrical conduction of the heart while an individual is performing normal day-to-day activities.
  - Echocardiography
    - Noninvasive procedure used to examine the structures of the heart

- Uses ultrasound technology to evaluate possible coronary artery disease, structural valve deficiencies, heart failure, and congenital heart anomalies. Can provide a measurement for ejection fraction, cardiac output, and valve functioning
- Stress testing
  - Induces cardiac stress by way of exercise or administration of medication to examine the heart in a state of activity rather than at rest
  - Used to diagnose heart disease and coronary artery disease
- Magnetic resonance imaging (MRI)
  - Uses magnetic resonant frequency to visualize the heart, myocardium, and great vessels
  - Can provide measurements of ejection fraction and ventricular function
- Technetium scanning
  - Injection of radioactive medication to visualize heart and coronary arteries
  - Used when there is debate about history of myocardial infarction, elevated cardiac enzymes with no clear cause, and ECG changes
- Cardiac catheterization with angiography
  - Invasive procedure using fluoroscopy to examine both sides of heart, chambers, valves, and vessels
  - Performed in a specially equipped surgical setting
  - Contrast dye injected into the heart chamber and cardiac cycles is visualized revealing any obstructions or abnormalities.
  - Risks include angina, coronary artery spasms, dysrhythmias, hypotension, and cardiac arrest.
- Cardiac enzyme evaluation
  - Blood tests to look at specific cardiac markers which may be elevated with heart muscle damage
- Cholesterol studies
  - Serum test to determine presence of coronary artery disease by looking at total cholesterol, low-density lipoprotein (LDL), high-density lipoprotein (HDL), and triglyceride levels
- Cardiac dysrhythmias
  - Abnormal heart rhythms from damage to the heart's conduction system
  - Can be caused by electrolyte imbalances
  - Stress, hypoxia, fever, drugs, and infection can affect the electrical activity of the heart.
  - Evaluated by ECG and/or Holter monitoring
  - Dysrhythmias interrupt the normal cardiac cycle and can impact cardiac output.
  - SA node dysrhythmias
    - Bradycardia
      - Heart rate less than 60 beats/min
      - Can be a normal finding in athletes
    - Tachycardia
      - Heart rate 100 beats/min or greater
      - Can be a normal finding with stress, exercise, fever, and infection
    - Sick sinus syndrome
      - Alternating patterns of high and low heart rates
      - May require treatment with cardiac pacemaker
  - Atrial node conduction dysrhythmias
    - Premature atrial contractions (PACs)
      - Ectopic, or extra beats, of the atria developing from excitable cells off the electrical conduction pathway of the heart

- May produce a feeling of heart palpitations
- Can be brought on by smoking, stress, and caffeine in the diet
  - Atrial fibrillation
    - Atrial heart rate of greater than 160 beats/min
    - Delayed conduction in the AV node
    - Causes pooling of blood in the atria, increasing the risk of thrombus formation
    - Pulse deficit may be present on assessment.
    - Can be asymptomatic
    - Anticoagulation medication administered to reduce risk of thrombus development
  - Atrial flutter
    - Atrial heart rate of 240 to 400 beats/min
- Atrioventricular node dysrhythmias
  - Heart block
    - Develops when conduction is stopped or delayed at the AV node or bundle of His.
    - Types
      - First degree
        - Prolonged time between atrial and ventricular contraction resulting in a prolonged PR interval on the ECG
      - Second degree
        - Longer delay in atrial and ventricular contraction than first-degree heart block, which results in a missed ventricular contraction by the heart
      - Third degree (total)
        - Absence of transmission of impulses from the atria to the ventricles
        - Ventricles contract at 30 to 45 beats/min, independent of the atrial contractions.
        - May cause fainting
        - Can lead to cardiac arrest
- Ventricular conduction abnormalities
  - Bundle branch block
    - Widened QRS complex on the ECG indicating a conduction problem in a bundle branch
  - Ventricular tachycardia
    - Increased rate of ventricular contraction
    - Reduces cardiac output
  - Ventricular fibrillation
    - Quivering contraction of ventricles preventing effective contraction and the ejection of blood from the heart
    - Rapidly leads to cardiac arrest
  - Premature ventricular contractions (PVCs)
    - Extra beats stemming from the ventricles
    - May be asymptomatic
    - Patterns of PVCs can develop into ventricular fibrillation and progress to cardiac arrest.
  - Cardiac asystole
    - All activity of the heart stops.
    - ECG reveals a flat line, indicating absence of all electrical conduction through the heart muscle.
    - Leads to death if not immediately corrected

- Requires immediate emergency treatment utilizing cardiopulmonary resuscitation and advanced cardiac life support
- Blood pressure
  - Measure of the amount of pressure against the arterial walls of the systemic circulatory structure
  - Dependent on cardiac output
  - Effected by peripheral resistance
  - Normal adult blood pressure should be around 120/70 mmHg when resting.
  - Measured using the brachial artery
  - Systolic pressure is the highest number; it measures the pressure by the blood ejecting from the left ventricle.
  - Diastolic pressure is the lower number; it indicates the amount of peripheral resistance and the workload of the left ventricle as the ventricles relax.
  - The difference between the systolic pressure and diastolic pressure is the pulse pressure. The pulse pressure represents the force the heart exerts with each contraction.
- Influences on blood pressure
  - Baroreceptors located in the aorta and carotid arteries sense changes in the blood pressure and activate the sympathetic nervous system (SNS) to respond.
  - Cardiac output
  - Heart rate
  - Pain
    - Patients with an increase in pain tend to have increased blood pressure.
  - Peripheral vascular resistance
    - Amount of friction or opposing blood flow in the vessel faced by blood as it progresses through the vascular system
    - Any obstruction in veins or arteries causes resistance and increases the blood pressure.
  - Sympathetic nervous system stimulation can cause widespread vasoconstriction or vasodilation. Vasoconstriction increases blood pressure. Vasodilation causes decreased blood pressure.
  - Stimulation of the parasympathetic nervous system causes bradycardia. Stimulation of the sympathetic nervous system causes tachycardia.
  - Arterial elasticity
  - Afterload
    - Stress in the left ventricle after ejection of blood from the heart
  - Preload
    - Amount of ventricular stretch at the end of diastole
  - Hormones
    - Antidiuretic hormone (ADH)
      - Also known as vasopressin
      - Increases blood volume by stimulating thirst and causing fluid reabsorption in the kidneys
    - Renin-angiotensin-aldosterone system (RAAS)
      - Major role in blood pressure regulation
      - Aldosterone, a product of RAAS, stimulates the kidney to reabsorb water, sodium, and chloride.
  - Lymphatic system
    - Consists of lymphatic vessels and lymph nodes
    - Three liters of fluid filter through the lymphatic system each day.

- Lymphatic vessels are contained in the same vasculature as the arteries and vessels of the cardiovascular and circulatory system.
- One-way valves control the flow of lymph through the one-way system toward the heart.
- Lymph is heavily filtered through the lymph nodes as it makes its way through the heart and body.
- Hypertension
  - Elevated blood pressure
  - Most common abnormality of the cardiac system
  - Three major categories:
    - Primary or essential hypertension
      - Idiopathic
      - New guidelines (ACC/AHA, 2017):
        - Normal: less than 120/80 mmHg
        - Elevated: systolic between 120 and 129 mmHg and diastolic less than 80 mmHg
        - Stage 1: systolic between 130 and 139 mmHg or diastolic between 80 and 89 mmHg
        - Stage 2: systolic at least 140 mmHg or diastolic at least 90 mmHg
        - Hypertensive crisis: systolic over 180 mmHg and/or diastolic over 120 mmHg
      - Increased arteriolar vasoconstriction leading to decreased blood flow to the kidneys
    - Secondary hypertension
      - Hypertension as the result of another disease process, such as kidney disease, sleep apnea, tumors of the adrenal gland
    - Malignant hypertension
      - Diastolic greater than 140 mmHg
      - Rapidly progresses
      - Causes many complications, such as encephalopathy, papilledema, cardiac failure, uremia, retinopathy, cerebrovascular accident
  - Increased blood pressure causes narrowing of the arterial walls and increases the risk of thrombi formation.
  - Increased blood pressure can cause damage to vital organs such as the eyes, kidneys, and brain.
  - Uncontrolled hypertension can lead to stroke, congestive heart failure, renal failure, and blindness.
  - Risk factors for developing hypertension include
    - Male gender
    - African-American race
    - Obesity
    - Increased age
    - Stress
    - High sodium diets
    - Alcohol consumption
  - Signs and symptoms of hypertension
    - May be asymptomatic
    - Morning headache
    - Fatigue
    - Elevated blood pressure
- Abnormalities of the heart
  - Congenital heart defects
    - Anatomic defects that develop within the first 8 weeks of embryonic life

- Includes defects in valve structure, septal defects, and anomalies in the shape, size, and position of great vessels
- Severity of defects can vary in degree.
- Most congenital heart anomalies seem to be a combination of environmental influence and genetics.
- Major cause of death in neonates
- Congenital heart defects may lead to developmental deficits.
- Signs and symptoms of congenital heart defects
    - Tachycardia
    - Tachypnea
    - Cyanosis
    - Pallor
    - Delayed growth and development
    - Development of clubbed fingers
    - Toddlers and children may frequently assume a squatting position to compensate for changes in blood flow.
- Ventricular septal defect
    - Most common type of congenital heart defect
    - Hole in the opening of the interventricular septum
    - Varies in size and exact location
    - Very small defects can increase the risk of developing infective endocarditis.
    - Large openings create a left-to-right shunt of blood, essentially reversing the normal flow of blood through the heart.
    - Pulmonary hypertension eventually forms owing to the high amount of oxygenated blood entering the pulmonary system.
    - Cyanosis is often present.
- Tetralogy of Fallot
    - Complicated defect with four abnormalities causing cyanosis at the time of birth
    - Pulmonary valve stenosis, ventricular septal defect (VSD), dextroposition of the aorta over the VSD, and right ventricular hypertrophy are the four disorders encompassed with tetralogy of Fallot.
- Rheumatic heart disease
    - Associated with an infection from rheumatic fever caused by group A beta-hemolytic streptococcus
    - Rheumatic fever is most likely to occur in children aged 5 to 15 years.
    - Rheumatic heart disease results when scar tissue from rheumatic fever occurs from the inflammation of the heart layers.
    - Signs and symptoms
        - Fever
        - Fatigue
        - Tachycardia
        - Leukocytosis
        - Nose bleed
        - Abdominal pain
        - Heart murmur
        - Possible heart dysrhythmias

- Pericarditis
  - Inflammation of the pericardium
  - May be an acute or chronic condition
  - Usually develops as a secondary disorder with viral infections, renal failure, cancer, lupus, or rheumatic fever
  - Sometimes develops after heart surgery or myocardial infarction
  - Inflammation can cause the development of a pericardial effusion, which can be life threatening with a compression effect on the heart impairing the heart's ability to expand and fill causing a decreased cardiac output.
    - Severely decreases cardiac output called cardiac tamponade
  - Signs and symptoms
    - Chest pain
    - Tachycardia
    - Dyspnea
    - Cough
    - Weakness
    - ECG changes
    - Friction rub on auscultation of the heart
    - Cardiac tamponade signs and symptoms may include neck vein distention, pulsus paradoxus, and distant heart sounds with auscultation.
- Infective endocarditis
  - Also known as bacterial endocarditis
  - People born with congenital valve defects are more susceptible to the development of endocarditis.
  - Those with a history of mitral valve prolapse, rheumatic fever, and artificial valve replacement are at an increased risk of developing infective endocarditis.
  - Intravenous drug users have an increased risk of developing acute infective endocarditis.
  - Bacteria attack the endocardium and form masses known as vegetations on the valve cusps. These vegetations are made of fibrin, platelets, microbes, and cells.
  - Vegetations impair the normal opening and closing of the valves.
  - Pieces of the vegetative masses may break away causing emboli, infarction, and the infection of other organs with the bacteria.
  - Types (2)
    - Subacute type
      - Develops when impaired heart valves are infected with bacteria such as *Streptococcus viridans*
    - Acute type
      - Normal heart valves become infected with highly virulent bacteria such as *Staphylococcus aureus.*
  - Some patients should be treated with an antibiotic prior to dental procedures and invasive procedures to decrease the risk of developing endocarditis.
  - Those at risk of developing endocarditis should have sources of infection treated immediately.
  - Signs and symptoms of infective endocarditis
    - New heart murmur
    - Painful nodes on the fingers

- ○ Abscesses on the body
- ○ Fever
- ○ Possible sudden onset of fever, chills, and drowsiness
- ○ Development of congestive heart failure
- ○ Enlarged spleen
- Myocarditis
    - Inflammation of the myocardium layer of the heart muscle usually caused by a viral infection, but can result from medication reactions
    - May be caused by bacteria, parasites, and fungi
    - Interferes with the electrical conduction system of the heart causing tachycardia and arrhythmias
    - Reduces the ability of the heart to pump blood
    - Untreated myocarditis can cause heart failure, heart attack, stroke, and sudden death.
    - Signs and symptoms
        - ○ General symptoms of a viral infection, such as fever, nausea, vomiting, sore throat, headache, or joint or muscle aches
        - ○ Chest pain
        - ○ Tachycardia
        - ○ Arrhythmias
        - ○ Shortness of breath
        - ○ Edema in lower extremities
- Valve disorders
    - Aortic valve stenosis
        - ○ Narrowing of the aortic valves caused by calcium build-up on the valve, rheumatic fever, or congenital abnormality
        - ○ Decreases the amount of blood that can adequately circulate through the heart
        - ○ Weakens the heart muscle
        - ○ Can range in severity from mild to severe and can progress to heart failure
        - ○ Signs and symptoms
            - ○ Vary according to level of severity
            - ○ Heart murmur
            - ○ Chest pain
            - ○ Dizziness
            - ○ Fainting
            - ○ Shortness of breath
            - ○ Heart palpitations
            - ○ Decreased appetite
            - ○ Weight loss
    - Heart valve regurgitation
        - Leaking heart valves cause backflow of blood through the valves during closure or leaking through the leaflets of the valves when they should be completely closed.
        - May develop suddenly or slowly over time
        - Types
            - ○ Mitral valve regurgitation
                - ○ Leakage of blood backward through mitral valve with each heart contraction
                - ○ Allows blood to flow in two directions
                - ○ Causes increased pressure in pulmonary veins
                - ○ Can result in fluid build-up in the lungs

- May experience heart palpitations, especially when lying on the left side
- Can cause enlarged heart and heart failure, depending on severity
- Aortic valve regurgitation
  - Develops from an infection or congenital heart defect
  - Allows blood to flow in two directions
  - Leads to thickened heart muscle and decreased ability of the heart to pump blood
- Pulmonary valve regurgitation
  - Rare
  - Leaky valve allows blood to flow back into the heart chamber before going to the lungs
  - Associated with long-term untreated hypertension and tetralogy of Fallot
  - Murmur may be detected in physical examinations
  - Patient may be asymptomatic
- Tricuspid valve regurgitation
  - Caused by enlarged lower chamber of the right side of the heart or valve problems exhausting the entire cardiac muscle system
  - May develop as a result of rheumatic fever or infective endocarditis
  - Blood flows backward through the tricuspid valve with each contraction of the right ventricle.
  - Eventually causes enlargement of the right atrium
  - Can be asymptomatic or produce pulsing neck veins, enlarged liver, fatigue, edema in the lower extremities
- Cardiomyopathy
  - Abnormal muscle of the heart
  - The exact cause of cardiomyopathy is unknown, but genetics, hypertension, tissue damage from a myocardial infarction, and metabolic disorders are thought to contribute to the development of the condition.
  - Can lead to the development of blood clots, valve problems, heart failure, and cardiac arrest
  - Types
    - Dilated
      - Most common type
      - Left ventricle is less forceful.
      - Enlargement of left ventricle
      - Most often found in middle-aged males
      - Associated with heart disease, infection, drug and alcohol use, or chemotherapy
    - Hypertrophic
      - Abnormal thickening of the heart muscle
      - Usually impacts the left ventricle
      - Linked to genetic mutations
    - Restrictive
      - Least common type
      - Idiopathic
      - Heart muscle becomes rigid and loses elasticity, which decreases the heart's ability to expand and fill with blood.
    - Arrhythmogenic right ventricular dysplasia
      - Rare
      - Right ventricle is replaced by scar tissue causing dysrhythmias.
      - Linked to genetic mutations

- Angina
  - Type of chest pain caused by an oxygen deficit to the muscles of the heart
  - May occur when the heart is working harder than normal or when blood flow or oxygen levels to the muscle of the heart fall below normal.
    - Atherosclerosis may be a factor in angina.
  - Can be caused by a spasm of the coronary arteries
  - No damage occurs to the heart muscle with angina unless the episodes are frequent, prolonged, or especially severe.
  - Usually relieved quickly with rest and administration of nitroglycerin
  - Classic or exertional angina is when vasospasms are induced by stress, exercise, and/or eating large meals. Exposure to extreme temperatures may also be a precipitant for classic angina symptoms.
  - Variant angina is diagnosed when vasospasm causing chest pain occurs at rest. Unstable angina is a more serious form and may be the result of thrombi. This may forewarn of an impending myocardial infarction. Patients usually complain of prolonged pain when resting with a recent onset of the development of chest pain.
  - Signs and symptoms of angina
    - Substernal chest pain triggered by physical or emotional stress
    - Pain described as tightness or pressure that may radiate to neck and left arm
    - Pallor
    - Nausea
    - Diaphoresis
    - Episodes are usually sporadic and may last from seconds to minutes.
- Arteriosclerosis
  - Used to describe a variety of arterial changes
  - Thickening and hardening of the arterial walls with loss of elasticity of arterioles and arteries
  - Narrowing of the arterial walls causes ischemia and tissue death in brain, heart, and kidneys.
  - Most commonly occurs in individuals over the age of 50
  - Can be related to diabetes
- Atherosclerosis
  - Presence of plaques in the arteries known as atheromas
  - Atheromas are made of lipids, living and dead cells, and fibrous particles, which often form thrombi and attach to walls of arteries.
  - Atheromas may block openings from main arteries to branching arteries.
  - Areas of bifurcation in the arteries, such as the coronaries, carotids, iliac, and the aorta, are more likely to develop atheromas.
  - Factors that increase the risk of atherosclerosis are classified as modifiable and nonmodifiable.
    - Factors
      - Obesity
      - Diet high in fat
      - Elevated cholesterol level
      - Cigarette smoking
      - Sedentary lifestyle

- ○ Diabetes
- ○ Uncontrolled hypertension
- ○ Use of oral contraceptives in conjunction with smoking cigarettes
- ▪ Nonmodifiable factors
  - ○ Age greater than 40 years
  - ○ Male gender
  - ○ Genetic factors
- ▪ Diagnostic testing for atherosclerosis includes monitoring serum cholesterol levels, cardiac stress test, and nuclear studies.
- • Myocardial Infarction (MI)
  - ▪ Death of myocardial tissue owing to lack of blood flow
  - ▪ Also known as a heart attack
  - ▪ Occurs when a coronary artery is completely obstructed, resulting in cell death of a portion of the wall of the heart
  - ▪ Cell death in the myocardium results in specific cardiac enzymes being released into the vascular system. These cardiac enzymes are used as part of the diagnostics for MI.
  - ▪ Most commonly caused by thrombi from atherosclerosis
  - ▪ MI can result in sudden death, congestive heart failure, and cardiogenic shock.
  - ▪ Necrotic heart tissue has the potential to rupture 3 to 7 days after the MI.
  - ▪ Thromboembolism, a possible complication from an MI, can travel to vital organs, resulting in severe damage and/or death.
  - ▪ Warning signs of an impending heart attack include
    - ▪ Feelings of anxiety, fear, and/or impending doom
    - ▪ Fatigue
    - ▪ Nausea
    - ▪ Diaphoresis
    - ▪ Sudden onset of shortness of breath
    - ▪ Chest pressure or burning, more notable with activity
  - ▪ Signs and symptoms of an MI
    - ▪ Sudden and severe chest pain radiating to neck, jaw, and/or left arm
    - ▪ Pain unrelieved by rest or nitroglycerin
    - ▪ Females may have milder symptoms and complain more of a sensation of indigestion as opposed to crushing chest pain.
    - ▪ Diaphoresis
    - ▪ Dizziness
    - ▪ Weakness
    - ▪ Shortness of breath
    - ▪ Low-grade temperature
    - ▪ Nausea
    - ▪ Anxiety, fear
    - ▪ Rapid and weak pulse
    - ▪ Decreased blood pressure
  - ▪ Diagnostic tests to determine presence of myocardial infarction
    - ▪ ECG changes
    - ▪ Elevation of lactate dehydrogenase (LDH)-1

- -1 and creatine kinase MB (CK-MB)
- Elevated troponin level, which is considered a most significant indicator of myocardial damage
- Possible alteration in serum potassium and sodium levels
- Elevated erythrocyte sedimentation rate
- Leukocytosis
- Elevated C-reactive protein (CRP) indicating an inflammatory response
- Changes in arterial blood gases
- Ventricular function changes may be evident with pulmonary artery pressure monitoring.
- Prognosis is dependent on the severity of the heart attack, location of the injury, and the time between the onset of symptoms and the start of treatment.
- Heart Failure
  - Heart failure occurs when the heart is unable to pump blood to meet the demands of the vital organs and tissues of the body.
  - Chronic illness
  - Usually appears as a comorbid complication from another disease process
  - May be the result of a valve abnormality or an MI
  - Could develop in conjunction with long-term hypertension and lung disease
  - Often classified as left-sided or right-sided heart failure depending on the cause
  - Pulmonary valve stenosis or lung disease initially has an impact on the right ventricle of the heart, resulting in right-sided heart failure.
  - MIs and hypertension often have an impact on the left ventricle of the heart, resulting in left-sided heart failure.
  - Signs and symptoms of heart failure
    - Fatigue
    - Dizziness
    - Generalized weakness
    - Shortness of breath, more noted with activity
    - Intolerance to cold weather
    - Difficulty with exercise
    - Hypoxia
    - Tachycardia
  - Left-sided heart failure signs and symptoms (Fig. 14.1)
    - Orthopnea
    - Chronic cough
    - Possible hemoptysis
    - Crackles auscultated in the lungs
    - Paroxysmal nocturnal dyspnea
    - Secondary pneumonia
  - Right-sided heart failure symptoms (Fig. 14.2)
    - Distended neck veins
    - Visual disturbances
    - Headache
    - Ascites
    - Hepatomegaly
    - Splenomegaly
    - Dependent edema

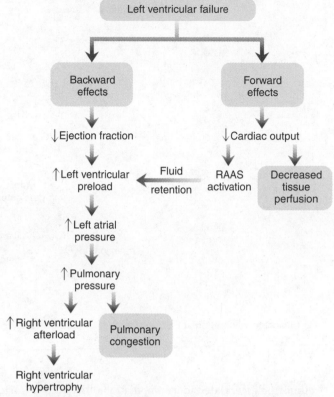

FIG. 14.1 Clinical manifestations of isolated left-sided heart failure. (From Banasik, J. L., & Copstead, L. C. [2019]. *Pathophysiology* [6th ed.]. St. Louis: Elsevier.)

- Aortic aneurysms
  - Dilation and weakening of the arterial wall
  - Develops owing to turbulent blood flow at the site caused by hypertension, atherosclerosis, thrombi, or trauma
  - Syphilis has also been identified as a causative factor of aneurysms.
  - Usually occur in the thoracic aorta or the abdominal aorta
  - The aneurysm may be in the form of a sac or a fusiform.
  - Dissecting aneurysms are a tear in the wall allowing blood to pulse between arterial wall layers.
  - Signs and symptoms of aneurysm
    - May be asymptomatic for long periods of time
    - Detected as a pulsating mass
    - Bruit heard over the site of the aneurysm with auscultation
    - Can cause dysphagia or pain, depending on location of aneurysm
    - Many aneurysms rupture causing severe hemorrhage, shock, and death.
- Dyslipidemia
  - Abnormal serum levels of lipoproteins, including lipids, phospholipids, cholesterol, and triglycerides
  - Dyslipidemia affects half of the population in the United States.

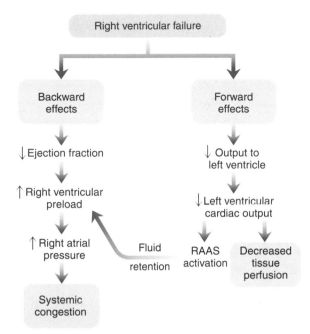

FIG. 14.2 Clinical manifestations of isolated right-sided heart failure. (From Banasik, J.L., & Copstead, L.C. [2019]. *Pathophysiology* [6th ed.]. St. Louis: Elsevier.)

- ▪ Abnormalities related to a combination of nutritional factors and genetics
- ▪ Conditions such as diabetes and renal disorders contribute to dyslipidemia.
- ▪ Medications such as diuretics, antihypertensives, and steroids can cause dyslipidemia.
- ▪ Increased levels of low-density lipoproteins in the blood indicate a risk of coronary artery disease.
- ▪ Low levels of high-density lipoproteins are an indicator of coronary artery disease. HDLs transport cholesterol for removal from the body.
- ▪ Increased serum very low-density lipoproteins (VLDL) triglyceride levels and increased lipoprotein are indicators of cardiac disease.
- • Peripheral vascular disease
  - ▪ Abnormalities of veins and arteries of the circulatory system outside the heart
  - ▪ Evaluated using Doppler studies and arteriogram
  - ▪ Signs and symptoms
    - ▪ Burning, tingling pain in legs and feet
    - ▪ Numbness of extremities
    - ▪ Weak or absent peripheral pulses
    - ▪ Fatigue
    - ▪ Weakness in legs
    - ▪ Intermittent claudication
      - ○ Leg pain with exercise
    - ▪ Legs may be pale and cyanotic with elevation and then red when standing, sitting, or dangling.
    - ▪ Absence of hair on legs
    - ▪ Thick, hard toenails

- Skin of affected area cold to touch
- May have ulcers, wounds, and gangrene from lack of blood supply
- Raynaud disease
  - Rare disorder of the blood vessels with unknown cause
  - Seen more often in colder climates
  - More common in females
  - Usually in the fingers and toes
  - Causes the blood vessels to constrict with cold temperatures or feelings of stress
  - With constriction, affected areas turn white and blue.
  - When the blood flow returns, the skin turns red and throbs or tingles.
  - In severe cases, loss of blood flow can cause sores or tissue death.
- Thrombophlebitis
  - Vein inflammation that leads to thrombus formation
  - Can lead to pulmonary embolism
  - Caused by stasis of blood flow from immobility, tight clothing, or any means of restricting blood flow
  - Can be caused by endothelial cell injury in cases of inflammatory response, trauma, intravenous injection, or chemical exposure
  - Increased blood coagulation from dehydration, pregnancy, or platelet disorders may increase the risk of developing thrombophlebitis.
  - Signs and symptoms of thrombophlebitis
    - Warmness and redness in the leg at the site of the inflamed vein
    - Aching and burning pain in the leg
    - May have edema distal to the site of the thrombus
    - Fever
    - Leukocytosis
- Varicose veins
  - Irregularly dilated superficial or deep veins
  - Most commonly found in lower extremities
  - Can develop in the esophagus (esophageal varices) and rectum (hemorrhoids)
  - Often develop from long periods of standing where pressure is exerted on already weakened vein walls
  - Pregnancy, genetics, and trauma to the veins make the development of varicosities more likely to occur.
  - The damaged wall prevents normal backflow of the blood, causing further vein wall dilation, aching pain, and possible thrombi formation.
  - Signs and symptoms of varicose veins
    - Irregular, purplish bulging veins on the extremities
    - Edema of the affected foot and leg
    - Fatigue
    - Aching sensation in affected leg and foot
    - Shiny, hairless skin on the lower legs
    - Possible venous ulcers on lower legs
- Lymphedema
  - Caused by removal of lymph nodes or damage to the node
  - Edema forms in arms and/or legs
  - Untreated can lead to cellulitis and inflammation of the lymph vessels
  - Classified as primary or secondary

- Often a result of radiation treatment for cancer, blockage of a lymph node or vessel from a tumor, infection, or surgery
- Inflammation of the lymph node or lymphatic pathway prevents lymph from draining causing a build-up of fluid.
- No cure
  - Preventative measures include rest and elevation of affected arms and legs, avoiding heat, hygiene measures, and protecting the affected extremity from injury.
- Shock
  - Extremely low blood pressure resulting from decreased circulating blood volume
  - Less cardiac output leads to reduced oxygen and nutrients for the cells. This causes anaerobic cell metabolism and, an increase in lactic acid in the body, and the development of acidosis.
  - Classified based on cause
    - Hypovolemic
      - Caused by significant loss of circulating blood in the body
    - Cardiogenic
      - The heart is unable to pump blood through the circulatory system. Often seen with MI or cardiac dysrhythmias.
    - Obstructive
      - Interference with blood flow through the cardiac system by a pulmonary embolism or cardiac tamponade
    - Distributive or vasogenic shock
      - Caused by pooling of blood in the periphery
    - Neurogenic
      - Develops owing to drugs, spinal cord injury, severe pain, and fear
    - Septic
      - Develops with severe infections, usually from gram-negative bacteria
      - Signs and symptoms include tachycardia, increased respiratory rate, signs of infection, fever, and flushed skin.
      - Antimicrobials are administered along with glucocorticoids to treat infection and inflammation.
    - Anaphylactic
      - Occurs with severe allergic reactions when rapid vasodilation releases large amounts of histamine
      - Antihistamines and corticosteroids are administered to treat anaphylaxis.
  - Stages of shock
    - Compensatory
      - Early signs of shock may be agitation, restlessness, and extreme thirst.
      - Oliguria, tachycardia, and skin changes to cool, moist, and pale develop as compensation to hypotension.
    - Progressive
      - Signs and symptoms of progressive shock are increased weakness, dizziness, lethargy, weak pulse, respiratory alkalosis, and hypoxemia.
      - Progresses to metabolic acidosis
    - Irreversible
      - Body's response system weakens and is unable to compensate metabolic acidosis, leading to widespread cellular death and multisystem failure

APPLICATION AND REVIEW

2. What assessment data suggest a client who experienced abdominal trauma should be closely monitored for possible hypovolemic shock?
   1. Client confused to both time and place
   2. Blood pressure 92/46 mm Hg
   3. Oral temperature 101.8° F (38.7° C)
   4. Reports of nausea and vomiting

3. The nurse is caring for a client suspected of experiencing anaphylactic shock. Which question should the nurse ask the client?
   1. "Have you had any chest pain recently?"
   2. "Are you allergic to anything?"
   3. "Do you have a history of pulmonary emboli?"
   4. "Have you had an infection with a fever recently?"

4. Which client is at greatest risk for developing neurogenic shock?
   1. A 53-year-old male client who is obese
   2. A 26-year-old female client who is a paraplegic
   3. A 12-year-old female client with second-degree burns
   4. A 60-year-old male client with a known allergy to bee stings

5. What is the most serious complication associated with varicose veins of the lower extremities?
   1. Calf and foot edema
   2. Absence of hair on affected lower leg
   3. An area on the calf that is warm to the touch
   4. Presence of a small venous ulcer on the affected foot

6. Which sites are characteristic locations for the development of varicose veins? **Select all that apply.**
   1. Esophagus
   2. Lower legs
   3. Upper arms
   4. Rectum
   5. Scalp

7. Which sign or symptom is associated with the most serious complication of thrombophlebitis?
   1. Leukocytosis
   2. Acute dyspnea
   3. A positive Homan sign
   4. Aching and burning sensations

8. Which finding would indicate to the nurse that a client has developed a varicose vein in the left lower extremity?
   1. Bilateral edema of the lower extremities
   2. Bulging, purple vein on affected leg
   3. Oral temperature is 100.2° F (37.8 ° C)
   4. Affected leg turns white then blue when exposed to a cold environment

9. Which client is at greatest risk for developing thrombophlebitis?
   1. A client who is 20 weeks pregnant
   2. An older adult client who has congestive heart disease (CHF)
   3. A middle-aged adult client who is a sales clerk at a grocery store
   4. A young adult client who is in the manic phase of bipolar disorder

10. Which clients would be at increased risk for developing Raynaud disease? **Select all that apply.**
    1. Client who is a female
    2. Client who is over 60 years of age
    3. Client who is a retired waitress
    4. Client who has a history of asthma
    5. Client who lives in southern Maine

11. The nurse is teaching a client about Raynaud disease. Which statement, if made by the client, indicates that teaching was successful?
    1. "The first color change that occurs is blue."
    2. "The cause of this disease is genetic."
    3. "This disease is more prevalent in warmer climates."
    4. "Attacks can be caused by emotional stress."

12. The nurse is caring for a client who has a possible diagnosis of peripheral vascular disease. Which diagnostic procedures would the nurse expect to be done? **Select all that apply.**
    1. X-rays
    2. Arteriogram
    3. Doppler studies
    4. Complete blood count (CBC)
    5. Magnetic resonance imaging (MRI)

13. What assessments should the nurse perform when collecting data on a client who has a possible diagnosis of peripheral vascular disease (PVD)? **Select all that apply.**
    1. Check the condition of toenails.
    2. Evaluate the legs for excess hair growth.
    3. Observe skin color with legs in a dependent position.
    4. Assess for numbness in the legs and feet.
    5. Ask about the presence of leg pain when walking

14. What is the most serious complication of peripheral vascular disease (PVD) resulting from impaired blood supply?
    1. Intermittent claudication
    2. Venous ulcers
    3. Gangrene
    4. Leg pain

15. What information collected during a nursing interview supports the diagnosis of an aortic aneurysm?
    1. Treated for syphilis 5 years ago
    2. Being medicated for hypotension
    3. Unable to auscultate bruit over aorta
    4. No family history of aortic aneurysms

16. What assessment data support the diagnosis of right-sided heart failure? **Select all that apply.**
    1. Ascites
    2. Orthopnea
    3. Hepatomegaly
    4. Dependent edema
    5. Distended neck veins

See Answers on pages 296–298.

ANSWER KEY: REVIEW QUESTIONS

1. **1 Pulmonary circulation, which delivers blood to the lungs for oxygenation, is controlled by the right side of the heart.**

   2 The delivery of oxygenated blood around the body is managed by the left side of the heart. **3** Oxygenated blood is not delivered to the lungs, but rather transported away from the lungs. **4** The circulating of oxygenated blood around the body is managed by the left side of the heart.

   Client Need: Physiological Adaptation; **Cognitive Level:** Understanding; **Integrated Process:** Teaching and Learning

2. **2 Hypovolemic shock is a result of significant blood loss—either internally or externally. A low blood pressure could be a sign of low blood volume.**

    1 Although a client's level of confusion should be monitored, it is not a definitive indicator of hypovolemic shock. 3 A fever is associated with septic shock. 4 Nausea is not a symptom associated with hypovolemic shock.

    Client Need: Physiological Adaptation; **Cognitive Level:** Analysis; **Nursing Process:** Analysis

3. **2 Anaphylactic shock occurs with severe allergic reactions when rapid vasodilation releases large amounts of histamine.**

    1 Cariogenic shock can be caused by a myocardial infarction characterized by chest pain. 3 Obstructive shock can be triggered by a pulmonary embolism that blocks blood flow. 4 Septic shock presents with a fever resulting from a gram-negative bacterial infection.

    Client Need: Physiological Adaptation; **Cognitive Level:** Applying; **Nursing Process:** Assessment

4. **2 Triggers for neurogenic shock include drugs, spinal cord injury, severe pain, and fear.**

    1 Age, gender, and weight are triggers for cardiogenic shock associated with cardiac dysfunction. 3 Severe burns can trigger distributive shock. 4 Allergic reactions are the trigger for anaphylactic shock.

    Client Need: Physiological Adaptation; **Cognitive Level:** Applying; **Nursing Process:** Assessment

5. **3 Varicose veins result in irregularly dilated deep veins that prevent normal backflow of blood that can trigger thrombi formation. The development of a warm and often reddened area of the affected calf is characteristic of a thrombus and needs immediate medical attention.**

    1, 2, 4 Edema, absence of hair, and presence of ulcers on the affected leg are normal occurrences for this condition.

    Client Need: Physiological Adaptation; **Cognitive Level:** Analysis; **Nursing Process:** Analysis

6. Answers: 1, 2, 4.

    1, 2, 4 Although varicose veins are most common in the lower legs, they are also found in the esophagus (esophageal varices) and the rectum (hemorrhoids).

    3, 5 The scalp and upper arms are not affected by varicose veins.

    Client Need: Physiological Adaptation; **Cognitive Level:** Understand; **Integrated Process:** Teaching and Learning.

7. **2 Thrombophlebitis (inflammation of a vein) can lead to pulmonary emboli causing acute respiratory distress. This complication requires immediate medical attention.**

    1 Leukocytosis occurs when the white blood cell count is above the normal range in the blood. It is frequently a sign of an inflammatory response, most commonly the result of infection. Although requiring intervention, it is not as critical as acute respiratory distress. 3 Calf pain is associated with the presence of thrombosis. 4 Burning and aching sensations in the affected leg are classic signs of the disorder. Although requiring intervention, it is not as critical as acute respiratory distress.

    Client Need: Physiological Adaptation; **Cognitive Level:** Analysis; **Nursing Process:** Analysis

8. **2 A varicose vein will appear as irregular, purplish bulging veins on the affected extremity.**

    1 Edema would be present on the affected leg, not on both legs. 3 A fever would not be expected with a varicose vein; a fever is more likely with thrombophlebitis. 4 Raynaud disease results in color changes to the extremity.

    Client Need: Physiological Adaptation; **Cognitive Level:** Analysis; **Nursing Process:** Assessment

9. **1 Increased blood coagulation from dehydration, pregnancy, or platelet disorders may increase the risk of developing thrombophlebitis.**

    2 The older, adult client diagnosed with CHF does not have the risk factor presented by pregnancy and its increase in blood coagulation. 3 Although standing for long periods, a risk present for varicose veins, is increased by the clerk's job, it does not have the risk factor presented by pregnancy and its increase in blood coagulation. 4 Mania is not a risk factor for thrombophlebitis.

    Client Need: Physiological Adaptation; **Cognitive Level:** Analysis; **Nursing Process:** Assessment

10. **Answers: 1, 5.**

    1 Raynaud disease is a rare disorder of the blood vessels with unknown cause seen more commonly in females. **5** Raynaud disease seen more often in colder climates causes the blood vessels to constrict with cold temperatures.

    2 Age is not a factor in the development of Raynaud disease. **3** The physical requirements of being a waitress do not necessarily increase the risk of developing Raynaud disease. **4** The physiology of asthma does not necessarily increase the risk of Raynaud disease, although stress has been known to cause vasoconstriction.

    Client Need: Physiological Adaptation; **Cognitive Level:** Applying; **Nursing Process:** Analysis

11. **4 Raynaud disease causes the blood vessels to constrict with cold temperatures or feelings of stress.**

    1 With constriction of the vessels, affected areas turn white and blue. When the blood flow returns, the skin turns red and throbs or tingles. **2** Raynaud disease is a rare disorder of the blood vessels with unknown cause. **3** Raynaud disease is seen more often in colder climates.

    Client Need: Physiological Adaptation; **Cognitive Level:** Apply; **Nursing Process:** Planning

12. **Answers: 2, 3.**

    2, 3 Peripheral vascular disease involves abnormalities of veins and arteries of the circulatory system outside the heart. Diagnosis is based on the results of Doppler studies and an arteriogram.

    1 An x-ray would not provide the information necessary related to the veins and arteries needed to make such a diagnosis. **4** A CBC provides information on components of the blood, not on the condition of the blood vessels. **5** The MRI would not provide the information necessary related to the veins and arteries needed to make such a diagnosis.

    Client Need: Physiological Adaptation; **Cognitive Level:** Understanding; **Integrated Process:** Teaching and Learning

13. **Answers: 1, 3, 4, 5.**

    1 PVD involves abnormalities of veins and arteries of the circulatory system outside the heart that result in toenails that are thick and hard. **3** Legs may be red when standing, sitting, or dangling. **4** Numbness in the affected leg is a characteristic of PVD. **5** PVD can trigger intermittent claudication that causes leg pain with exercise.

    2 Absence of hair on the affected extremity is associated with PVD.

    Client Need: Physiological Adaptation; **Cognitive Level:** Applying; **Nursing Process:** Assessment

14. **3 Gangrene is the death of tissue resulting from an insufficient blood supply. Gangrene requires urgent care. Treatment includes antibiotics and removing dead tissue.**

    1 Intermittent claudication results in exercise-induced leg pain. Although painful and requiring management, it is not as acutely serious as gangrene and the effect of necrotic tissue on the health of the body. **2** Although venous ulcers can occur and require treatment, they are not as acutely serious as gangrene and the effect of necrotic tissue on the health of the body. **4** Leg pain, although serious does not have the acute seriousness as does gangrene and its effect on the health of the body.

    Client Need: Physiological Adaptation; **Cognitive Level:** Analysis; **Nursing Process:** Analysis

15. **1 An aortic aneurysm, which involves the dilation and weakening of the arterial wall, has been associated with a history of syphilis.**

    2 Hypertension, rather than hypotension, is a possible factor in the pathology of an aortic aneurysm. **3** A bruit (sound reflecting turbulence of flow) is characteristically heard at the site of an aneurysm. **4** There is some support for a genetic predisposition for aortic aneurysms.

    Client Need: Physiological Adaptation; **Cognitive Level:** Applying; **Nursing Process:** Assessment

16. **Answers: 1, 3, 4, 5.**

    1, 3, 4, 5 The pathology of right-sided heart failure results in ascites (collection of fluid in the abdominal cavity), hepatomegaly (an enlarged liver), dependent edema (swelling of the legs and feet), and distended neck veins.

    2 Orthopnea (difficult breathing in a reclining position) is characteristic of left-sided heart failure.

    Client Need: Physiological Adaptation; **Cognitive Level:** Understanding; **Integrated Process:** Teaching and Learning

RESPIRATORY SYSTEM OVERVIEW (Fig. 15.1)

- The respiratory system and the cardiovascular system work in conjunction to provide oxygenated blood to body tissues and vital organs.
- The lungs function to exchange environmental gases with the blood system.
- The respiratory system is the only source of oxygen to the body.
- Ventilation, perfusion, and diffusion are necessary processes for the exchange of gases.
- The lungs are protected from infection by cellular processes and structural protection.
- Alterations in respiratory system performance may develop if airways are obstructed, lungs are prevented from fully expanding, an interruption in pulmonary blood flow occurs, or damage to the main structures for gas exchange, the alveoli.
- Signs and symptoms, such as dyspnea, cough, abnormal sputum, hemoptysis, and an abnormal breathing pattern, may be related to an alteration in normal pulmonary system function.

Two Divisions

- The upper respiratory system consists of the nasal passages, sinuses, nasopharynx, pharynx, larynx, tonsils, and glottis.
- The lower respiratory system is in the thorax and it contains the lower trachea, right and left bronchus, bronchial tree, lungs, pleural membranes, alveolar ducts, alveoli, and mediastinum.
- Conducting airways
  - The respiratory system consists of upper and lower airways and the lungs contained in the chest cavity. The diaphragm and the blood vessels, which infuse these airways and lungs, are considered part of the pulmonary system.
  - The two lungs are divided into lobes.
    - The right lung contains an upper, middle, and lower lobe.
    - The left lung contains an upper and lower lobe.
- Bronchi are conducting airways that deliver air to each lobe of the lungs.
- Bronchi are supported by lung tissue which prevents collapse.
- The heart, esophagus, and great vessels are contained in the space between the lungs known as the mediastinum.
- Upper airway
  - Consists of oropharynx and nasopharynx
  - Coated with mucus and cilia
  - Blood supply to the upper airways warms and humidifies air and removes extraneous particles before air enters into the lungs.
  - With nasal obstruction, the mouth and oropharynx provide ventilation. The mouth and oropharynx are unable to adequately filter and humidify air in comparison to the nasopharynx.
- Larynx
  - Connects upper and lower airways
  - Consists of endolarynx and its cartilage structures

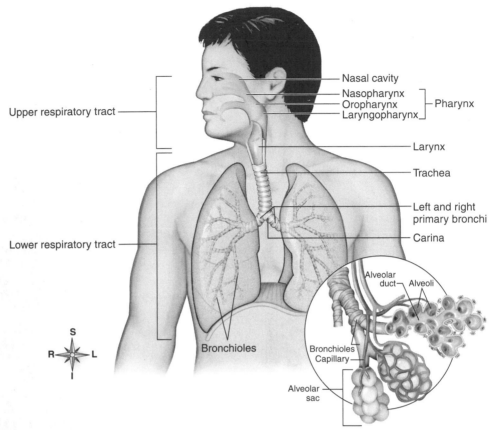

FIG. 15.1　Structural plan of the respiratory system. (From Patton, K. T., & Thibodeau, G. A. [2018]. *The human body in health and disease* [7th ed.]. St. Louis: Mosby.)

- The false vocal cords and true vocal cords form the endolarynx.
- The glottis is formed by the space between the sets of vocal cords.
- The epiglottis, thyroid, and cricoid are large cartilages that form the laryngeal box. Smaller cartilages also form the box and are connected by ligaments.
- Ligaments and muscles support the larynx with breathing movements, speech, and swallowing.
- Trachea
  - Connects bronchi and the larynx
  - Divides at the carins to form the right and left bronchi
  - Owing to the size and angle of the right bronchus, aspirated fluids and substances, along with foreign particles, verge to the right in most cases.
  - The hila are the roots of the lungs and where the right and left main bronchi enter the lungs.
  - The bronchi are covered with cilia and goblet cells which secrete mucus.
  - Cilia cells continually push mucus toward the pharynx where it exits the respiratory system through coughing or swallowing.

- After entering the lungs, the bronchi branch into segmental and subsegmental bronchi ending in terminal bronchioles.
- Bronchioles end in alveolar ducts which contain alveolar sacs containing alveoli.
- Gas exchange
  - Gas exchange occurs in the acinus which consists of bronchioles, alveolar ducts, and alveoli.
  - Gas exchange primarily occurs in the alveoli where the exchange of oxygen and carbon dioxide occur.
  - Adult lungs contain about 480 million alveoli. Lungs of the neonate contain about 50 million alveoli.
  - The alveoli contain epithelial cells that provide structure and another type that secretes surfactant.
  - Surfactant is important in gas exchange in that it decreases surface tension and facilitates expansion, which prevents collapse, known as atelectasis.
  - Surfactant plays a role in protecting lungs from the inflammatory response and decreasing the amount of bacteria in the lung.
  - Alveolar macrophages perform phagocytosis and allow removal of foreign substances in the lung through the lymphatic system.
  - Ventilation/perfusion ratio (VQ ratio)
    - Ratio between the amount of air getting to the alveoli and the amount of blood being sent to the lungs.
    - V = Alveolar ventilation in mL/min
    - Q = Cardiac output in mL/min

Gas Transportation

- Oxygen and carbon dioxide are the gases transported through the blood and to the vital organs and tissues.
- Oxygen is difficult to diffuse. It is the dissolved form of oxygen that is used in the body, and only about 1% of total oxygen taken into the body is able to transition to the dissolved form.
- Hemoglobin is the measure of oxygen saturation of the blood. The blood is considered fully saturated with oxygen when all four of the heme molecules in the hemoglobin have become saturated with oxygen.
- Carbon dioxide easily diffuses across membranes and is the waste product of cellular metabolism in the body.
- The majority of carbon dioxide enters red blood cells where it is ultimately converted to bicarbonate ions and maintains the blood pH through the blood buffer system.

Lung Compliance

- Compliance is the capability of the lungs to expand when breathing.
- Lung compliance is determined by the surface tension of the alveolar and the elasticity of the chest wall.
  - Increased compliance is an indicator that the chest wall has lost some elasticity, or elastic recoil, and inflates too easily.
    - Normal aging can cause increased compliance.
  - Decreased compliance occurs when the chest wall or lungs is difficult to inflate owing to a lack of elasticity.
    - Decreased compliance occurs with disease processes such as fibrosis, pneumonia, pulmonary edema, and acute respiratory distress syndrome (ARDS).

- Elasticity
  - The lungs have elastin fibers that allow expansion during inspiration and return during expiration.
  - Elastic recoil is the natural inclination of the lung to return to a resting state after a breath. This allows a passive expiration without the use of accessory muscles.
  - If disease processes, such as emphysema or other conditions that affect conducting airways or impact elastic recoil, accessory muscles will need to be used to force air out of the lung.
- Surfactant
  - Surfactant has a soap detergent effect that pushes liquid molecules apart and decreases alveolar surface tension, which allows alveolar ventilation or distention.
  - Without adequate surfactant, alveoli collapse and gas exchange will not occur.

Breathing

- Controlled by medulla oblongata
- Requires muscles to perform movement for inspiration and expiration (Fig. 15.2)

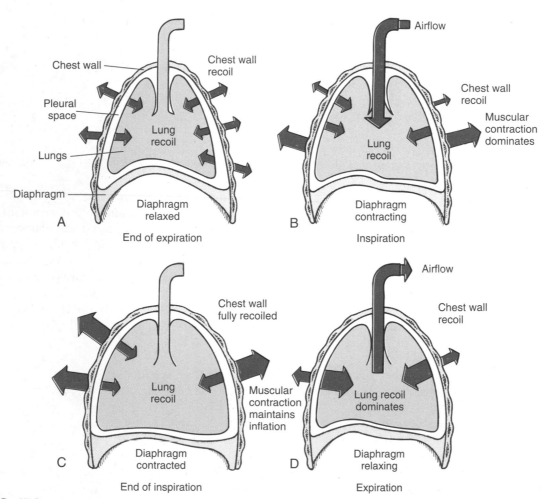

FIG. 15.2 Interaction of forces during inspiration and expiration. (From McCance, K. L., & Huether, S. E. [2019]. *Pathophysiology: The biologic basis for disease in adults and children* [8th ed.]. St. Louis: Elsevier.)

- The primary muscle for ventilation to occur is the diaphragm.
  - A contracted diaphragm pulls air into the lungs through negative pressure.
  - Ordinary expiration requires no muscle involvement. Occasionally, abdominal and internal intercostal accessory muscles can assist to push high levels of air out of the lungs.
- The chest and lungs must have a degree of elasticity to perform the movement required for breathing.
- The conducting airways must be able to resist airflow.
  - Measured by pulmonary function tests
    - Used to evaluate presence of lung disease, flow rates, and lung volume
  - Can be affected by size of airways and the properties of the gas entering the airways
  - Normally very low
  - Bronchodilation decreases resistance to airflow.
  - Bronchoconstriction increases resistance to airflow.
- The work of breathing is estimated by muscular effort. In normal cases, the work of breathing is minimal.

Role in pH Balance

- CO_2 or carbon dioxide, the waste product from cellular metabolism, diffuses into the red blood cells.
- Once inside the red blood cell, carbon dioxide is converted to carbonic acid and then into bicarbonate ions.
- The ratio of 20 bicarbonate ions to 1 part carbonic acid works to sustain a blood pH of 7.35 to 7.45.
- Lungs
  - Increased rate of breathing increases pH by blowing off more carbonic acid.
  - Decreased rate of breathing decreases pH by retaining more carbonic acid.

APPLICATION AND REVIEW

1. What structures should the nurse assess to best monitor a client diagnosed with a lower respiratory infection? **Select all that apply**.
   1. Lungs
   2. Glottis
   3. Tonsils
   4. Trachea
   5. Mediastinum
2. What structures are associated with gas exchange? **Select all that apply**.
   1. Alveoli
   2. Trachea
   3. Bronchi
   4. Bronchioles
   5. Endolarynx
3. A client is hospitalized with diaphragmatic trauma. The nurse will be most concerned with which process associated with breathing? **Select all that apply**.
   1. Ventilation
   2. Perfusion
   3. Diffusion
   4. Exchange

See Answers on pages 318–320.

Respiratory Abnormalities

- Asthma
  - Reversible airway obstruction involving the bronchial airways
  - Can be severe

- Acute cases are single episodes and are often associated with the common cold.
- Irreversible lung damage and chronic asthmatic disease can occur if the condition is not controlled.
- Clients can have a single type or a combination of the two types of asthma.
  - Basic types (2)
    - Extrinsic asthma
      - Inhalation of an antigen causes a type 1 hypersensitivity reaction
      - May be a family history of asthma or other allergic type conditions
      - Usually begins in childhood and clients grow out of the disease in adolescence
    - Intrinsic asthma
      - Adult onset
      - Various stimuli can trigger asthma attacks.
        - Exposure to second-hand smoke
        - Stress
        - Exercise
        - Cold temperatures
        - Some drugs
  - With both types of asthma the body responds with an inflammatory response in the bronchi and bronchioles that increases production of thick mucus and bronchoconstriction, which creates a partial or total airway obstruction.
  - Air trapping can occur with partial airway obstruction causing lung hyperinflation and prevents air from fully exiting the lungs. This makes it difficult to expectorate excess mucus or to inhale air.
  - Total obstruction of the airways occurs when mucus completely fills the passages. This causes atelectasis and prevents gas exchange, resulting in severe hypoxia.
  - Severe asthma attacks not responding to treatment are known as status asthmaticus and can lead to death.
  - Signs and symptoms
    - Cough
    - Shortness of breath
    - Labored breathing with use of accessory muscles
    - Inability to speak
    - Feeling of chest tightness
    - Wheezing
    - Hypoxia
    - Thick mucus production
    - Tachycardia
    - Pulsus paradoxus, a difference in blood pressure with inspiration and expiration, may occur.
    - Respiratory alkalosis may develop initially with rapid breathing and then progress to respiratory acidosis owing to decreased ability to take oxygen into the lungs.
    - Can progress to respiratory failure if not treated
  - Nocturnal asthma
    - Symptoms such as chest tightness, wheezing, and shortness of breath that develop at night and make asthma symptoms more difficult to control in the waking hours. Nocturnal asthma can have a severe impact on sleep quality, which can contribute to poor health.

- Exercise-induced asthma
  - Also referred to as exercised-induced bronchoconstriction
  - Vigorous exercise produces coughing, wheezing, and shortness of breath.
- Occupational asthma
  - Caused by substances in the workplace that result in swelling of the lungs and narrowing of the bronchial passages
  - Thought to be an allergic type reaction to substances
  - Signs and symptoms include shortness of breath, cough, and wheezing.
  - Repeated exposure to the allergen can result in permanent lung damage.
- Drug-induced asthma
  - Can be caused by drugs that block the COX-1 enzyme
  - Common drugs, such as aspirin, ibuprofen, naproxen, and beta-blockers, may cause drug-induced asthma in some patients.
  - Extreme caution should be used with patients who have an existing asthma diagnosis.
- Stages of an asthma attack
  - Stage one
    - Swelling of the airway mucosa
    - Bronchoconstriction
    - Increased mucus section in the airway passage
  - Stage two
    - Prolonged inflammation, bronchoconstriction, and damage to the epithelial cells
    - Partial or total obstruction of the airways
    - Hypoxia
- Aspiration
  - Passage of foreign material such as food, fluid, emesis, or drugs into lungs
  - More often involves right lung owing to structural design of the airways
  - Aspiration of foreign objects affects all age groups. More prominent in small children and adults with impaired gag reflex
  - Signs and symptoms
    - Dependent on the characteristics of the aspirate
    - Coughing
      - Aspiration caused by dysphagia may produce cough with eating or swallowing saliva.
    - Choking
    - Wheezing
    - Shortness of breath
    - Stridor
    - Inability to speak
    - Total or partial obstruction of the larynx
    - Cardiac distress
- Obstructive sleep apnea
  - Tissues of the pharynx collapse during sleep, obstructing airflow.
  - Clients with obstructive sleep apnea awake frequently because of the inability to breathe.
  - Some clients may not be aware this occurs during their sleep. About 3% to 5% of the population is thought to have sleep apnea.
  - Those with a body mass index (BMI) greater than 30 are at greater risk of developing sleep apnea.
  - Diagnosed with sleep studies.

- Signs and symptoms
  - Loud snoring
  - Gasping for air during sleep
  - Daytime drowsiness
  - Fatigue
- Complications
  - Type 2 diabetes
  - Congestive heart failure
  - Stroke
  - Pulmonary hypertension
  - Erectile dysfunction
  - Depression
  - Chronic fatigue
- Chronic obstructive pulmonary disease (COPD)
  - Also known as chronic obstructive lung disease (COLD)
  - Chronic disease causing irreversible damage to the lungs as a result of airway obstruction and tissue degeneration in the lungs
  - Diagnosed using chest imaging, symptomology, and pulmonary function testing
  - COPD can cause right-sided heart failure or cor pulmonale.
    - Caused by chronic bronchitis and emphysema
      - Emphysema is most commonly caused by cigarette smoking.
      - Destroys walls and septae of the alveoli, resulting in continuous inflation of air sacs, which result in the following
        - Decreased surface area for gas exchange
        - Decreased perfusion and diffusion of available gases
        - Narrow and weak airway walls that easily collapse
        - Inability to passively expel air, which causes use of accessory muscles to push trapped air out of the body
        - Flat diaphragm
        - Hyperinflation of the lungs that produces a barrel chest appearance over time
  - Chronic emphysema causes large holes or blebs in the lung that can erupt causing development of pneumothorax. Clients with chronic emphysema respond to higher levels of carbon dioxide and lower levels of oxygen as the drive to breathe. They may have frequent infections, pulmonary hypertension, and heart failure as the disease progresses.
  - Signs and symptoms of emphysema
    - Shortness of breath
    - Barrel chest appearance
    - Hyperresonant on percussion of chest
    - Tripod position (sitting, leaning forward with hands on knees or table)
    - Decreased appetite and weight loss
    - Fatigue
    - Clubbed fingers
    - May have elevated hematocrit as a result of chronic hypoxemia, which is known as secondary polycythemia
    - Clients with chronic emphysema may be described as "pink puffers" to describe the trio of symptoms of shortness of breath, over-inflation, and hyperventilation.

- Chronic bronchitis
  - Progressive and irreversible damage to the bronchi caused by smoking or exposure to pollutants
  - Causes thickening of bronchial walls with increased mucus production with low oxygen levels
  - Signs and symptoms of chronic bronchitis
    - Severe shortness of breath, which can interfere with eating and activities of daily living
    - Weight loss
    - Productive cough
    - Increased respiratory rate
    - Thick, purulent sputum and respiratory secretions
    - Hypoxia leading to cyanosis and hypercapnia
    - Secondary polycythemia
    - Signs of heart failure
- Bronchiectasis
  - Abnormal widening of the bronchi, usually medium-sized, which form sac-like structures in the airways that obstruct airflow
  - Fluid may pool around the sac-like or elongated (fusiform) areas that then become inflamed and infected.
  - Bronchiectasis is usually a secondary condition developing with cystic fibrosis or COPD.
  - May be the result of aspiration, congenital impairments in the bronchial wall, or childhood infectious processes
  - Signs and symptoms
    - Chronic productive cough producing 1 to 2 cups of purulent sputum per day
    - Weight loss
    - Hemoptysis
    - Anemia
    - Bad breath
    - Fatigue
    - Rales and rhonchi auscultated in the lungs

APPLICATION AND REVIEW

4. A nurse is caring for a client with chronic bronchitis. Which finding would the nurse expect?
   1. Coughing up thick mucous secretions
   2. Weight gain of 10 pounds
   3. Substernal chest pain on inspiration
   4. Asymmetric chest expansion
5. The nurse is caring for a client with chronic emphysema. Which clinical manifestation would the nurse expect?
   1. Clubbing of fingers
   2. Slow, irregular respirations
   3. Subcutaneous hemorrhages
   4. Decreased red blood cell count
6. A nurse is caring for a client with a history of chronic obstructive pulmonary disease (COPD). Which complication is most commonly associated with COPD?
   1. Cardiac problems
   2. Joint inflammation
   3. Kidney dysfunction
   4. Peripheral neuropathy

See Answers on pages 318–320.

Restrictive Lung Disorders

- Pneumoconiosis
  - Develops from long-term inhalation of irritants, such as asbestos, where the particles are tiny and able to enter the alveolar ducts and sacs over time
  - Lungs become fibrotic and alveoli are unable to perform gas exchange.
  - May be seen with occupations such as mining
  - Cigarette smoking can worsen the condition.
  - Asbestos exposure increases the chance of developing lung cancer.
  - Signs and symptoms
    - Shortness of breath worsening over time
    - Cough

Upper Respiratory Tract Infections

- Infectious rhinitis
  - Also known as the common cold
  - Viral infection of the upper airways
  - Most common viruses: parainfluenza, rhinovirus, adenovirus, and coronavirus
  - Spread by respiratory droplets in the air or on surfaces
  - Highly contagious
  - Self-limiting infection
  - Signs and symptoms
    - Headache
    - Fever (usually low grade), which may indicate the infection has spread to the larynx, pharynx, or bronchioles
    - Fatigue
    - Sneezing
    - Watery eyes
    - Nasal congestion
    - Rhinorrhea (runny nose), which may result in mouth breathing
    - Cough
- Sinusitis
  - Usually results as a secondary infection from infectious rhinitis or untreated allergies
  - Caused most commonly by streptococci, *Haemophilus influenza*, or pneumococci
  - Signs and symptoms
    - Pain and pressure sensation around sinus cavities
    - Increased temperature
    - Sore throat
    - Congested nasal passages
- Laryngitis
  - Inflammation of the vocal cords resulting in hoarseness or absence of voice
  - Most often caused by a viral infection and may be accompanied by a runny nose or sore throat
  - Usually self-limiting and resolves within a few days
  - Laryngitis lasting longer than a week should be evaluated for underlying disease processes.
- Croup
  - Also known as laryngotracheobronchitis
  - Common infection in childhood

- Most common causative agents are viral.
  - Adenoviruses and parainfluenza viruses are the usual source.
- May worsen at night
- Signs and symptoms
  - Barking cough (croup)
  - Inflammation of the larynx and subglottis
  - Drainage from the throat, which may cause obstruction
  - Hoarse voice
  - Stridor with inspiration
  - Fever
- Acute bronchitis
  - Short-term inflammation of the bronchial tree most often caused by a virus
  - Generally lasts around 2 weeks; usually self-limiting
  - May be accompanied by sore throat, runny nose, and cough
  - Cough may be productive with clear or yellow sputum.
  - Recommended treatment includes over-the-counter medications, humidified air, and cough medications.
  - May develop into pneumonia or other bacterial infection requiring antibiotics
- Influenza
  - Also known as flu
  - Incubation period of 1 to 4 days; can be transmitted to others before symptoms appear
  - Can result in death
  - There are three groups of viral influenza.
    - Type A, which is the most common
    - Type B
    - Type C
  - Types of influenza frequently mutate making immune defense for the body difficult to obtain.
  - Annual vaccination to prevent flu is highly recommended. Immunity develops within 2 to 3 weeks after receiving vaccine.
  - Signs and symptoms
    - Rapid onset with fever
    - Fatigue
    - Body aches
    - Commonly accompanied by viral pneumonia
    - May develop secondary bacterial pneumonia

APPLICATION AND REVIEW

7. A nurse is caring for a child with croup. Which clinical finding alerts the nurse that immediate action is required?
   1. Irritability
   2. Hoarseness
   3. Barking cough
   4. Use of accessory muscles
8. Which clinical findings does a nurse expect when assessing a child with acute laryngotracheobronchitis (croup). **Select all that apply.**
   1. Fever
   2. Crackles
   3. Hoarseness
   4. Barking cough
   5. Inspiratory stridor

See Answers on page 318–320.

Lower Respiratory Tract Infections

- Pneumonia
  - May occur as an acute or secondary infection of the lungs
  - May develop with aspiration of foreign bodies or fluid into the lung.
  - Can be caused by fungus, virus, or bacteria
    - Most common bacterial agents are pneumococcus and *Staphylococcus aureus*.
    - Immune compromised individuals are more at risk of developing pneumonia.
    - Hospitalized individuals are at risk of developing hospital-acquired (nosocomial) pneumonia.
    - Types of pneumonia
      - Lobar pneumonia
        - Commonly caused by pneumococcus
        - Found in one or more lobes of the lung
        - Can cause empyema
      - Bronchopneumonia
        - Occurs more commonly in lower lobes of the lungs
        - Usually caused by multiple microorganisms
        - Slower onset
        - Usually produces purulent, green, or yellow sputum
      - Primary atypical pneumonia
        - Causes inflammation of the interstitial lung tissue
        - Causative agents
          - Mycoplasma pneumonia
            - Aerosol transmission
            - Causes repeated coughing
            - Treated with erythromycin or tetracycline
          - Viral
            - Influenza A and B, adenoviruses, or respiratory syncytial virus (RSV)
            - Vague symptomology, usually self-limiting course
- Legionnaire disease
  - Caused by the gram-negative *Legionella pneumophila* bacteria, which grows in warm, moist environments such as spas and heating and cooling systems
  - Usually develops as a nosocomial infection
  - Requires special culture medium to diagnose
  - Can cause lung necrosis resulting in death
    - Pneumocystis carinii pneumonia
      - May be seen in clients diagnosed with acquired immunodeficiency syndrome (AIDS)
      - Often results in death owing to lung necrosis
      - Clients with AIDS may be given prophylaxis treatment to prevent occurrence.
      - Signs and symptoms of pneumonia
        - High fever
        - Rapid onset
        - Chills
        - Increased white blood cell count
        - Fatigue
        - Shortness of breath
        - Increased respiratory and heart rate
        - Pain around lungs on the affected side

- ○ Rales in affected lung field
  - ○ Person may have diminished breath sounds in affected area if consolidation has occurred because of the inflammatory response
  - ○ Cough with rusty appearing sputum
  - ○ Confusion and altered level of consciousness may develop if pneumonia is having an impact on gas exchange and oxygenation
- Tuberculosis (TB)
  - Global disease with some drug resistant strains
  - Transmitted by respiratory droplets from a person with active TB
  - Often found in low socioeconomic areas and in overcrowded conditions such as prisons
    - Higher rates in patients with human immunodeficiency virus (HIV) and the homeless
  - Primarily caused by *Mycobacterium tuberculosis*, which may live in sputum, inside or outside the body, for several weeks
  - Primary infection from TB occurs when the TB bacteria first enter the lungs forming a tubercle. Healthy individuals can resist disease formation and the tubercle will remain walled off in the lung. As long as the individual has a healthy immune response there is exposure, but no active disease. The immune response takes about 6 to 8 weeks to complete.
  - A tuberculin skin test (TST) is used to diagnose TB exposure.
  - Chest x-rays and sputum cultures are used to determine if an individual has active TB.
  - Extrapulmonary or miliary TB affects large areas of the lungs and may spread through the circulation to other parts of the body.
  - Secondary TB is considered an active infection and may be referred to as reinfection. New tubercles may form in this stage. Cavitation, large caverns in the lung, may also form during active infection. These can progress into the bronchi and affect the blood supply to the lung. Clients may cough up blood and through salivation and swallowing can infect the digestive tract with TB.
  - Active infection is highly contagious.
  - Signs and symptoms
    - May be asymptomatic
    - Night sweats
    - Fever, usually appearing as low-grade in the afternoon hours
    - Fatigue
    - Loss of appetite
    - Weight loss
    - Cough, increasing in severity as disease progresses
    - Purulent sputum, sometimes containing blood
    - Patients with positive sputum cultures should wear a mask, avoid long periods of close contact with others, and practice covering their mouth with coughing and sneezing.
    - Hospitalized clients should be placed in airborne precautions; individuals entering the room need to wear a particulate filter respirator or mask.
- Lung cancer
  - Third most common type of cancer in the United States. Tumors found in the lungs are rarely benign.
  - Tumors in the lung are staged based on the tumor size-node involvement metastases (TNM) classification system as are other forms of cancer.

- Smoking is a factor in the development of 90% of lung cancers. This includes cases related to second-hand smoke exposure.
- Individuals who smoke and are exposed to carcinogens through work have an increased risk of developing lung cancer.
- Primary lung cancer results directly from tumor formation in the lung.
- Secondary lung cancer is a result of tumor cells from other body parts lodging in the lungs.
- Lung cancer most typically spreads to brain, bone, and liver if not controlled.
- Computed tomography (CT) scans, magnetic resonance imaging (MRI), x-ray, bronchoscopy, and mediastinoscopy are used to diagnose the presence of lung cancer.
- Types
  - Bronchogenic carcinoma
    - Most common type
    - Develops from epithelium of the bronchi
  - Squamous cell carcinoma
    - Often enters into airway after arising from the lining of the bronchus near the hilum
  - Adenocarcinomas
    - Arise from glands
    - Often reside on the lung periphery
    - Difficult to detect in early stages
  - Bronchoalveolar cell carcinomas
    - Produce fewer symptoms
    - Found in periphery of lung
    - Difficult to detect
  - Small cell carcinoma
    - Also known as "oat cell" carcinoma
    - Rapid growth
    - Located near main bronchus in center of lung
    - Spreads quickly to other parts of the body
  - Large cell carcinoma
    - Made of many undifferentiated cells
    - Rapid growth results in early metastasis to other areas of the body.
  - Mesothelioma
    - Affects pleura of the lung
    - Fatal unless diagnosed very early
    - Caused by asbestos exposure
- Signs and symptoms
  - Early signs
    - Productive cough
    - Shortness of breath
    - Wheezing
    - Hemoptysis
    - Chest pain
    - Facial or arm edema
    - Headache
    - Difficulty swallowing
    - Voice changes
    - Development of pneumothorax, effusion, or hemothorax

- Systemic signs and symptoms
  - Fatigue
  - Anemia
  - Weight loss
- Signs and symptoms can involve other body systems if metastasis has occurred.
- Pleural effusion
  - Defined as fluid in the pleural space
  - Diagnosed with lung and chest imaging and thoracentesis
  - Causes
    - Abscess
    - Tumors or lesions
    - Lymphatic fluid
    - Leaking blood vessel beneath the lung pleura
      - May accumulate rapidly
      - Fluid may appear as exudate or more clear
        - Empyema indicates a pleural effusion with pus.
        - Hemothorax is pleural effusion with blood.
        - Chylothorax is caused from the accumulation of chyle, a milky substance from the lymphatic system.
  - Signs and symptoms
    - Depend on cause
    - Some pleural effusions may be small and produce no symptoms.
    - Shortness of breath
    - Decreased breath sounds
    - Pleural friction rub may be auscultated
    - Dullness detected with percussion over effusion
    - Impaired gas exchange
    - Mediastinal shifts
    - Cardiac dysthymias
- Empyema
  - Infected pleural effusion resulting from an inability of the lymphatic system to drain lymph fluid from the pleural space
  - Diagnosed with sputum cultures, chest imaging, and thoracentesis
  - Occurs more commonly in older adults and children suffering from complications of surgery, pneumonia, and tumors.
  - Stages (3)
    - Exudative stage
    - Fibrinopurulent stage
    - Organizing stage
  - Signs and symptoms
    - Fever
    - Tachycardia
    - Pleural pain
    - Cough
    - Cyanosis
- Pneumothorax
  - Gas or air in the pleural space
  - Caused by trauma to the visceral pleura, parietal pleura, and chest wall

- Entering air into the pleural space disrupts the negative pressure of the lung and prevents lung expansion.
- Signs and symptoms
  - Shortness of breath
  - Chest pain
  - Tachycardia
- Types
  - Spontaneous (primary)
    - Unexpected occurrence in healthy adult
    - Usually impacts men between age 20 and 40 years
    - Caused by rupture of blisters or blebs on the visceral pleura usually occurring at the apex of the lungs
    - Smoking can be a factor in the occurrence.
    - Some genetic links have been discovered.
    - Many affected have been found to have disease-like lung changes resembling emphysema despite no history of smoking.
  - Traumatic (secondary)
    - Caused by chest trauma, such as gunshot wounds, knife wounds, or rib fractures from accidents
    - Can be caused by surgical procedures
    - COPD can cause large blebs to rupture causing traumatic pneumothorax development.
    - May result from ventilator settings with positive end-expiratory pressure (PEEP)
    - Iatrogenic pneumothorax, which is considered a type of secondary pneumothorax, is caused by transthoracic needle aspiration.
  - Primary and secondary pneumothorax are classified as open or tension.
    - Open pneumothorax allows air to be drawn in the pleural space during inspiration and forced back out on expiration through the damaged area.
    - Tension pneumothorax allows air to be drawn in the pleural space during inspiration, but does not allow the air to escape. This is a medical emergency as the expanding chest compresses the lung, prevents gas exchange from occurring, and forces deviation of the trachea to the unaffected side. The heart and great vessels can be displaced with a tension pneumothorax.
- Flail chest
  - Develops when the thorax is fractured by trauma such as falls or motor vehicle accidents.
  - Medical emergency
  - Changes from flail chest can kink the inferior vena cava and interfere with venous blood flow to the heart, reducing cardiac output.
  - Usually involves fractures of several ribs or severe trauma to the sternum
  - Chest wall has no structural support, resulting in paradoxical chest movement during inspiration and expiration.
  - During inspiration the flail chest section moves inward instead of outward and prevents lung expansion. The other lung may also be compressed and the influx of air from the damaged lung may flow into the unaffected lung.
  - With expiration the flail chest is pushed outward and the paradoxical movement of the ribs impacts airflow.

- Signs and symptoms
  - Paradoxical chest movement
  - Chest pain
  - Difficulty breathing
- Infant respiratory distress syndrome (IRDS)
  - Associated with infant lung immaturity and premature birth
  - Common cause of neonatal death
  - Lungs do not have adequate surfactant.
  - Signs and symptoms
    - Difficulty breathing at birth or shortly after birth
    - Respiratory rate greater than 60 breaths/min
    - Use of accessory muscles to breathe with nasal flaring
    - Rales auscultated in lung fields
    - Low body temperature
- Pulmonary edema
  - Caused by water in the lung
  - Medical emergency
  - Development can begin with a pulmonary capillary wedge pressure of 20 mmHg
  - Signs and symptoms
    - Shortness of breath
    - Edema
    - Anxiety
    - Sensation of drowning
    - Wheezing
    - Coughing
    - Production of frothy, sometimes blood–tinged sputum
  - Causes
    - Most commonly left-sided heart failure
    - Inhalation of toxic gases
    - Injury to pulmonary vessels in adult respiratory distress syndrome (ARDS)
    - Blocked lymphatic drainage from the lung
- Acute respiratory distress syndrome (ARDS)
  - Also known as adult respiratory distress syndrome (ARDS), wet lung, stiff lung, postperfusion lung, and shock lung
  - Causes
    - Shock
    - Aspiration
    - Smoke inhalation
    - Sepsis
  - Occurs within 1 to 2 days after a preceding event and often leads to multiple organ failure and death
  - Changes in lung tissue from a precipitating event lead to increased permeability of the alveolar membrane, increased immune response to the lung, and a decreased ability for the cells in the lungs to produce adequate surfactant for gas exchange. This results in lung failure and increased fluid in the lung causing heart failure to develop.
  - Poor prognosis for recovery with an 80% to 90% chance of death if caused by sepsis

- Signs and symptoms
  - Frothy sputum
  - Confusion and restlessness
  - Shortness of breath with rapid, shallow respirations
  - Cyanosis
  - Decreased PaO_2
  - Tachycardia
  - Auscultation indicates fluid in the lungs.

APPLICATION AND REVIEW

9. The nurse is caring for a client who has experienced a near-drowning in the ocean. For which potential complication should the nurse assess the client?
   1. Alkalosis
   2. Renal failure
   3. Hypervolemia
   4. Pulmonary edema
10. A client's sputum smears for acid-fast bacillus (AFB) are positive, and transmission-based precautions are instituted. What should the nurse teach family members to do?
    1. Avoid contact with objects in the room
    2. Limit their contact with nonexposed people
    3. Put on a gown and gloves before going into the room.
    4. Wear a high-efficiency particulate respirator when visiting
11. The nurse is caring for a client with adult respiratory distress syndrome (ARDS). Which finding would the nurse expect?
    1. Restlessness
    2. Bradycardia
    3. Constricted pupils
    4. Clubbing of the fingers

See Answers on pages 318–320.

Perfusion and Ventilation Abnormalities

- Atelectasis
  - Collapse of the lung or part of the lung
  - Prevents appropriate gas exchange, which leads to hypoxia.
  - Mainly a complication of other disease processes, which should be treated quickly to avoid lung necrosis
  - Types of atelectasis
    - Postoperative atelectasis
      - Occurs 24 to 72 hours after surgery
      - More common with abdominal surgeries; development owing to impaired ventilation because of abdominal distention or pain
      - Can result from breathing changes from surgical anesthesia, prolonged immobility in surgery, and diminished cough response
    - Contraction atelectasis
      - Results from decreased lung expansion owing to fibrous disease in the lungs or pleura
    - Compression atelectasis
      - Develops when pressure is applied to part of the lung preventing entrance of air, or when air or fluid prevents lung expansion
      - Obstructive or resorption atelectasis
        - Caused from total airway obstruction by a tumor or mucus

- Signs and symptoms of atelectasis
  - May be asymptomatic depending on amount of lung affected
  - Increased heart rate
  - Shortness of breath
  - Increased respiratory rate
  - Chest pain
  - Chest may appear asymmetric
  - Mediastinum may shift to unaffected side if atelectasis is caused by compression
  - Diminished lung sounds

Role of the Respiratory System in Acid–Base Balance

- The respiratory system controls the rate of respirations in order to maintain pH balance of the blood.
- Normal pH is 7.35 to 7.45.
- Chemoreceptors recognize changes in pH and $PaCO_2$.
- Respirations increase when serum carbon dioxide levels increase in an attempt to rid the body of more acid in the form of carbon dioxide.
- Respirations decrease when alkalosis develops in an attempt to retain acid in the form of carbon dioxide and normalize the acid–base balance in the body.
- Responds to changes in pH balance within minutes or hours.

Respiratory Acid–Base Imbalances

- Respiratory acidosis
  - Results from an increase in carbon dioxide levels from a respiratory origin
  - Laboratory results: Decreased pH, Increased $PaCO_2$
  - Causes
    - Airway obstruction
    - Chest injuries
    - Sedation
    - Pneumonia
    - Any condition that depresses the respiratory system
    - Patients with COPD may experience chronic respiratory acidosis.
  - Signs and symptoms of respiratory acidosis
    - Lethargy
    - Blurred vision
    - Headache
    - Tremors
    - Convulsions
    - Coma possible
    - Hypotension
    - Cardiac conduction changes are possible
- Respiratory alkalosis
  - Develops from a decrease in carbon dioxide levels from a respiratory origin
  - Laboratory results: Increased pH, decreased $PaCO_2$
  - Causes of respiratory alkalosis
    - Hyperventilation
    - High fever
    - Anxiety

- Aspirin overdose
- Tumors or head injuries, which impact the respiratory control center in the brain
- Signs and symptoms of respiratory alkalosis
  - Dizziness
  - Tachypnea
  - Carpopedal spasm
  - Confusion
  - Tingling of the extremities
  - Convulsions
  - Coma

APPLICATION AND REVIEW

12. A nurse is caring for a client who had abdominal surgery. Which finding would indicate to the nurse that the client has developed postoperative atelectasis?
    1. Pleural friction rub
    2. Heart rate of 48 beats/min
    3. Tracheal deviation
    4. Respiratory rate of 26 breaths/min
13. A client is diagnosed postoperative as having atelectasis. Which nursing assessment supports this diagnosis?
    1. Productive cough
    2. Clubbing of the fingertips
    3. Crackles at the height of inhalation
    4. Diminished breath sounds on auscultation
14. What complication is prevented when a nurse addresses the needs of a client who is hyperventilating?
    1. Cardiac arrest
    2. Carbonic acid deficit
    3. Reduction in serum pH
    4. Excess oxygen saturation

See Answers on pages 318–320.

ANSWER KEY: REVIEW QUESTIONS

1. **Answers: 1, 4, 5.**
   1, 4, 5 The lower respiratory system is contained in the thorax and it contains the lower trachea, right and left bronchus, bronchial tree, lungs, pleural membranes, alveolar ducts, alveoli, and mediastinum.
   2, 3 The upper respiratory system consists of the nasal passages, sinuses, nasopharynx, pharynx, larynx, tonsils, and glottis.
   Client Need: Physiological Adaptation; **Cognitive Level:** Applying; **Nursing Process:** Planning
2. **Answers: 1, 4.**
   1, 4 Gas exchange occurs in the acinus, which consists of bronchioles, alveolar ducts, and alveoli.
   2 The trachea connects bronchi and the larynx; it is not associated with gas exchange. **3** Bronchi facilitate the movement of air into the lungs; they are not associated with gas exchange. **5** The false vocal cords and true vocal cords form the endolarynx.
   Client Need: Physiological Adaptation; **Cognitive Level:** Understanding; **Integrated Process:** Teaching and Learning
3. **1 The primary muscle needed for ventilation to occur is the diaphragm; a contracted diaphragm pulls air into the lungs through negative pressure.**
   2 The diaphragm is not associated with the perfusion (delivery of blood/oxygen) of body tissue. **3, 4** Diffusion is the exchange of gases between the capillaries and alveoli.
   Client Need: Physiological Adaptation; **Cognitive Level:** Analysis; **Nursing Process:** Analyzing

4. **1 Thick, purulent sputum is an expected clinical manifestation of chronic bronchitis.**

    2 Weight loss, not weight gain, is an expected finding in clients with chronic bronchitis. **3** Chest pain on inspiration is a finding in clients with pericarditis or pleurisy. **4** Asymmetric chest expansion occurs in clients with a pneumothorax.

    Client Need: Physiological Adaptation; **Cognitive Level:** Analysis; **Nursing Process:** Analysis

5. **1 Hypoxia leads to poor peripheral circulation; clubbing occurs because of tissue hypertrophy and additional capillary development in the fingers.**

    2 Respirations generally are rapid to compensate for oxygen deprivation. **3** Subcutaneous hemorrhage is not a physiologic response in clients with chronic hypoxia resulting from emphysema. **4** Emphysema is likely to produce polycythemia or increased red blood cell count.

    Client Need: Physiological Adaptation; **Cognitive Level:** Applying; **Nursing Process:** Assessment

6. **1 COPD causes increased pressure in the pulmonary circulation. The right side of the heart hypertrophies (cor pulmonale), causing right ventricular heart failure.**

    2 The skeletal system is not directly related to the pulmonary system; joint inflammation does not occur because of COPD. **3** This system is not as closely related to the pulmonary system as is the cardiac system; kidney problems usually do not occur because of COPD. **4** Peripheral neuropathy does not occur because of COPD.

    Client Need: Physiological Adaptation; **Cognitive Level:** Understanding; **Integrated Process:** Teaching and Learning

7. **4 Use of accessory muscles is not an expected finding in croup; it indicates respiratory distress.**

    1 Irritability is an expected finding in croup. **2** Hoarseness is an expected finding in croup. **3** A barking cough is an expected finding in croup.

    Client Need: Physiological Adaptation; **Cognitive Level:** Applying; **Nursing Process:** Assessment

8. **Answers: 1, 3, 4, 5.**

    1 Fever is a common finding with acute laryngotracheobronchitis. **3** Hoarseness is caused by edema of the mucosa of the larynx. **4** The cough is tight, with a barking, metallic sound owing to laryngeal edema. **5** Children with acute laryngotracheobronchitis experience inspiratory stridor because of laryngeal edema.

    2 Crackles are not characteristic of acute laryngotracheobronchitis.

    Client Need: Physiological Adaptation; **Cognitive Level:** Applying; **Nursing Process:** Assessment

9. **4 Additional fluid from surrounding tissues will be drawn into the lung because of the high osmotic pressure exerted by the salt content of the aspirated ocean water; this results in pulmonary edema.**

    1 Hypoxia and acidosis may occur after a near-drowning. **2** Renal failure is not a sequela of near-drowning. **3** Hypovolemia occurs because fluid is drawn into the lungs by the hypertonic saltwater.

    Client Need: Physiological Adaptation; **Cognitive Level:** Applying; **Nursing Process:** Assessment

10. **4 Tubercle bacilli are transmitted through airborne droplets; therefore, airborne precautions are necessary, and a particulate filter respirator or mask is needed.**

    1 Transmission occurs through the airborne route, not by contact. **2** Contact of family members with others does not have to be limited as long as airborne precautions are employed by family members when visiting the client. **3** Transmission occurs through the airborne route; gowns and gloves are unnecessary.

    Client Need: Physiological Adaptation; **Cognitive Level:** Applying; **Integrated Process:** Teaching and Learning

11. **1 Inadequate oxygenation of the brain may produce restlessness or behavioral changes.**

    2 The pulse increases with cerebral hypoxia. **3** The pupils dilate with cerebral hypoxia. **4** Clubbing of the fingers is the result of increased vascularization and reflects a response to prolonged hypoxia.

    Client Need: Physiological Adaptation; **Cognitive Level:** Applying; **Nursing Process:** Assessment

12. **4 Postoperative atelectasis may cause an increase in respiratory rate; normal adult respiratory rate is 12 to 20 breaths/min.**

    1 A pleural friction rub would be expected with pleural effusion, not with atelectasis. **2** Atelectasis may cause an increased heart rate, not decreased. **3** Tracheal deviation would be expected with compression atelectasis, not postoperative atelectasis.

    Client Need: Physiological Adaptation; **Cognitive Level:** Applying; **Nursing Process:** Implementation

13. **4 Atelectasis refers to the collapse of alveoli; breath sounds over the area are diminished.**

    1 A productive cough most often is associated with inflammation or infection, not atelectasis. **2** Clubbing of the fingertips is a late sign of chronic hypoxia related to prolonged obstructive lung disease. **3** Crackles are associated with fluid in the alveoli, which occurs with heart failure and pulmonary edema.

    Client Need: Physiological Adaptation; **Cognitive Level:** Applying; **Nursing Process:** Assessment

14. **2 Hyperventilation causes excessive loss of carbon dioxide, leading to carbonic acid deficit and respiratory alkalosis.**

    1 Cardiac arrest is unlikely; the client may experience dysrhythmias, but will lose consciousness and begin breathing regularly. **3** Hyperventilation causes alkalosis; the pH is increased. **4** Excess oxygen saturation cannot occur; the usual oxygen saturation of hemoglobin is 95% to 98%.

    Client Need: Physiological Adaptation; **Cognitive Level:** Applying; **Nursing Process:** Planning

Endocrine System Disorders 16

OVERVIEW

Hormones (Table 16.1)

- Complex chemical substances that trigger or regulate an organ or group of cells
- Hormones serve as chemical messengers in the body and help maintain homeostasis.
- Hormones are released into bodily fluids, such as blood, which carry them to target cells.
- Target cells respond to a hormone when they express a specific receptor for that hormone.
- Hormones also play a role in the regulation of cell death, the immune system, reproductive development, mood swings, and hunger cravings.
- In the adrenal gland, epinephrine and norepinephrine regulate responses to stress; in the thyroid gland, thyroid hormones regulate metabolic rates.

Polypeptides

- Protein compounds
- Made of many amino acids
- Connected by peptide bonds
- Anterior pituitary gland hormones
  - Growth hormone
  - Thyroid-stimulating hormone
  - Corticotrophin-releasing hormone
  - Follicle-stimulating hormone
  - Luteinizing hormone
  - Prolactin
- Posterior pituitary hormones
  - Antidiuretic hormone
  - Oxytocin
- Parathyroid hormones
  - Parathormone or parathyroid hormone
- Pancreatic hormones
  - Glucagon
  - Insulin

Steroids

- Derived from cholesterol
- Adrenocortical hormones secreted by the adrenal cortex
  - Aldosterone
  - Cortisol
- Sex hormones secreted by the gonads
  - Female
    - Estrogen
    - Progesterone

TABLE 16.1   Structural Categories of Hormones

Structural Category	Examples
Water Soluble	
Peptides	Growth hormone
	Insulin
	Leptin
	Parathyroid hormone
	Prolactin
Glycoproteins	Follicle-stimulating hormone
	Luteinizing hormone
	Thyroid-stimulating hormone
Polypeptides	Adrenocorticotropic hormone
	Antidiuretic hormone
	Calcitonin
	Endorphins
	Glucagon
	Hypothalamic hormones
	Lipotropins
	Melanocyte-stimulating hormone
	Oxytocin
	Somatostatin
	Thymosin
	Thyrotropin-releasing hormone
Amines	Epinephrine
	Norepinephrine
Lipid Soluble	
Thyroxine (an amine but lipid soluble)	Both thyroxine (T_4) and triiodothyronine (T_3)
Steroids (cholesterol is a precursor for all steroids)	Estrogens
	Glucocorticoids (cortisol)
	Mineralocorticoids (aldosterone)
	Progestins (progesterone)
	Testosterone
Derivatives of arachidonic acid (autocrine or paracrine action)	Leukotrienes
	Prostacyclins
	Prostaglandins
	Thromboxanes

From Huether, S. E., McCance, K. L., Brashers, V. L., & Rote, S. R. (2017). *Understanding pathophysiology.* (6th ed.). St. Louis: Elsevier.

- Male
  - Testosterone

Amines

- Derived from tyrosine, an essential amino acid found in most proteins
  - Thyroid hormones
    - Thiiodothyronine (T_3) and thyroxine (T_4)
    - Catecholamines

- Epinephrine
- Norepinephrine
- Dopamine

Homeostasis

- Tendency of the body to regulate the internal environment and maintain equilibrium, usually through feedback systems to help stabilize health and functioning
- Every organ in the body contributes to homeostasis.
- A complex set of chemical, thermal, and neural factors interact in complex ways, both helping and hindering the body while it works to maintain homeostasis.
  - Stimulus: produces a change to a variable (the factor being regulated).
  - Receptor: detects the change.
  - The receptor monitors the environment and responds to change (stimuli).
  - Input: information travels along the (afferent) pathway to the control center. The control center determines the appropriate response and course of action.
  - Output: information sent from the control center travels down the (efferent) pathway to the effector.
  - Response: a response from the effector balances out the original stimulus to maintain homeostasis.
- Negative feedback mechanisms
  - Almost all homeostatic control mechanisms are negative feedback mechanisms.
  - Changes the variable back to its original state or ideal value
  - The control of blood sugar (glucose) by insulin is a good example of a negative feedback mechanism.
    - When blood sugar rises, receptors in the body sense a change.
    - In turn, the control center (pancreas) secretes insulin into the blood, effectively lowering blood sugar levels.
    - Once blood sugar levels reach homeostasis, the pancreas stops releasing insulin.
- Positive feedback mechanisms
  - A positive feedback mechanism is the exact opposite of a negative feedback mechanism.
  - In a positive feedback system, the output enhances the original stimulus.
  - An example of a positive feedback system is childbirth.
    - During labor, oxytocin is released, which intensifies and speeds up contractions.
    - The increase in contractions causes more oxytocin to be released and the cycle goes on until the baby is born.
    - Delivery of the baby ends the release of oxytocin and ends the positive feedback mechanism.

Hypothalamus

- Controls the body temperature, water balance, appetite, pituitary secretions, autonomic functions (sleeping and waking cycles), and emotions

Pituitary Gland (a.k.a the hypophysis or master gland)

- Sits in the sella turcica, which is a depression in sphenoid bone at the base of the brain.
- Blood vessels and nerves carry messages from the hypothalamus to the pituitary gland
- Two main regions of the pituitary gland
  - Anterior pituitary (adenohypophysis) hormones
    - Thyroid-stimulating hormone (TSH)

- Growth hormone (GH)/somatotropin
- Adrenocorticotropic hormone (ACTH)
- Follicle-stimulating hormone (FSH)
- Luteinizing hormone (LH)
- Melanocyte-stimulating hormone (MSH)
- Posterior pituitary hormones
  - Antidiuretic diuretic hormone (ADH)
  - Oxytocin

Problems With the Pituitary

- Hypopituitarism
  - Proportionate dwarfism
    - The body parts are in proportion but shortened.
    - GH deficiency
  - Central diabetes insipidus (DI)
    - Insufficiency of ADH
    - Kidneys cannot reclaim water.
    - Large amounts of dilute urine excreted
    - Causes of central DI
      - Traumatic brain injury
      - Aneurysms
      - Infection
      - Problem with the ADH-producing cells due to an autoimmune disease
      - Loss of blood supply to the pituitary gland
      - Surgery
        - Tumors in or near the pituitary gland
    - Signs and symptoms
      - Polydipsia (frequent drinking of liquids)
      - Polyuria (frequent urination; 8 to 12 liters of urine/day)
      - Nocturia (urinating at night time)
      - Dehydration
      - Hypernatremia
      - Hyperosmolarity
  - Hyperpituitarism
    - Gigantism
      - Excess secretion of growth hormone
      - Children and adolescents
      - Skeletal growth is excessive (8 to 9 feet tall).
    - Acromegaly
      - Excess secretion of growth hormone in adults
      - Epiphyseal plates are closed.
      - Causes
        - Pituitary tumor
      - Signs and symptoms
        - Connective tissue and bony proliferation
          - Acromegaly features
          - Enlarged tongue
        - Enlarged and overactive sebaceous and sweat glands

- Coarse skin and hair
- Enlarged bones of head, hands, face, and feet (irreversible)
- Nerves get entrapped in bones.
  - Neuralgia
- Headaches (pituitary tumor enlarges)
  - Seizures
  - Vision problems
- Barrel-chest appearance
- Hypertension
- Left ventricular hypertrophy
- Cardiomyopathy
- Sexual dysfunction
- Amenorrhea
- Diabetes mellitus
- Hyperphosphatemia
- Hyperprolactinemia
- Syndrome of inappropriate secretion of antidiuretic (SIADH)
  - Excess secretion of ADH
  - Enhanced renal water retention
  - Leads to dilutional hyponatremia, hyposomolarity, and concentrated urine
  - Causes
    - Outside central nervous system (CNS) include production of ADH by tumors elsewhere in the body and surgery
    - CNS causes include encephalitis, meningitis, intracranial hemorrhage, trauma, and tumors.
    - Medications (especially in the elderly), such as hypoglycemic, narcotics, antidepressants, antipsychotic, chemotherapeutic agents, nonsteroidal anti-inflammatory drugs (NSAIDs), general anesthesia
  - Signs and symptoms
    - Thirst
    - Impaired taste
    - Anorexia
    - Dyspnea on exertion
    - Fatigue
    - Decreased sensorium
    - Vomiting
    - Abdominal cramps
    - Weight gain from water retention
    - Confusion
    - Lethargy
    - Muscle twitching
    - Permanent neurologic damage
- Hyperprolactinemia
  - Causes
    - Prolactinoma (benign pituitary tumor)
    - Renal failure, polycystic ovarian disease, primary hypothyroidism, breast stimulation, stress
    - Medications: antipsychotics, chlorpromazine, metoclopramide, tricyclic antidepressants, methyldopa

- Signs and symptoms
  - Galactorrhea in nonpregnant/nursing women
  - Headache
  - Visual changes
  - Amenorrhea
  - Hirsutism
  - Osteopenia, osteoporosis
- Diagnosis
  - TSH level
  - Magnetic resonance imaging (MRI) scan of head

APPLICATION AND REVIEW

1. After surgical clipping of a cerebral aneurysm, the client develops the syndrome of inappropriate secretion of antidiuretic hormone. Which clinical manifestation would the nurse expect?
   1. Decreased urine output
   2. Decreased urine specific gravity
   3. Increased serum sodium level
   4. Increased blood urea nitrogen
2. Which client statements suggest an association with hormone dysfunction? **Select all that apply**.
   1. "My knees hurt when I run."
   2. "I have to get my vision checked."
   3. "My friends tell me I'm really moody."
   4. "I seem to get a lot of infections lately."
   5. "I've got this craving for salsa and chips."
3. A malfunctioning posterior pituitary gland would affect which hormones? **Select all that apply**.
   1. Oxytocin
   2. Glucagon
   3. Corticotropin
   4. Parathormone
   5. Antidiuretic hormone
4. Which clinical manifestations may be associated with a dysfunctional hypothalamus? **Select all that apply**.
   1. Edema
   2. Anorexia
   3. Insomnia
   4. Fractures
   5. Hypothermia
5. The nurse is caring for a client with a condition that causes ineffective messaging from the hypothalamus. Which assessments by the nurse would be appropriate? **Select all that apply**.
   1. Height
   2. Fluid intake
   3. Head diameter
   4. Urinary output
   5. Respiratory rate
6. Which clients are at an increased risk for developing syndrome of inappropriate antidiuretic hormone (SIADH)? **Select all that apply**.
   1. A 4-year-old client recovering from general anesthesia after abdominal surgery
   2. A 55-year-old client being medicated with a nonsteroidal anti-inflammatory drug (NSAID) for arthritis
   3. A 72-year-old client who is prescribed antipsychotic medication
   4. A 22-year-old client who is experiencing an intracranial hemorrhage
   5. A 15-year-old client who has a two-pack a day smoking habit

See Answers on pages 337–340.

Pancreas

- Nestled in the curve of the duodenum
- Lies horizontally behind the stomach extending to the spleen
- Nerves from both the sympathetic and parasympathetic divisions of the autonomic nervous system innervate the pancreatic islets.
- Endocrine function
  - Secreted hormones from islet cells or islet of Langerhans
  - Flow directly into the blood stream
  - Stimulated by blood glucose levels
  - Alpha cells
    - Produce glucagon to raise blood sugar by triggering the breakdown of glucagon to glucose
  - Beta cells
    - Produce and secrete insulin, which lowers blood sugar by stimulating the conversion of glucose to glycogen
    - Secretes amylin, which is a peptide hormone secreted with insulin in response to nutrient stimuli
      - Delays gastric emptying and suppresses glucagon secretion after meals
      - Has a satiety effect to reduce food intake
    - Secretion of insulin is regulated by chemical, neural, and hormonal control.
    - Delta cells secrete gastrin and somatostatin.
      - Produces somatostatin, which inhibits the release of growth hormone, corticotropin and other hormones
    - Acinar cells
      - These cells make up most of the pancreas.
      - Regulate pancreatic exocrine function
    - Pancreatic polypeptide (PP) cells
      - Secrete pancreatic polypeptide, which regulates carbohydrates
    - Epsilon cells
      - Secretes ghrelin
      - Newly found in the human fetus and continues to be present through adulthood; thought to support the pancreas
  - Exocrine function
    - 1000 mL of digestive juices a day
    - Secretes digestive enzymes
      - Trypsin, chymotrypsin, carboxypeptidase, and elastase
        - Protein-digesting enzymes
        - Secreted in inactive forms to spare the pancreas

Problems With the Pancreas

- Diabetes mellitus
  - Type 1
    - Genetic susceptibility
    - A trigger (may be viral) causes the production of antibodies that destroy the beta cells in the pancreas.
    - The pancreas no longer makes insulin.
    - Leads to hyperglycemia and the cells begin to starve
    - When there is no glucose to use, the body will break down fats (lipolysis) and protein catabolism.

- Signs and symptoms
  - Extreme thirst (polydipsia)
  - Extreme appetite
  - Weight loss
  - Frequent urination (polyuria)
  - Ketones in the urine (from fat metabolism)
  - Fruit breath odor
  - Drowsiness
  - High blood glucose
  - Rapid, hard, or heavy breathing (Kussmaul respirations)
  - Stupor to unconsciousness
  - Requires lifelong exogenous insulin
- Type 2
  - Genetic susceptibility
  - Insulin resistance
  - Obesity and sedentary lifestyle hasten the diabetes.
  - Pancreas can produce insulin, but it is insufficient or it is ineffective.
  - Signs and symptoms
    - May be no signs or symptoms
    - Frequent urination (polyuria)
    - Nighttime urination (nocturia)
    - Extreme thirst (polydipsia)
    - Wounds that are slow to heal
    - Dehydration
    - Dry skin
    - Fatigue
    - Unexplained weight loss
    - Sudden vision changes
- Gestational diabetes
  - Diabetes during pregnancy
  - Screening for diabetes with an oral glucose tolerance test at 24 weeks
  - Careful glucose control is imperative during pregnancy.
  - If signs and symptoms continue postnatally, the mother needs medical management.
  - Mothers are at high risk for type 2 diabetes.

Problems With the Thyroid Gland

- Hypothyroidism
  - Hashimoto thyroiditis
    - Autoimmune disorder that causes damage to the thyroid gland
    - Thyroid gland is unable to make thyroid hormones
    - It affects as many as 10 million people in the United States
    - Women affected 10 times more than men
    - Affects approximately 10% of women over age 30 have Hashimoto thyroiditis
    - There is no cure but can be managed with medication
    - Cause is unknown
    - Risk factors include
      - Family history of thyroid disease or other autoimmune diseases

- Pregnancy: thyroid problems occur in some women the first year after a pregnancy and approximately 20% of those women develop Hashimoto thyroiditis years later.
  - Ingestion of excess iodine
  - Exposure to radiation (treatment cancer)
  - Drugs
    - Amiodarone can inhibit the synthesis and release of thyroid hormone and the conversion of peripheral conversion of tetraiodothyronine (T4) to T_3.
    - Anti-thyroid medications used to treat overactive thyroid glands.
    - Interferon-alpha
    - Interleukin-2
    - Lithium slows the production and release of thyroid hormones.
- Symptoms
  - Enlarged thyroid called a goiter
    - Neck looks swollen
    - May make swallowing difficult
  - Weight gain
  - Fatigue
  - Slowed heart rate
  - Joint and muscle pain
  - Paleness or puffiness of the face
  - Constipation
  - Infertility
  - Hair thinning or loss; brittle hair
  - Depression
  - Heavy or irregular menstrual periods
- Myxedema
  - Myxedema is the result of long-standing hypothyroidism.
  - Result of the abnormal composition of the dermis and other tissues secondary to hypothyroidism.
    - Connective tissue fibers are separated by large amounts of protein and mucopolysaccharide
    - This complex binds water and causes nonpitting edema, boggy edema around the eyes, hands, feet, and in the supraclavicular fossae.
    - There is thickening of the mucus membranes, larynx, and pharynx, which leads to hoarseness, thick voice, and slurred speech.
  - Myxedema coma
    - It is rare condition but can be life-threatening
    - Requires emergent evaluation, diagnosis, and treatment
    - The person with hypothyroidism has very low levels of thyroid hormones and symptoms become worse.
    - These conditions contribute to myxedema coma.
      - Not taking thyroid medication as prescribed
      - Lung infection
      - Urinary tract infection
      - Surgery
      - Trauma

- o Heart failure
- o Stroke
- o Drugs
  - o Prolonged iodide use
  - o Phenothiazines
  - o Amiodorone
  - o Lithium
  - o Tranquilizers
- ▪ Signs and symptoms
  - o Weakness
  - o Feeling cold
  - o Swelling of the body, especially face, tongue, and lower legs
  - o Low body temperature
  - o Difficulty breathing
  - o Confusion
  - o Nonresponsiveness
- Hyperthyroidism (a.k.a. thyrotoxicosis)
  - Excess amounts of thyroid hormone from the thyroid gland
  - Signs and symptoms of hyperthyroidism
    - ▪ Related to the effects of increased circulating thyroid hormones
      - ▪ Thinning hair
      - ▪ Exophthalmos
      - ▪ Enlarged thyroid (nodular, warm)
      - ▪ Tachycardia
      - ▪ Heart failure
      - ▪ Weight loss
      - ▪ Diarrhea
      - ▪ Warm skin
      - ▪ Sweaty palms
      - ▪ Hyperreflexia
      - ▪ Pretibial edema
  - Types of hyperthyroidism
  - Graves disease
    - ▪ Most common cause of hyperthyroidism
    - ▪ More common in females
    - ▪ Cause unknown, but likely multifactorial
    - ▪ Autoimmune disease; a type II hypersensitivity
      - ▪ Thyroid-stimulating immunoglobulins (TSI) override the regulatory mechanisms, increase the levels of thyroid hormone, and enlarges the thyroid gland.
        - o TSIs specifically causes the pretibial edema (dermopathy) and the eye changes (ophthalmopathy).
        - o Dermopathy symptoms include
          - o Pretibial edema
          - o Clubbing appearance of the fingers
        - o Ophthalmopathy symptoms include
          - o Hyperactivity of the sympathetic division of the autonomic nervous system leading to lag in moving the eye upward and the upper lid downward
          - o Enlargement of the ocular muscles

- These changes lead to exophthalmos, periorbital edema, and extraocular muscle weakness, which causes diplopia.
- Eye irritation, lacrimation, photophobia, decreased visual acuity, papilledema, and visual field impairment
- The exposed cornea can become inflamed or ulcerated.
- The aforementioned signs and symptoms of hyperthyroidism are also present in Grave disease.
- Nodular thyroid disease
  - Several hyperfunctioning nodules of the thyroid gland that lead to hyperthyroidism
  - A single hyperfunctioning nodule is called a toxic adenoma.
  - Classic symptoms of hyperthyroidism usually develop slowly.
  - There is no pretibial edema or exophthalmos.
  - Can be malignant
- Thyrotoxic crisis (thyroid storm)
  - Rare but can lead to death within 48 hours.
  - Caused by the thyroxine (T3) and triiodothyronine (T4) exceeding the body's demand
  - Usually happens in undiagnosed or partially treated Graves disease and is subject to the following conditions
    - Stress
    - Infection
    - Pulmonary or cardiac problems
    - Trauma
    - Surgery (especially thyroid surgery)
    - Obstetric complications
    - Dialysis
  - Signs and symptoms
    - Hyperthermia
    - Tachycardia and tachyarrhythmias
    - High-output heart failure
    - Tachyarrhythmias
    - Agitation
    - Delirium
    - Nausea, vomiting and diarrhea

APPLICATION AND REVIEW

7. Which clinical findings should the nurse assess when caring for a client diagnosed with hyperthyroidism? **Select all that apply.**
   1. Lethargy
   2. Tachycardia
   3. Weight gain
   4. Constipation
   5. Exophthalmos
8. Which statements should be included in a discussion about the pancreas? **Select all that apply**.
   1. The beta cells in the pancreas are associated with the lowering of blood sugar.
   2. The alpha cells in the pancreas support the breakdown of glucose to glycogen.
   3. The pancreas secretes hormones from the islet of Langerhans.
   4. The pancreas is associated with the endocrine system.
   5. The pancreas lies behind the stomach.

9. Which exocrine functions are provided by the pancreas? **Select all that apply**.
   1. Secretion of trypsin
   2. Secretion of insulin
   3. Secretion of elastase
   4. Production of digestive juices
   5. Regulation of endocrine function

10. What information should be included in a discussion about type 1 diabetes mellitus? **Select all that apply**.
    1. It can trigger protein catabolism.
    2. It can be triggered by pregnancy.
    3. It is believed to have a genetic risk factor.
    4. It ultimately results in the starvation of cells.
    5. It supports the destruction of beta cells.

11. Which statements, if made by a client, should alert the nurse to further assess for signs and symptoms of type 1 diabetes mellitus? **Select all that apply**.
    1. "I can't seem to lose weight."
    2. "I'm almost never thirsty."
    3. "I always feel sleepy."
    4. "I'm always hungry."
    5. "I urinate a lot."

12. How do type 1 and type 2 diabetes mellitus differ?
    1. Only type 1 presents with thirst as a symptom.
    2. Only type 2 presents with frequent urination.
    3. Only type 1 presents with unexplained weight loss.
    4. Only type 2 is accelerated by a sedentary lifestyle.

13. A female client who develops hyperglycemia during pregnancy asks, "Will I be diabetic now?" Which response by the nurse is best?
    1. "This does increase your risk of developing diabetes."
    2. "It's only a likelihood if diabetes runs in your family."
    3. "Symptoms generally go away once the baby is delivered."
    4. "Your primary health care provider will discuss the risks with you."

14. Which statements, if made by a client, support a diagnosis of hyperthyroidism? **Select all that apply**.
    1. "My hair is getting very thin."
    2. "My palms are always sweaty."
    3. "I have diarrhea at least twice a week."
    4. "I'm always cold and need a sweater."
    5. "I'm told my thyroid is getting bigger."

See Answers on pages 337–340.

Parathyroid Gland (Fig. 16.1)

- Smallest endocrine gland
- Embedded on the posterior surface of the thyroid in each corner
- Produces parathyroid hormone (PTH)
- PTH helps regulate calcium balance
- Adjusts the rate at which calcium and magnesium ions are lost in the urine
- Increases the movement of phosphate ions from the blood to the urine for excretion

Problems With the Parathyroid Gland

- Hypoparathyroidism
  - Caused most often by damage to the parathyroid gland during thyroid surgery
  - Hypomagnesemia can cause a decrease in PTH secretion and function.
    - Alcoholism
    - Malnutrition

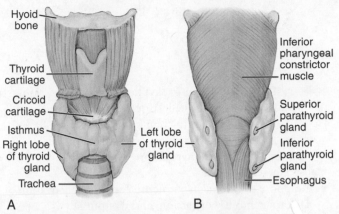

FIG. 16.1 Thyroid and parathyroid glands. **A,** Anterior view. **B,** Posterior view. (From Fehrenbach, M. J., & Herring, S. W. [2016]. Illustrated anatomy of the head and neck [5th ed.]. Philadelphia: Saunders.)

- Idiopathic or autoimmune forms also
- Causes decreased calcium levels and increased phosphate levels
- Decreases renal clearance of phosphate resulting in hyperphosphatemia
- Signs and symptoms
  - Lower threshold for nerve and muscle excitement
    - Tetany (muscle spasm, hyperreflexia)
    - Chvostek sign: tapping the cheek results in twitching of the upper lip
    - Trousseau sign: carpopedal spasm caused by inflating the blood-pressure cuff to a level above systolic pressure for 3 minutes.
  - Dry skin
  - Hair loss
  - Damaged teeth
  - Horizontal ridges in the nails
  - Cataracts
  - Bone deformities
    - Tibial bowing
  - Clonic-tonic seizures
  - Laryngeal spasms
  - Death by asphyxia
  - Tooth deformities, cataracts, and bone deformities do not resolve after treatment.
- Hyperparathyroidism
  - Types of hyperparathyroidism
    - Primary hyperparathyroidism
      - Adenoma or gland hyperplasia
      - Excess secretion of PTH by one or both parathyroid glands
      - Common endocrine disorder
      - Calcium level increased because of bone resorption and gastrointestinal absorption of calcium.
      - Signs and symptoms
        - Hypercalcemia and hypophosphatemia
        - May be asymptomatic

- ○ Nausea and vomiting
- ○ Anorexia
- ○ Fatigue
- ○ Headache
- ○ Depression
- ○ Pathologic fractures, kyphosis, and compression fractures of vertebral bodies from increased osteoclastic and osteocytic activity
- ○ Increased risk of calcium kidney stones
- ○ Increased risk of urinary tract infection (UTI)
  - ▪ Secondary hyperparathyroidism
- Caused by renal disease
  - ▪ Response to chronic hypocalcemia and renal activation of vitamin D
  - ▪ Dietary deficiency of calcium and vitamin D
  - ▪ Ingestion of certain medications
  - ▪ Signs and symptoms
    - ▪ Increased bone resorption
    - ▪ Symptoms of hypocalcemia
    - ▪ Symptoms of hyperphosphatemia
- Tertiary hyperparathyroidism
  - ▪ Excess secretion of PTH and hypercalcemia that occurs after long-standing hyperparathyroidism

Adrenal Glands

- Two glands each on the top of a kidney
- Two parts
- Adrenal cortex
  - Three layers
    - ▪ Zona glomerulosa
      - ▪ Outermost zone
      - ▪ Produces mineralocorticoids (aldosterone)
      - ▪ Maintains fluid balance by increasing sodium reabsorption
    - ▪ Zona fasciculate
      - ▪ Middle and largest layer
      - ▪ Produces the glucocorticoids
        - ○ Cortisol (hydrocortisone)
        - ○ Cortisone
        - ○ Corticosterone
      - ▪ Produces sex hormones
        - ○ Estrogen
        - ○ Androgen
        - ○ Glucocorticoids help maintain metabolism and resistance to stress.
    - ▪ Zona reticularis
      - ▪ Innermost layer
      - ▪ Produces gonadocorticoids which
        - ○ Dehydroepiandrosterone (DHEA)
        - ○ DHEA sulfate

- Adrenal medulla
  - Innermost layer of the adrenal gland
  - Part of the sympathetic nervous system
  - Produces two catecholamines
    - Epinephrine
    - Norepinephrine
  - Both are important in the autonomic nervous system.
  - Adrenal medulla is considered a neuroendocrine structure.

Adrenal Gland Disorders

- Addison disease
  - Primary adrenal insufficiency
  - Decreased mineralocorticoid, glucocorticoid, and androgen secretion
  - Uncommon; occurs in both males and females
  - Signs and symptoms
    - Weakness and fatigue
    - Weight loss
    - Hyperpigmentation of the skin especially in the creases of the hands
    - Darkening of scars
    - Areas of vitiligo (white skin; loss of melanin)
    - Orthostatic hypotension (blood pressure drops when standing up)
    - Irregular pulse
    - Unable to tolerate stress
    - Crave salty foods
    - Fasting hypoglycemia
- Addisonian crisis
  - Causes
    - Addison disease not yet diagnosed
    - When there is no response to hormone replacement therapy
    - Experiences stress without adequate glucocorticoid replacement
    - Stop hormone replacement abruptly
    - Experiences trauma
    - Adrenalectomy
  - Signs and symptoms are a progression of the symptoms of Addison disease
    - Anorexia, nausea, vomiting, and diarrhea
    - Hypotension $\rightarrow$ vascular collapse $\rightarrow$ shock
- Cushing syndrome (hypercortisolism)
  - Causes
    - Excess endogenous secretion of ACTH
    - More common in females than males
    - Loss of circadian rhythm patterns of ACTH and cortisol secretion
    - No increased ACTH or cortisol release secondary to stress
  - Signs and symptoms
    - Weight gain
    - Accumulation of adipose tissue in the trunk, face, and cervical areas
      - Moon face

- Buffalo hump
- Truncal obesity
  - Glucose intolerance from cortisol-induced insulin resistance and increase gluconeogenesis in the liver
  - Polyuria from hyperglycemia
  - Protein wasting from the catabolic effect of cortisol on peripheral tissues
  - Muscle weakness
  - Osteoporosis
    - Pathologic fractures
  - Back pain
  - Loss of collagen makes skin loose
    - Purple striae
  - High blood pressure
  - Sodium and potassium loss
  - Increased androgen levels
    - Facial hair
    - Acne
    - Limited menstrual cycles
- Diagnosis
  - Blood tests
    - Hyperglycemia
    - Glycosuria
    - Hypokalemia
    - Metabolic alkalosis
    - Confirmatory tests
    - Elevated urinary free cortisol level
    - Late night salivary cortisol levels
- Pheochromocytoma
  - Tumor of adrenal medulla
  - Rare, 10% malignant with extensive metastasis
  - Sympathetic para gangliomas
  - Excessive production of norepinephrine
  - Large tumors secrete epinephrine and norepinephrine.
  - Signs and symptoms
    - Hypertension
    - Headache
    - Pallor
    - Diaphoresis (sweating)
    - Tachycardia palpitations
    - Glucose intolerance
    - Tumor is vascular and can rupture.
  - Signs and symptoms worsened by
    - Exercise
    - Eating too many foods with tyrosine
    - Caffeine ingestion
    - Pressure on the tumor
    - Induction of anesthesia

APPLICATION AND REVIEW

15. The nurse is caring for a client who has Addison disease. Which discharge instruction should the nurse emphasize for this client about an Addisonian crisis?
    1. Decrease glucocorticoid medication during emotional stress
    2. Hypertension and hyperglycemia are expected during a crisis.
    3. Never abruptly stop taking glucocorticoid medication
    4. Emotional stress cannot cause a crisis to occur.

16. A client experiencing adrenal insufficiency reports feeling weak and dizzy, especially in the morning. What should the nurse determine is the most probable cause of these symptoms?
    1. A lack of potassium
    2. Postural hypertension
    3. A hypoglycemic episode
    4. Increased extracellular fluid volume

17. A dysfunction in which hormones would likely affect the client's response to stress. **Select all that apply**.
    1. Epinephrine
    2. Progesterone
    3. Norepinephrine
    4. Growth hormone
    5. Thyroid-stimulating hormone

18. What is the most common direct cause of hypoparathyroidism?
    1. General malnutrition
    2. Complication of thyroid surgery
    3. Ineffective absorption of sunlight
    4. Effects of alcohol on the parathyroid

19. How does the nurse perform an assessment associated with the Chvostek sign?
    1. Tapping the cheek to monitor for the twitching of the upper lip
    2. Gently striking the jaw to monitor for involuntary opening of the mouth
    3. Inflating a blood pressure cuff for 3 minutes to monitor for hyperflexion in the wrist
    4. Inflating a blood pressure cuff to pressure 3 points above systolic pressure to monitor for finger pain

See Answers on pages 337–340.

ANSWER KEY: REVIEW QUESTIONS

1. **1 Antidiuretic hormone (ADH) causes water retention, resulting in decreased urine output.**
   2 ADH acts on nephrons to cause water to be reabsorbed from glomerular filtrate, leading to an increased specific gravity of urine. **3** The client is overhydrated so that serum sodium is decreased. **4** Blood volume may increase, causing dilution of nitrogenous wastes in the blood.
   Client Need: Physiological Adaptation; **Cognitive Level:** Applying; **Nursing Process:** Planning

2. **Answers: 3, 4, 5.**
   3, 4, 5 Hormones play a role in the regulation of cell death, the immune system, reproductive development, mood swings, and hunger cravings.
   1 Joint pain, triggered by exercise, is not generally associated with hormone dysfunction. **2** Vision changes are not generally associated with hormone dysfunction.
   Client Need: Physiological Adaptation; **Cognitive Level:** Analysis; **Nursing Process:** Analysis

3. **Answers: 1, 5.**

   1 Posterior pituitary hormones include oxytocin. **5** Posterior pituitary hormones include ADH.

   2 Glucagon is a pancreatic hormone. **3** Corticotropin is an anterior pituitary gland hormone. **4** Parathormone is a parathyroid hormone.

   Client Need: Physiological Adaptation; **Cognitive Level:** Understanding; **Integrated Process:** Teaching and Learning

4. **Answers: 1, 2, 3, 5.**

   1, 2, 3, 5 The hypothalamus controls the body temperature (hypothermia), water balance (edema), appetite (anorexia), and autonomic functions (sleeping and waking cycles).

   4 Bone formation/strength is not related to the hypothalamus.

   Client Need: Physiological Adaptation; **Cognitive Level:** Applying; **Nursing Process:** Analysis

5. **Answer: 1, 2, 3, 4.**

   1 Blood vessels and nerves carry messages from the hypothalamus to the pituitary gland. A problem with this connection would affect pituitary production of growth hormone, triggering proportionate dwarfism. **2** Blood vessels and nerves carry messages from the hypothalamus to the pituitary gland. A problem with this connection would affect pituitary production of ADH resulting in diabetes insipidus (DI) causing large amounts of dilute urine to be excreted. **3** Blood vessels and nerves carry messages from the hypothalamus to the pituitary gland. A problem with this connection would affect pituitary production of growth hormone triggering gigantism with its associated acromegaly. **4** Blood vessels and nerves carry messages from the hypothalamus to the pituitary gland. A problem with this connection would affect pituitary production of ADH resulting in diabetes insipidus (DI) causing polydipsia (frequent drinking of liquids).

   5 Respiratory rate is not directly associated with hypothalamus or pituitary function.

   Client Need: Physiological Adaptation; **Cognitive Level:** Analysis; **Nursing Process:** Analysis

6. **Answers: 1, 2, 3, 4.**

   1 Excess secretion of ADH can be triggered by general anesthesia. **2** Excess secretion of ADH can be triggered by NSAID use. **3** Excess secretion of ADH can be triggered by antipsychotic medication therapy. **4** Excess secretion of ADH can be triggered by an intracranial hemorrhage.

   5 Smoking tobacco is not associated with SIADH.

   Client Need: Physiological Adaptation; **Cognitive Level:** Analysis; **Nursing Process:** Analysis

7. **Answers: 2, 5.**

   2 Tachycardia is associated with hyperthyroidism and is caused by an increase in the basal metabolic rate. **5** Exophthalmos is associated with hyperthyroidism and results from the accumulation of fluid behind the eyeball.

   1 Lethargy is associated with hypothyroidism; hyperactivity occurs with hyperthyroidism. **3** Weight gain occurs with hypothyroidism; weight loss occurs with hyperthyroidism because of the high metabolic rate. **4** Constipation is associated with hypothyroidism; frequent loose stools occur with hyperthyroidism.

   Client Need: Physiological Adaptation; **Cognitive Level:** Applying; **Nursing Process:** Assessment

8. **Answers: 1, 3, 4, 5.**

   1 The beta cells in the pancreas produce insulin that lowers blood sugar. **3** The pancreas secretes hormones from the islet of Langerhans. **4** The pancreas does have endocrine functions. **5** The pancreas lies horizontally behind the stomach extending to the spleen.

   2. Alpha cells produce glucagon to raise blood sugar by triggering the breakdown of glucagon to glucose.

   Client Need: Physiological Adaptation; **Cognitive Level:** Understanding; **Integrated Process:** Teaching and Learning

9. **Answers: 1, 3, 4.**

   1 Exocrine functions performed by the pancreas include the secretion of the digestive enzyme trypsin. **3** Exocrine functions performed by the pancreas include the secretion of the digestive enzyme elastase. **4** Exocrine functions performed by the pancreas include the secretion of the digestive juices.

2 Insulin secretion is considered an endocrine function. **5** The regulation of endocrine function is not an exocrine function.

Client Need: Physiological Adaptation; **Cognitive Level:** Understanding; **Integrated Process:** Teaching and Learning

10. **Answers: 1, 3, 4, 5.**

    1 Type 1 diabetes causes protein catabolism when there is no longer enough glucose to be utilized. **3** Type 1 diabetes is believed to create a genetic susceptibility passed from generation to generation. **4** Type 1 diabetes leads to hyperglycemia and the cells begin to starve. **5** Type 1 diabetes causes the production of antibodies that destroy the beta cells in the pancreas.

    2 Gestational diabetes is triggered by the stressors of pregnancy.

    Client Need: Physiological Adaptation; **Cognitive Level:** Understanding; **Integrated Process:** Teaching and Learning

11. **Answers: 3, 4, 5.**

    3 Drowsiness is a symptom of type 1 diabetes. **4** Extreme appetite is a symptom of type 1 diabetes. **5** Frequent urination is a symptom of type 1 diabetes.

    1 Weight loss is a symptom of type 1 diabetes. **2** Extreme thirst is a symptom of type 1 diabetes.

    Client Need: Physiological Adaptation; **Cognitive Level:** Analysis; **Nursing Process:** Assessment

12. **4 Type 2 diabetes is hastened by obesity and a sedentary lifestyle.**

    1, 2, 3 Both type 1 and type 2 diabetes can present with thirst, frequent urination, and unexplained weight loss.

    Client Need: Physiological Adaptation; **Cognitive Level:** Understanding; **Integrated Process:** Teaching and Learning

13. **1 Females who develop diabetes during pregnancy are at high risk for developing type 2 diabetes.**

    2 Although diabetes is believed to have a genetic component, this response does not address the client's concern effectively. **3** Although the symptoms may resolve, the risk for type 2 diabetes is considered high. **4** The nurse should provide the client with a response; the nurse can then offer to have the discussion continue with the primary care provider.

    Client Need: Physiological Adaptation; **Cognitive Level:** Analysis; **Integrated Process:** Teaching and Learning.

14. **Answers: 1, 2, 3, 5.**

    1 Thinning hair can be a sign of hyperthyroidism. **2** Sweaty palms can be a sign of hyperthyroidism. **3** Diarrhea can be a sign of hyperthyroidism. **5** An enlarged thyroid can be a sign of hyperthyroidism.

    4 Heat intolerance rather than cold intolerance can be a sign of hyperthyroidism.

    Client Need: Physiological Adaptation; **Cognitive Level:** Analysis; **Nursing Process:** Assessment

15. **3 Clients with Addison disease must take glucocorticoids regularly to enable them to adapt physiologically to stress and prevent an Addisonian crisis, a medical emergency-like shock.**

    1 Glucocorticoid medications should be increased during emotional stress. **2** Hypotension and hypoglycemia are expected findings during an Addisonian crisis. **4** Both emotional and physiologic stress can cause an Addisonian crisis.

    Client Need: Physiological Adaptation; **Cognitive Level:** Applying; **Nursing Process:** Planning

16. **3** Deficiency of glucocorticoids causes hypoglycemia in the client with Addison disease. Clinical manifestations of hypoglycemia include nervousness; weakness; dizziness; cool, moist skin; hunger; and tremors.

    1 Hypokalemia is evidenced by nausea, vomiting, muscle weakness, and dysrhythmias. **2** Weakness with dizziness on arising is postural hypotension, not hypertension. **4** An increased extracellular fluid volume is evidenced by edema, increased blood pressure, and crackles.

    Client Need: Physiological Adaptation; **Cognitive Level:** Analysis; **Nursing Process:** Analysis

17. **Answers: 1, 3.**

    1, 3 In the adrenal gland, epinephrine and norepinephrine regulate responses to stress.

    2 Progesterone is associated with female reproduction. **4** In the thyroid gland, thyroid hormones regulate metabolic rates.

    Client Need: Physiological Adaptation; **Cognitive Level:** Understanding; **Integrated Process:** Teaching and Learning

18. **2 Damage to the parathyroid gland during thyroid surgery is the most common cause of hypopara-thyroidism.**
    1 While malnutrition can cause a decreased secretion of parathyroid hormone (PTH) by causing hypomagnesemia, it is not a direct cause of hypoparathyroidism. **3** Sunlight is not a factor in the development of hypoparathyroidism. **4** While alcoholism can cause a decreased secretion of PTH by causing hypomagnesemia, it is not a direct cause of hypoparathyroidism.
    Client Need: Physiological Adaptation; **Cognitive Level:** Understanding; **Integrated Process:** Teaching and Learning

19. **1 Chvostek sign assessment involves tapping the cheek and observing for twitching of the upper lip.**
    2 Gently striking the jaw to monitor for involuntary opening of the mouth is not reflective of a Chvostek sign assessment. **3** A Trousseau sign is elicited by placing a blood pressure cuff on the arm, inflating the cuff slightly above the systolic pressure, leaving the cuff inflated 2 to 3 minutes, and deflating. A carpal spasm is a positive response. **4** Inflating a blood pressure cuff to pressure 3 points above systolic pressure to monitor for finger pain is not reflective of a Chvostek sign assessment.
    Client Need: Physiological Adaptation; **Cognitive Level:** Applying; **Nursing Process:** Assessment

Gastrointestinal System Disorders 17

DIGESTIVE SYSTEM OVERVIEW

- Also known as the gastrointestinal (GI) tract, alimentary tract, or gut
- Extends through entire torso of the body
- Functions of digestive tract
  - Processes and digests food contents
  - Absorbs nutrients, electrolytes, and fluid
  - Excretes waste products
- Composed of upper and lower sections
  - Upper section
    - Mouth
    - Pharynx
    - Esophagus
    - Stomach
  - Lower portion
    - Small intestine
    - Large intestine
    - Rectum
    - Anus
- Accessory glands and organs
  - Consists of salivary glands, liver, gallbladder, and pancreas
  - Essential for secreting digestive enzymes and metabolizing products necessary for the body to function

Digestion and Absorption

- Nutrients in digested food are broken into simple molecules, which are then absorbed into the general blood circulation and ultimately transported to the liver.
- Carbohydrates
  - Digestion
    - Mouth and small intestine
    - Simple sugars (monosaccharides)
  - Absorption
    - Jejunum and ileum
      - Glucose and galactose
        - Cotransport mechanism bound to transport protein (with sodium)
      - Fructose
        - Facilitated diffusion
- Proteins
  - Digestion
    - Into peptides in stomach and small intestine
    - Into amino acids in small intestine
  - Absorption
    - Sodium cotransport system in small intestine

- Lipids or fats
  - Primarily triglycerides
  - Digestion
    - Bile converts into tiny droplets.
    - Enzymes breakdown into monoglycerides and free fatty acids.
  - Absorption
    - Diffuse across cell membrane
    - May form into triglycerides again
      - Bound to protein to form chylomicrons
      - Eventually reach liver or adipose cells via the lymph and blood system
    - Short chain fatty acids
      - Diffuse directly into the general circulation
- Fat-soluble vitamins (A, D, E, and K)
  - Digestion
    - Not necessary
  - Absorption
    - Absorbed with the fatty acid
- Very small lipid-soluble molecules (alcohol)
  - Absorption
    - Simple diffusion across the membrane into the blood
      - Results in quick high blood alcohol levels
    - Food in the stomach delays absorption.
- Water-soluble vitamins (B and C) and minerals (iron, copper, zinc)
  - Diffuse directly into the blood
- Vitamin B_{12}
  - Absorption
    - Requires binding to intrinsic factor
- Electrolytes (e.g. potassium)
  - Absorption
    - Active transport
    - Diffusion
- Water
  - Absorption
    - Osmosis
- Drugs
  - Digestion
    - Enzymes break down some drugs
  - Absorption
    - Primarily small intestine
    - Small acidic molecules (aspirin) in stomach
    - Small molecules in oral mucosa
    - Some interfere with the absorption of other drugs.
    - Food in stomach or intestine can delay absorption.

Oral Cavity

- First section of upper GI section
  - Mouth is separated from the nasal cavity by soft and hard palates.

- Initiates mechanical breakdown of food
  - Mastication process by teeth
  - Saliva
  - Produced by parotid, sublingual, and submandibular glands
  - Secreted into mouth by salivary ducts
  - Softens and lubricates food bulk
- Digestive process begins
  - Carbohydrate digestion
    - Amylase in saliva
- Movement of food to pharynx
  - Facilitated by tongue and cheeks

Pharynx

- Located behind the oral cavity
- Role in digestion
  - Receives food products from the oral cavity
  - Receptors of the trigeminal and glossopharyngeal nerves located in the pharynx activate the swallowing center in the medulla of the brain.
    - The swallowing center controls the process of moving food or fluid down the esophagus into the stomach.
    - Prevents aspiration of food contents into the lungs

Esophagus

- Muscular tube that connects the pharynx to the stomach
- Esophageal structure
  - Upper portion: skeletal muscle
  - Gradually replaced by smooth muscle
  - Lined with mucous membranes for lubrication
- Role in digestion
  - Esophageal wall expands and peristalsis is initiated to pass food contents to the stomach.
  - Distal portion of the esophagus drops through an opening (hiatus) in the diaphragm to merge with the stomach in the abdominal cavity.
  - Esophageal sphincter relaxes to allow the food contents to enter the stomach.
  - Esophageal sphincter pressure usually prevents reflux of gastric contents back into the esophagus.
  - Esophagus tube normally only opens during swallowing.

Stomach

- Function
  - Muscular elastic sac serves as a reservoir for food and liquid
  - Holds up to 1 to 1.5 liters
  - Reshapes into folds or rugae when empty
- Role in digestion
  - Breakdown of food aided by secretions of gastric glands
    - Gastric glands located on fundus of stomach
      - Secretes hormone gastrin when food enters stomach

- Gastrin activates parietal cells and chief cells in glands.
- Parietal and chief cells
  - Produce enzymes hydrochloric acid and pepsinogen (pepsin in its active form)
    - Hydrochloric acid and pepsin kill microorganisms that enter the stomach from the normal flora of the mouth.
    - Produce mucus to protect stomach lining from acidic enzymes
  - Protein digestion begins.
    - Results in creamy fluid called chyme
- Role in absorption of nutrients
  - Parietal cells produce intrinsic factors.
    - For absorption of vitamin B_{12} in the small intestine
- Chyme passes slowly into the small intestine through the pyloric sphincter into the duodenum.
- Digestion and virtually all absorption of nutrients continue in the small intestine.

Small Intestine

- Consists of three sections in the lower GI section
  - Duodenum
  - Jejunum
  - Ileum
- Peristalsis
  - Gastric contents or chyme move slowly along the small intestine proximal to distal in direction.
  - Chyme is propelled forward by the mixing of ingredients and intestinal wall movements.
- Digestion
  - Duodenum continues the digestion process by adding enzymes.
    - Pepsidases, nucleotidases, lipase, sucrase, maltase, and lactase enzymes
    - Make chyme more alkaline in pH
    - Goblet cells in the intestine secrete large amount of mucus to protect the intestine and alkaline the acidic chyme.
- Absorption
  - Ileum
    - Site for the majority of absorption of nutrients
  - Structures in small intestine
    - Mucosa with transverse folds lined with numerous villa and microvilla
      - Tiny projections in small intestine
      - Increase surface area for greater absorption
      - Contain capillary networks, nerves, and lymphatic vessels for absorption of nutrients and lipids

Large Intestine

- Structure
  - Ileocecal valve designates the transition from the ileum of the small intestine to the large intestine.
  - Cecum is a pouch located at this point from which the appendix extends down.
  - Superior from the cecum is the ascending colon moving to the transverse colon and the descending colon, which passes down the left side of the torso.
  - Large intestine terminates as the sigmoid colon, rectum, and the anus.

- Peristalsis
  - Slow in the colon to promote absorption of fluid and formation of formed feces
- Absorption
  - Nutrients
    - Primarily completed in small intestine
  - Fluids and electrolytes
    - Large amounts absorbed in the colon
  - Fluid and acid–base balances are adjusted in the large intestine by absorbing large volumes of bicarbonate and sodium.
- Role of bacteria
  - Aids in synthesizing vitamin K for clotting factors produced in the liver
  - Assists in the breakdown of certain food materials for excretion
    - Causes intestinal gas
- Excretion
  - Large pouches (haustra) in the intestinal wall allow for distention as solid materials are collected.
  - Large bulk of solid materials in the colon increases peristalsis and the rate of passage of fecal material.
  - Strong peristalsis in the transverse and descending colon occurs several times a day.
  - Feces consist of fiber, sloughed mucosal cells, bacteria, and other indigestible material.

Rectum/Anus

- Store fecal material
- Defecation
  - Distention of the rectal wall stimulates the defecation reflex.
  - Sensory nerves' impulses cause pelvic muscles to contract.
  - Voluntary relaxation of the internal and external sphincter to defecate

Liver

- Location
  - Right upper quadrant of the abdomen
  - Under the diaphragm
- Structure
  - Fibrous capsule
  - Divided into four lobes
  - Lobes are divided into lobules.
    - Contain rows of hepatocytes (liver cells)
      - Can regenerate in a healthy liver
    - Hepatocytes close contact with blood-filled channels (sinusoids)
      - Channels carry blood from hepatic artery.
        - Provide oxygen to hepatocytes
        - Carry blood from the portal vein.
        - Transport nutrients from the stomach and intestine to the hepatocytes
    - Hepatic artery and hepatic portal vein branches and bile duct are located near the perimeter of the lobule.
- Function of cells in liver
  - Manage most metabolic actions
    - Absorb iron, copper, vitamins (A, B_{12}, D, K), and folic acid

- Monitor and replace blood components
  - Iron and amino acids
- Maintain blood glucose levels
  - Converting glucose to glucagon
  - Glycogenesis
  - Glucagon is stored in the liver.
  - Stored when blood glucose levels are high
- Breakdown glucagon to glucose
- Glycogenolysis
- Glucose manufactured from carbohydrate molecules
  - Response to low blood glucose levels
    - Synthesize and control plasma protein clotting factors
    - Synthesize cholesterol
      - For production of
        - Cortisol, sex hormones, and bile salts
    - Inactivates aldosterone and estrogen
      - For excretion
    - Removes ammonia from the blood
      - Converts to urea
      - Excreted by kidneys
    - Detoxifies drugs and alcohol
      - Makes less harmful
      - More soluble for excretion
    - Removes nonfunctioning erythrocytes
      - Reuses protein and iron from hemoglobin
    - Produces bile
      - For digestion
      - Breakdown of fats and fat-soluble vitamins for absorption in small intestine
      - Bicarbonate ions in bile neutralize gastric acid in the small intestine so pancreatic and intestinal enzymes are effective.
      - For removing bilirubin and excess cholesterol
- Releases a large volume of blood into circulation when volume is low

Gallbladder

- Location
  - Right side of abdomen
  - Under the liver
- Function
  - Storage for bile
    - Enters common bile duct via left and right hepatic ducts

Pancreas

- Location
  - Behind the stomach
  - Head of pancreas next to duodenum
- Function
  - Secretion of digestive enzymes
    - Trypsin, chymotrypsin, carboxypeptidase, and ribonuclease

- Amylase
  - Carbohydrates
- Lipase
  - Fats
- Enzymes are inactive until they enter the duodenum.
- Secretion of electrolytes
- Secretion of water
- Secretion of bicarbonate ions
  - Neutralizes hydrochloric acid in the duodenum
- Drain into main pancreatic duct via smaller ducts
- Structure
  - Pancreatic duct
    - Joins common bile duct
    - Drains into duodenum

Layers of Gastrointestinal Wall

- The GI system has primarily five continuous layers with some variations throughout the system.

Mucosa

- Location
  - Inner layer of intestinal wall
- Function
  - Contains mucus-producing cells
    - Mucus
      - Facilitates movement of GI contents
      - Provides protection for the tissues
  - Epithelial cells
    - Breakdown quickly as GI contents scrape mucosal wall
    - Rapidly replaced
  - Contain villa

Submucosa

- Location
  - Layer lies next to the mucosa
- Structure
  - Consists of
    - Connective tissue
    - Blood vessels
    - Nerves
    - Lymphatic tissue
    - Secreting glands
- Function
  - Supports mucosa layer

Muscle

- Location
  - Lies above the submucosal layer

- Structure
  - Circular and longitudinal smooth muscle fibers
- Function
  - Provides peristalsis of contents in GI tract

Serosa

- Location
  - Outer most layer of GI tract
- Structure
  - Loose connective tissue
  - Smooth membrane
    - Cells secrete serous fluid.
      - Lubricates tissue to reduce friction

Peritoneum

- Large continuous double-layered serous membrane
  - One layer lines abdominal cavity.
  - One layer lines the organs.
    - Stomach, small and large intestine, liver, gallbladder, pancreas, and spleen
- Function
  - Supports organs
  - Allows nerves, blood vessels, and lymph vessels to reach organs

Parietal Peritoneum

- Outer layer of peritoneum
  - Serous membrane
  - Covers the abdominal wall
  - Covers the upper surface of the uterus and bladder
- Pain receptors
  - Senses pain from the abdominal wall

Visceral Peritoneum

- Inner layer of peritoneum
  - Serous membrane
  - Wraps around internal organs
    - Stomach, spleen, liver, sections of the intestines, uterus, and ovaries

Peritoneal Cavity

- Location
  - Area between parietal and visceral peritoneum
- Function
  - Potential space with serous fluid
    - Allows movement of organs (stomach)
    - Excess fluid drains through the lymphatic system.
    - Peritoneal dialysis
      - Permeability and vascular characteristics
- Membrane capable of spreading infection or tumor cells to abdominal cavity or general circulation owing to permeability

Mesentery
- Particular fold of the peritoneum
- Function
  - Holds intestines in place
    - Attaches jejunum and ileum to posterior abdominal wall
    - Supports and allows flexibility of intestines
    - Facilitates peristalsis
    - Transports blood vessels and nerves to intestinal wall

Gastrointestinal Abnormalities
Cleft Lip
- Characteristics
  - Common developmental deformity
    - Occurs at 2 to 3 months' gestation
  - Mild or severe deformity
    - One or both sides of lip
    - May also have cleft palate
- Etiology
  - Failure of the upper lip to fuse
  - Failure of the maxillary processes to fuse with naval elevations

Cleft Palate
- Characteristics
  - Common developmental deformity
    - Occurs at 2 to 3 months' gestation
  - Opening between oral and nasal cavity
    - Problems with feeding because of poor sucking
    - Respiratory problems owing to risk of aspiration
    - Poor speech development
- Etiology
  - Failure of hard palate and soft palate to fuse

Pyloric Stenosis
- Location of pyloric sphincter
  - Between stomach and duodenum
- Function
  - Controls flow of food contents from stomach to duodenum
- Stenosis
  - Sphincter becomes tough and enlarged.
  - Blocks food contents from entering the duodenum
- Infants
  - Congenital deformity
    - Evident at weeks of birth
  - Characteristics
    - Narrowing and obstruction of pyloric sphincter
    - Hypertrophied and palpable hard mass
  - Signs and symptoms
    - Regurgitation of food

- Projectile vomiting
- Stools are small and infrequent
- No weight gain
- Infant irritable and hungry
- Adults
  - No apparent cause
  - Signs and symptoms
    - Delayed gastric emptying
    - Fullness and vomiting
    - Weight loss

Dysphagia

- Difficulty swallowing
  - May be associated with pain
  - Severe or mild
    - Inability to swallow large solid pieces
    - Inability to swallow liquids
  - Causes
    - Neurologic
      - Brain damage due to stroke, trauma
      - Infection
      - Achalasia
        - Esophageal sphincter does not open to stomach because of muscular nerve damage.
        - Food contents back up into the esophagus.
    - Muscular
      - Parkinson disease, muscular dystrophy, muscular sclerosis
    - Mechanical obstruction
      - Congenital atresia
        - Upper esophagus ends and does not connect with the lower esophagus and stomach.
  - Signs and symptoms
    - Vomiting
    - Coughing or choking
    - Respiratory dysfunction or distress due to aspiration
- Esophageal stenosis and esophageal stricture
  - Causes
    - Developmental defect
    - Radiation therapy
    - Esophageal ulcers
    - Esophageal fibrosis

Esophageal Diverticuli

- Out-pouching of esophageal wall
- Collect food and obstruct flow
- Signs and symptoms
  - Dysphagia
  - Cough
  - Regurgitation
  - Aspiration

- Tumors
  - Internal
  - External

Gastroesophageal Reflux Disease

- Intermittent backflow of gastric contents into the esophagus
- Causes
  - Incompetent lower esophageal sphincter (LES)
  - Decreased competency of LES
  - Increased intraabdominal pressure
  - Delayed gastric emptying
- Signs and symptoms
  - Heartburn
    - 30 to 60 minutes after a meal
    - Usually occurs at night
- Chronic gastroesophageal reflux disease (GERD)
  - Inflammation
  - Ulcers
  - Fibrosis
  - Strictures
    - Symptom relief
      - Avoid
        - Caffeine
        - Fatty food
        - Alcohol
        - Cigarette smoking
        - Certain medications (e.g., nonsteroidal anti-inflammatory drugs [NSAIDs])

Hiatal Hernia

- Portion of the stomach sticks through an opening (hiatus) of the diaphragm into the thoracic cavity
- Types
  - Sliding hernia
    - Most common
    - Stomach slides into opening when the patient is supine.
    - Slides back into position when standing
  - Rolling hernia or paraesophageal hernia
    - Fundus moves through hiatus
      - Stomach wall blood vessels compressed
      - May lead to ulceration
- Risk of reflux and dysphagia
  - Food packs into herniated portion of stomach
  - May cause esophageal obstruction
- Risk of chronic esophagitis
  - Caused by inflammation
    - May lead to fibrosis and stricture
    - Incompetent LES increases risk
- Contributing factors
  - Short esophagus

- Weak diaphragm
- Increased pressure in abdomen (e.g., pregnancy)
- Signs and symptoms
  - Heartburn
  - Sour taste in mouth
  - Belching
    - Occurs after meals
    - Increased with lying down after meals, bending over, or coughing
    - Caused by GI reflux
  - Dysphagia
    - Caused by inflammation
    - Esophageal pressure from food in the herniated pouch
  - Signs and symptoms relief
    - Small frequent meals
    - Remain upright after meals

Vomiting

- Also called emesis
  - Expulsion of stomach and sometimes intestinal contents
  - Controlled by vomiting center in the medulla
    - Activated by
      - GI tract irritation or distention
      - Noxious smells or unpleasant sights
      - Pain or stress
      - Motion sickness
      - Increased intracranial pressure
      - Drugs or toxins
- Characteristics of vomitus
  - Bloody or hematemesis
  - Coffee ground
  - Red blood
  - Yellow or greenish
    - Bile from duodenum
  - Deep brown color
    - Contents from lower intestine
  - Undigested food
    - Delayed gastric emptying

Anorexia

- Loss of appetite
- Often precedes nausea and vomiting

Gastritis

- Inflammation of the stomach mucosa
  - Acute
  - Mucosal lining is red and edematous.
  - Lining with ulcers and bleeding if more severely damaged

- Causes
  - Bacterial or viral infection
  - Food or medication allergies
  - Spicy foods
  - Mucosal irritating medications
  - Aspirin
  - Alcohol
  - Intake of toxic substances
  - Radiation
  - Chemotherapy
- Signs and symptoms
  - Poor appetite
  - Nausea/vomiting
  - Hematemesis
    - With ulcerated or bleeding mucosa
  - Epigastric pain, cramps, and fever
  - With infectious process
    - New mucosal cell growth
  - Chronic
    - Atrophy of gastric mucosa
    - Unable to absorb vitamin B_{12}
- Risk factors
  - Elderly
  - Excessive alcohol intake
  - Peptic ulcers
  - Idiopathic
- Signs and symptoms
  - Mild abdominal pain
  - Poor appetite
  - New intolerance to spicy or fatty foods
  - May lead to peptic ulcer disease (PUD) or gastric cancer

Peptic Ulcer Disease

- Frequently seen in clinics and hospital settings
  - Can be disabling
- Characteristics
  - Breakdown of mucosal lining of stomach or duodenum
    - Common factor is the presence of bacteria *Helicobacter pylori*
      - *H. pylori* secretes cytotoxins and enzymes.
    - Long-term stress also a contributing factor
      - Can influence blood flow to mucosa
      - Slows down movement of chyme through the stomach and small intestine
      - Sustains glucocorticoid effects
      - Results in more ulcer-producing behaviors
        - Alcohol consumption
        - Cigarette smoking
        - Unhealthy food choices, such as high-fat, fried foods

- Mucosal defenses are compromised and ulcer develops.
  - Ulcers appear as single circular lesion with smooth borders.
    - Lesions pierce submucosal layers (Fig. 17.1)
    - May erode into a blood vessel and cause bleeding
    - Severity of bleeding depends on the size of the blood vessel
    - Iron deficiency anemia or occult blood may lead to a diagnosis of peptic ulcer disease.
    - Enzymes, such as pepsin, seep into the lesion and may cause further tissue damage.
      - May penetrate into the muscle layer
      - May perforate the entire wall
  - Common location in duodenum, but also may be present in the stomach or lower esophagus
- Duodenal ulcers
  - Develop from an increase in acid-pepsin secretion
    - Conditions that increase acid-pepsin secretion
      - Increase secretion of gastrin
      - Increase vagal stimulation
      - Increase in number of acid-secreting cells
      - Alcohol and caffeine
      - Increase gastric emptying
      - Faulty feedback mechanism
  - More common in those with type O blood
- Gastric ulcers
  - Develop from impaired mucosal lining defenses
    - Defenses may be damaged by
    - Poor blood supply
      - Anemia
      - Cigarette smoking (vasoconstriction)
      - Inhibits regrowth of mucus-producing epithelial cells
      - Increases glucocorticoid secretion
      - Medications
        - Prednisone
    - Other mucosal lining irritants
      - NSAIDs

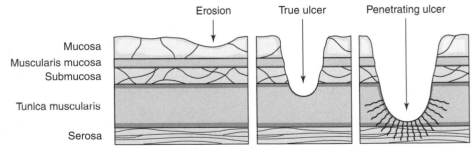

FIG. 17.1 **Lesions caused by peptic ulcer.** (From Monahan, F. D., Sands, J. K., Neighbors, M., Marek, J. F., & Green-Nigro, C. J. [2007]. *Phipps medical-surgical nursing: Health and illness perspectives* [8th ed.]. St. Louis: Mosby.)

- - ○ Aspirin
    - ○ Alcohol
    - Chronic gastritis
  - More common in elderly
- Signs and symptoms
  - Epigastric burning pain
    - 2 to 3 hours after a meal
    - At night
    - Relieved with food intake
    - Relieved with antacids
  - Nausea and vomiting
    - Vomiting with eating offending foods
    - Vomiting with alcohol intake
  - Weight loss
- Complications
  - Bleeding
    - Acute or chronic
      - Depending on blood vessel eroded by the ulcer
  - Peritonitis
    - GI contents and bacteria flow into the peritoneal cavity when the ulcer erodes the entire mucosal lining.
  - GI obstruction
    - Chronic ulcers
      - Scar tissue causes a stricture around the pylorus and duodenum.
- Diagnosis
  - Endoscopy
  - Barium x-ray
- Stress ulcers
  - Causes
    - Severe trauma
      - Burns
      - Head injury
    - Critical health conditions
      - Hemorrhage
      - Sepsis
- Cushing ulcers
  - Develop from brain trauma or surgery
    - Increase in vagal stimulation
    - Increase in acid secretion
  - Sign of stress ulcers
    - Bleeding
    - Rapid development of ulcer

Cholelithiasis

- Definition
  - Formation of solid masses or calculi (gallstones)
    - Consists of
      - Cholesterol

- Bilirubin
- Mixture of substances
- Develop owing to
  - Inflammation or infection of biliary structures
  - Sluggish bile flow
- May form in gallbladder, bile ducts, or cystic ducts
  - Small stones may be removed in the bile and cause no problems.
  - Large stones are prone to block the flow of bile in the cystic or common bile ducts.
    - Obstruction causes pain as the body attempts to remove the stone.
- Pain (biliary colic) located in the right upper quadrant and may radiate to the right shoulder.
- Nausea and vomiting may be present.
- Pain is present until the stone is removed from the duct.
- Pancreatitis may develop if pancreatic enzymes are blocked or if infected bile enters the pancreatic ducts.
- Risk factors for developing cholesterol gallstones
  - Female
  - Multiparity
  - Obesity
  - High cholesterol
  - Diet of fatty foods
  - Use of oral contraception or estrogen supplements
- Risk factors for developing bilirubin stones
  - Hemolytic anemia
  - Alcoholic cirrhosis
  - Biliary tract infections

Cholecystitis

- Definition
  - Inflammation of the gallbladder wall
    - Owing to gallstones
    - Infection
      - Often *Escherichia coli*
- Signs and symptoms
  - Chronic
    - Milder signs and symptoms than with acute episodes
    - Belching
    - Bloating
    - Mild epigastric pain
    - May be triggered by fatty foods

APPLICATION AND REVIEW

1. Although a nurse is unable to identify any obvious signs or symptoms of bleeding, a client repeatedly has tested positive for occult blood in the stool. What data in the client's history present the greatest concern?
   1. Pernicious anemia
   2. Anal fissure
   3. Peptic ulcer
   4. Hemorrhoids

2. The nurse is caring for a client who has acute cholecystitis with biliary colic. What clinical findings should the nurse expect when performing a health history and physical assessment? **Select all that apply.**
   1. Diarrhea with black feces
   2. Intolerance to foods high in fat
   3. Coffee-ground emesis
   4. Gnawing pain when the stomach is empty
   5. Pain in the mid epigastric quadrant of the abdomen

See Answers on pages 376–378.

Hepatitis

- Definition
  - Inflammation of the liver
    - Mild or severe inflammation of liver cells or hepatocytes
      - Severe inflammation results in liver cell death.
        - Obstructs flow of blood and bile through the liver
        - Seriously impacts liver cell functions
        - Greatly affects general health of the individual
- Causes of hepatitis
  - Steatohepatitis or fatty liver
  - Infections outside the liver (mononucleosis)
  - Chemical or drug toxicity (acetaminophen)
  - Viral hepatitis
    - Hepatitis A, B, C, D, E
    - Hepatocytes are damaged directly (hepatitis C).
    - Hepatocytes are damaged by the body's cell-mediated response to the virus.

Viral Hepatitis

- Viruses have different modes of transmission, incubation times, and effects on the liver; they manifest varying signs and symptoms.
- Hepatitis A (HAV)
  - Small RNA virus
  - Transmission
    - Oral-fecal route
    - Primarily contaminated water
  - Incubation period
    - Short: 2 to 6 weeks
  - Characteristics
    - Self-limiting infection
    - Not a chronic virus
    - Not a carrier type of virus
    - Contagious
      - During fecal shedding of virus
      - Occurs weeks before showing signs and symptoms of the virus
    - Immunity
      - Antibodies immunoglobulin (Ig) M followed by IgG-HAV
      - Stays in the blood and provides immunity

- Prevention
  - Vaccine
    - Travelers to problem countries
    - Individuals with liver disease
- Hepatitis B (HBV)
  - 2 billion cases world wide
  - 350 million carriers are able to transmit the virus
  - Double-stranded DNA virus
  - Transmission
    - Infected blood and other body secretions
  - Incubation period
    - Long: approximately 2 months
  - Characteristics
    - Many infected are asymptomatic.
    - Viral antigens stimulate antibody production.
      - Essential for diagnosing
      - Essential for monitoring chronicity of the virus
  - Risks of contracting HBV
    - Blood transfusion
    - Intravenous (IV) drug use
    - Hemodialysis
    - Exposure to blood and body fluids (health care workers)
    - Sexual transmission
    - Fetus from infected mother
    - Tattooing and body piercings
  - Prevention
    - HBV vaccine is available to health care workers, high risk groups, and children.
- Hepatitis C
  - Single-stranded RNA virus
  - Transmission
    - Blood and body fluids
  - Incubation
    - 6 to 9 weeks
  - Characteristics
    - 50% of cases are chronic.
    - Can be transmitted (carriers)
    - Risk factor for hepatocellular cancer (HCC)
  - Prevention
    - No vaccine available
- Hepatitis D (HDV)
  - Delta virus (incomplete RNA virus)
  - Transmission
    - Blood and body fluids
    - High incidence in IV drug users
  - Incubation
    - 2 to 20 weeks
  - Characteristics
    - HBV must be present to activate HDV.

- HBV is more severe when also infected with HDV.
- Chronic infection
- Hepatitis E (HEV)
  - Single-stranded RNA virus
  - Transmission
    - Fecal-oral route
  - Characteristics
    - Neither chronic nor carrier state
    - More cases in Asia and Africa
    - High mortality rate during pregnancy

Hepatitis Phases

- Inflammation of the liver from the hepatitis virus may be mild or severe.
- Liver cells may regenerate or scar tissue may develop in the liver. This obstructs bile and blood flow, disrupting cell organization in the liver lobule and leads to more liver damage.

Acute

- Mild to severe and often fatal
- Three stages in the course of the disease
  - Preicteric or prodromal stage
    - Initially: frequently fatigue, malaise, anorexia, nausea, and general muscle aching
    - May also experience fever, headache, aversion to cigarettes, and mild upper right quadrant pain
    - Blood levels of liver enzymes aspartate aminotransferase (AST) and alanine amino-transferase (ALT) are elevated.
  - Icteric stage
    - Presence of jaundice
    - Blood levels of bilirubin are elevated owing to biliary obstruction.
    - Stools become tan in color.
    - Urine becomes amber in color.
    - Pruritis
    - Hepatomegaly (enlarged liver) occurs causing aching pain.
    - In more severe cases, coagulopathy occurs as the manufacture of clotting factors made in the liver is impaired.
    - Icteric stage lasts longer with HBV.
  - Posticteric or recovery stage
    - Characterized by a reduction in signs and symptoms
    - May last for several weeks
    - Acute stage of hepatitis A is 8 to 10 weeks
    - Acute stage of hepatitis B is over 16 weeks

Chronic

- Chronic inflammation of the liver with hepatitis B, C, and D
  - Inflammation and necrosis must occur for more than 6 months.
  - Causes permanent liver fibrosis and cirrhosis
  - Increased risk of hepatocellular cancer

Fulminant

- Massive liver failure and liver necrosis that occurs very quickly
- Also called acute liver failure
- Can be caused by acetaminophen overdose, hepatitis, virus

Cirrhosis

- Destruction of liver tissue leading to liver failure
- Characteristics
  - Liver is large at first and becomes small as fibrosis continues.
  - Often patient is asymptomatic until cirrhosis is advanced.
  - 80% to 90% of liver is destroyed.
  - End stage of chronic liver diseases
- Diagnosis
  - Cause of cirrhosis and extent of disease determined by liver biopsy and blood tests.
- Fatality
  - 28,000 in this country die of liver cirrhosis yearly.
  - 50% of these deaths are from alcoholic cirrhosis.
- Causes of liver cirrhosis (4)
  - Alcoholic cirrhosis
    - Alcohol and metabolite, such as acetaldehyde, are toxic to liver cells.
    - Malnutrition may worsen the damaging effects on the liver cells.
    - Three stages of liver damage related to alcohol
      - The first stage involves a build-up of fat in the liver cells creating a fatty liver. This stage is characterized by an enlarged liver, but is usually asymptomatic and is reversed if alcohol intake is reduced.
      - The second stage called alcoholic hepatitis involves inflammation and cell necrosis and fibrous tissues form, which are an irreversible state. The individual may be asymptomatic or have mild symptoms such as anorexia, nausea, and liver failure. At this stage if there is binge drinking there may be enough acute inflammation to cause liver failure, encephalopathy, and death.
      - The third stage is referred to as end-stage cirrhosis. Liver function is greatly reduced as fibrous tissue replaces normal liver tissue. Early signs at this stage are impaired digestion and absorption.
  - Biliary cirrhosis owing to immune disorders or conditions where the flow of bile is obstructed
    - Bile stones
    - Mucus plugs in the bile ducts from cystic fibrosis
  - Postnecrotic hepatitis related to chronic hepatitis or prolonged exposure to toxic materials
  - Metabolic, caused by an excess storage of materials in the liver, such as iron (hemochromoatosis)
- Cirrhosis effects
  - Dysfunctional liver cells
  - Obstruction of blood and bile flow through the liver
    - Dysfunctional liver cells result in
- Decreased removal and conjugation of bilirubin
- Decreased production of bile
- Altered digestion and absorption of nutrients, especially fats and fat soluble vitamins

- Decreased production of blood clotting factors (prothrombin and fibrinogen)
- Decreased production of plasma proteins (albumin)
- Impaired glucose/glycogen metabolism
- Decreased storage of iron and vitamin B_{12}
- Impaired hormonal function
- Decreased elimination of toxic substances (ammonia and drugs)
- Ammonia is a substance that is created by protein metabolism in the liver.
- High blood levels of ammonia affect the central nervous system (CNS) and result in hepatic encephalopathy.
- Bile duct and blood flow obstruction effects
  - Reduced bile to the intestines affecting digestion and absorption
  - Elevated bilirubin levels in the blood with obstructive jaundice
  - Portal hypertension (high pressures in portal vein)
  - Spleen congestion (splenomegaly) increasing cell hemolysis
  - Intestinal and gastric wall congestion affecting digestion and absorption
  - Esophageal varices and hemorrhage
  - Ascites in peritoneal cavity
- Signs and symptoms of cirrhosis
  - Initial signs and symptoms
    - Fatigue
    - Anorexia
    - Weight loss
    - Anemia
    - Diarrhea
    - Dull pain in right upper quadrant
  - Later signs and symptoms
    - Ascites and peripheral edema
    - Bruising
    - Esophageal varices (may hemorrhage and lead to shock)
    - Jaundice
    - Encephalopathy
    - Asterixis (hand flapping tremor)
    - Confusion
    - Disorientation
    - Convulsions
    - Coma
    - Chronic encephalopathy: personality changes, memory lapses, irritability, and poor self-care habits
    - Skin spider nevi, testicular atrophy, impotence, gynecomastia, and irregular menses all owing to sex hormone imbalance
    - Frequent infections (respiratory and skin infections) owing to fluid in tissue that interferes with the delivery of nutrients and protein deficiency
    - Chronic itching of skin may also lead to skin infections.

Diarrhea

- Diarrhea is defined as frequent episodes of loose and watery stools.
- Blood, mucus, and/pus also may be present in the stools.

- Cramping pain may be present or nausea and vomiting may occur when the GI tract is infected and inflamed.
- Acute
  - Watery stools often caused by viruses (gastroenteritis) or bacteria (common cause of traveler's diarrhea)
- Chronic
  - Prolonged diarrhea is caused by conditions such as irritable bowel syndrome (IBS), inflammatory bowel disease, or chronic infections.
  - Results in the inability to digest and absorb foods
  - May result in dehydration, electrolyte imbalances, acidosis, and malnutrition
- Enterocolitis (diarrhea diseases) classifications
  - Large-volume diarrhea
    - Watery stools from fluid retained in the intestine
    - Caused by infections, quick gastric emptying when fluids cannot be absorbed, or increased osmotic pressure in the intestine, which decreases fluid absorption
    - Common cause is lactose intolerance where lactose is not digested or absorbed, creating increased osmotic pressure in the intestine.
  - Small volume diarrhea:
    - Stools may contain blood, mucus, or pus.
    - Occurs with inflammatory bowel disease
    - May be accompanied by cramping and urgency
  - Steatorrhea (fatty diarrhea)
    - Bulky, greasy diarrhea often accompanied with a foul odor
    - Result of malabsorption conditions such as celiac disease or cystic fibrosis
    - Fat is not digested or absorbed, which interferes with the digestion of other nutrients.
    - Results are bloating as food contents remain in the intestine.
    - Malnutrition often is present.
  - Blood may be present in diarrhea, normal stool, or constipation.
    - Bright red blood (frank blood) on the surface of stool refers to trauma in the intestinal wall or rectum/anus.
    - Occult blood is hidden in stool content and is usually caused by bleeding ulcers in the stomach or intestine.
    - Melena (dark colored stools) is caused usually by bleeding in the upper GI tract.
- Excessive gas results from swallowed air, digestion and bacterial impact on food contents, and certain ingested foods.
- Gas may cause abdominal distention and pain, plus flatus and belching.

Constipation

- Individuals have different bowel patterns, and constipation refers to less-frequent bowel movements than normal. The result is small dry hard stools.
- Causes of constipation
  - Age and decreased tone of intestinal muscles
  - Decreased intake of dietary fiber, which slows down peristalsis
  - Decreased intake of fluids
  - Ignoring the urge to defecate owing to inconvenience
  - Muscles weakness and inactivity
  - Neurologic conditions, such as muscular sclerosis, and spinal cord trauma
  - Opiate drugs and CNS depressants or anticholinergics that slow peristalsis

- Iron supplements and antacids without adequate fluid intake
- Bowel obstructions caused by tumors or strictures
- Hemorrhoids and diverticulitis may result from chronic constipation.
- Severe constipation may lead to a bowel impaction that can cause abdominal distention and pain.
- May be an acute or chronic problem
- Constipation periods may be interspersed with periods of diarrhea.

Intestinal Obstruction

Intestinal obstruction is defined as no flow of intestinal contents through the intestine.
- Primarily located in small intestine
- Mechanical obstruction of the intestine
  - Caused by adhesions
    - Common cause of mechanical obstruction
    - Adhesions can be caused by previous surgeries, radiation, or infection.
    - Adhesions may twist or constrict the intestine.
  - Caused by hernias
    - Hernias are a section of the intestine that poke through a weakness in the muscular wall and cause an intestinal obstruction.
  - Caused by tumors
    - Masses (growing or existing)
  - Other causes
    - Scar tissue causing a stricture
    - Intussusception when a portion of the intestine slides into the adjacent portion of the intestine
    - Volvulus or twisting
    - Hirschsprung disease causing nerve damage to a portion of the intestine
    - Inflammatory diseases (Crohn disease) causing a gradual obstruction
    - Foreign objects
  - Obstruction process
    - Initially GI contents (fluids/gas) build up proximal to the obstruction, causing distention.
    - Proximal intestine contracts forcefully in an attempt to move the contents forward.
    - Edema builds up in the intestine as fluids are secreted into the intestine.
    - Vomiting occurs
      - Significant loss of fluid and electrolytes
    - Intestinal ischemia and necrosis may occur.
      - Blood flow to the intestine is compromised by pressure and edema.
    - Decreased blood flow leads to decreased peristalsis.
      - Absence of bowel sounds
  - Intestinal bacterial endotoxins may be leaked into the peritoneal cavity (peritonitis) or in the general blood circulation.
    - Caused by an increasing permeable intestinal wall
  - Perforation of the intestinal wall may result, leading to peritonitis.
- Functional obstruction of the intestine
  - Neurologic innervation is impaired, resulting in impaired peristalsis.
    - Causes
      - Postoperative abdominal surgery
        - Temporary paralytic ileus
          - Caused by anesthesia and inflammation

- Ischemia
- Infection and inflammation as in pancreatitis and peritonitis
- Thrombosis in the mesentery of the intestine
- Hypokalemia
- Toxemia
- Signs and symptoms of intestinal obstruction
  - Mechanical obstruction
    - Colicky, wavy abdominal pain
    - Audible gas rumblings
    - Tinkly bowel sounds to no bowel sounds
  - Vomiting and abdominal distention
  - No stool or flatus
  - Diaphoresis and tachycardia
  - Dehydration and electrolyte imbalance, weakness, and confusion
  - Large bowel obstructions
    - Occur more slowly
    - Initially, signs and symptoms are mild but are more severe as the obstruction grows.

APPLICATION AND REVIEW

3. Which questions should the nurse ask to assess a client for a possible intestinal obstruction? **Select all that apply**.
   1. "Have you vomited in the last 3 days?"
   2. "Are you able to digest dairy products easily?"
   3. "How would you describe your abdominal pain?"
   4. "When did you have your last bowel movement?"
   5. "Are you feeling weak or unsteady when you walk?"
4. Which finding places a client at risk for developing intestinal adhesions?
   1. Allergic to several different foods
   2. Receiving radiation therapy for gastric cancer
   3. Long-term antipsychotic medication therapy
   4. History of gastroesophageal reflux disease (GERD)
5. What question should the nurse ask to best assess for a common complication of chronic constipation?
   1. "How often do you move your bowels?"
   2. "Do you eat a high-fiber diet?"
   3. "Do you have hemorrhoids?"
   4. "What color is your stool?"
6. The nurse is caring for a client who is diagnosed with second stage alcoholic cirrhosis. Which statement by the nurse would be appropriate?
   1. "You have what is referred to as a fatty liver."
   2. "Binge drinking will likely trigger liver failure."
   3. "Your liver is enlarged, but the symptoms can be reversed."
   4. "Your liver is replacing normal tissue with fibrous tissue."

See Answers on pages 376–378.

Pancreatitis
- Inflammation of the fragile tissues
  - Caused by autodigestion of pancreatic enzymes
    - Typsin, amylase, and lipase
    - Enzymes are prematurely activated.
      - Leads to bleeding and necrosis
      - Considered a medical emergency
- Characteristics
  - Pancreas lacks a fibrous capsule
    - Enzymes may leak into surrounding tissues.
- Local injury
  - Pancreatic pseudocysts or abscesses occur.
- Inflammation of peritoneal membrane
  - Inflammatory response
    - Includes
      - Vasodilation
      - Increased capillary permeability
      - Hypovolemia
      - Circulatory collapse
  - Intestinal bacteria leak through permeable membrane.
    - Leaks into peritoneum and general circulation
      - Sepsis
      - Adult respiratory distress syndrome (ARDS)
      - Acute renal failure
      - Death
- Causes of pancreatitis
  - Gallstones
    - Obstruct the bile and pancreatic enzymes flow into the duodenum
    - Bile backs up into the pancreatic duct prematurely activating trypsinogen into typsin.
  - Alcohol
    - Increases secretion of pancreatic enzymes
    - Contracts sphincter of Oddi, preventing flow out of the pancreas
- Acute
  - May follow a big meal or binge drinking
  - Occurs suddenly
  - Signs and symptoms
    - Severe epigastric pain
      - Radiates to back
      - Worsens in supine position
    - Low-grade temperature
      - Febrile as infection sets in
    - Peritonitis leads to
      - Paralytic ileus
      - Abdominal distention
- Chronic
  - Alcoholics may have chronic pancreatitis with acute episodes.
- Diagnosed with increased blood levels of amylase and lipase
- High mortality rate, especially those with comorbid conditions and the elderly

Appendicitis

This is an inflammation and infection of the appendix.
- Occurs mainly in young adults
- Causes
  - Obstruction by a gallstone
  - Hard stony mass of feces
  - Foreign material
  - By twisting
- Appendicitis process
  - Fluid builds up in the appendix
  - Inflammation and infection occur.
- Appendix is swollen.
  - Blood supply is compromised.
- Appendix tissues are ischemic and necrotic.
  - Increasing tissue permeability
- Bacteria leaks into the surrounding tissue.
  - Causing abscess formation
  - Localized peritonitis
- The appendix wall can develop gangrene.
  - Rupture may occur.
    - Generalized peritonitis may occur.
    - May be a serious medical emergency
- Signs and symptoms
  - Periumbilical pain as the appendix stretches
  - Increased pain in lower upper quadrant
  - Pain lessens temporarily if the appendix ruptures
  - Pain increases as peritonitis sets in
  - Low-grade temperature and leukocytosis
  - Nausea and vomiting

Peritonitis

This is the inflammation of the peritoneal membrane.
- Causes
  - Chemical irritation
    - Bile, chyme, enzymes, or other substances
      - Bile from perforated gallbladder
      - Chyme from perforated ulcer
      - Enzymes from pancreatitis
      - Blood or foreign material in peritoneal cavity
  - Bacteria
    - Penetrating trauma to intestine
    - Ruptured appendix
    - Intestinal blockage leading to wall permeability
    - Foreign object retained from abdominal surgery
    - Fallopian tube infection from pelvic inflammatory disease
  - Intestinal wall permeability allows chemical peritonitis to progress to bacteria peritonitis if it is not treated quickly.

- Peritonitis process
  - The peritoneum and omentum initially will produce a sticky exudate to seal off the area when there is abdominal wall inflammation.
  - Unless the original problem is treated, this is will be effective only temporarily.
- Signs and symptoms
  - Sudden extreme generalized abdominal pain
  - Vomiting
  - Decreased skin turgor and dry oral mucosa
  - Pallor and low blood pressure
  - Tachycardia
  - Fever and leukocytosis with infection
  - Distended and rigid abdomen
  - Decreased bowel sounds, which indicates a paralytic ileus

Diverticulitis

This is the inflammation of the diverticula.
- Diverticulum
  - Out-pouching of the mucosa in the muscle layer of the colon
  - Most frequently the sigmoid colon
- Diverticulosis
  - Asymptomatic diverticular disease
- Diverticulitis
  - Inflammation
- Risk factors
  - Elderly
  - Congenital weakness of the mucosa
  - Low residue diets
  - Irregular bowel habits
  - Chronic constipation
- Signs and symptoms
  - Left lower quadrant cramping and tenderness
  - Nausea and vomiting
  - Slight fever and elevated white blood cell count

Inflammatory Bowel Disease

- Crohn disease and ulcerative colitis
  - Both chronic inflammatory bowel diseases
  - Genetic and autoimmune diseases
  - Occurs in males and females
  - Crohn disease usually develops during adolescence.
  - Ulcerative colitis usually develops in the 20s or 30s.
  - Both diseases are marked with remission periods with acute exacerbations.
  - Both diseases vary in the severity of signs and symptoms.
- Crohn disease
  - Development
    - Occurs mostly in small intestine
      - Spotty arrangement (diseased tissue alongside healthy tissue)

- Initially presents as a shallow ulcer in the mucosa
  - Increased inflammation and fibrosis
- May impact all layers
  - Creates a thick wall
  - Results in smaller intestinal lumen
  - May become obstructed
  - Prevents digestion and absorption of nutrients (such as iron and vitamin B_{12})
- Increases gastric motility
  - Further decreasing digestion and absorption of nutrients
  - Further erosion of intestinal wall
    - Adhesions, abscesses, or fistulas may develop
- Signs and symptoms
  - Diarrhea and cramping abdominal pain
  - Right lower quadrant pain
  - Melena stools if ulcer erodes blood vessels
  - Anorexia, weight loss, anemia, and fatigue associated with malnutrition
  - Psychological symptoms can occur with long-term illness.
- Ulcerative colitis (Fig. 17.2)
  - Development
    - Inflammation usually begins in the rectum and moves proximal through the colon.
      - Mucosal and submucosal layers are inflamed.
        - Ulcers develop
      - Granulation tissue develops to try to heal the ulcer.
        - Ulcer is vascular, fragile, and bleeds easily.
        - Difficult to heal
      - Impaired tissue
        - Impairs digestion and absorption of fluids and electrolytes
    - Toxic megacolon may occur in acute periods
      - Inflammation impedes peristalsis
        - Leads to obstruction and dilation of colon (usually transverse colon)

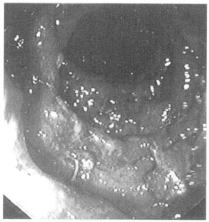

FIG. 17.2 **Ulcerative colitis.** (From Sleisenger, M. H., & Fordtran, J. S. [eds]. [1993]. *Gastrointestinal disease* [5th ed.]. Philadelphia: Saunders.)

- Increased risk of colorectal cancer
- Signs and symptoms
  - Watery stools with blood and mucus
  - Abdominal cramping
  - Rectal bleeding in severe periods leading to anemia
  - Fever and weight loss

Celiac Disease

This is a disease of malabsorption.
- Characteristics
  - Genetic defect of intestinal enzyme
    - Prevents digestion of gliadin
    - Breakdown product of gluten
      - Product of grains: rye, wheat, barley, and oats
  - An immunologic response
    - Results in villa atrophy in intestine
    - Promotes less enzyme production
    - Less absorption of nutrients
      - Malabsorption and malnutrition result in
        - Steatorrhea
        - Muscle wasting
        - Weight loss
        - Irritability
        - Malaise
- Diagnosis
  - Celiac blood panels
  - Duodenal biopsy

Irritable Bowel Syndrome

- IBS is characterized by abdominal pain and changes in normal bowel patterns.
- Types of IBS are based on
  - Primary signs and symptoms
    - Constipation or diarrhea
- GI motility and secretion abnormalities
  - Fast motility of contents through GI tract leads to diarrhea IBS.
  - Delayed motility of contents leads to constipation and bloating IBS.
  - Cause may be hypersensitivity or the serotonin effect on the GI nervous system.
- GI flora overgrowth
  - Methane gas production for flora overgrowth may cause constipation and bloating IBS.
    - Pain
- Increased sensitivity to visceral pain
  - Caused by abnormal motility and secretion and may also involve activated mast cells and T-lymphocytes' effects on the autonomic and CNS, causing an increased sensitivity to pain
  - Food allergies/intolerance
    - Certain food antigens activate the immune response in the mucosal lining may cause IBS symptoms.

- Psychological factors
  - IBS signs and symptoms may be caused by emotional stress, which in turn affects the autoimmune nervous system, the neuroendocrine pathway, and pain responses.
- Signs and symptoms
  - Lower abdominal pain
  - Diarrhea
  - Constipation
  - Alternating diarrhea and constipation
  - Gas
  - Bloating
  - Nausea
  - Fecal urgency and incomplete emptying of bowels
- Diagnosis
  - Diagnosis by excluding other structural or metabolic reasons for signs and symptoms
  - Test for
    - Food allergies
    - Bacterial or parasitic infections
    - Other problems such as lactose intolerance

APPLICATION AND REVIEW

7. What is the primary change in bowel elimination reported by an individual experiencing fast gastrointestinal (GI) tract motility?
   1. Bloating
   2. Diarrhea
   3. Hard stools
   4. Constipation
8. The nurse is caring for a client with possible irritable bowel syndrome (IBS) and diarrhea. What other possible diagnoses could present with similar signs and symptoms?
   1. Anal fissure
   2. Food allergy
   3. Parasite infection
   4. Lactose intolerance
   5. Salmonella infection
9. The nurse is caring for a client with celiac disease. Which food should the nurse teach the client to avoid?
   1. A rice cake with honey
   2. A bowl of corn flakes
   3. A cup of barley soup
   4. Tapioca pudding
10. What comorbid condition should the nurse provide information on to a client newly diagnosed with Crohn disease?
    1. Peptic ulcer
    2. Dumping syndrome
    3. Iron deficiency anemia
    4. Gastroesophageal reflux disease (GERD)

See Answers on pages 376–378.

Gastrointestinal Cancers

- Oral cancer
  - Squamous cell carcinoma most common
  - Characteristics
    - Appears as white lesion
      - Develops into nodular mass or ulcer
      - Spreads to regional lymph nodes and nodes in neck

- Common sites
  - Floor of the mouth
  - Sides of the tongue
  - Malignant tumors in mouth
- Poor prognosis
  - Tumors are painless.
  - Not easily seen
    - Lip cancers (usually lower lip) have a good prognosis.
      - Spreads locally
      - Easily discovered
  - Risk factors for oral cancers:
    - Age >40
    - Cigarette smoking
    - Pipe smoking
    - Alcohol abuse
    - Preexisting leukoplakia (benign white patches)
    - Ultraviolet (UV) light exposure
    - Poor nutrition (diet low in fruits and vegetables)
    - Weakened immune system (e.g., acquired immunodeficiency syndrome, immunosuppressants, graft-versus-host disease)
    - Genetic syndromes
- Esophageal cancer
  - Usually squamous cell
  - Characteristics
    - Located primarily in distal esophagus
    - Result of chronic irritation
  - RISK factors
    - Chronic esophagitis
    - Achalasia
    - Hiatal hernia
    - Alcohol abuse
    - Smoking/tobacco use
    - Obesity
    - Ages 45 to 70 years
    - Male gender
    - Barrett esophagus
      - Causes dysphagia late in disease
      - Poor prognosis
        - Diagnosed late in the disease process
  - Risk factors
    - Age
    - Increased risk between the ages of 45 and 70 years
    - Gender
    - Males are 3 to 4 times more likely than females to develop esophageal cancer.
    - Race
    - Blacks are twice as likely as whites to develop squamous cell esophageal cancer.
    - Tobacco use

- Heavy alcohol consumption over a long period of time
- Barrett's esophagus
- Diet that is low in fruits and vegetables
- Obesity
- Accidental ingestion of lye in childhood
- Achalasia
- Gastric cancer
  - Characteristics
    - Lesion that begins as an ulcer.
      - Irregular center
      - Raised margin
    - Early lesion lies in mucosa and submucosa
    - Advanced cancer
      - Invades into muscular layer
      - Extends into the serosa
      - Spreads to lymph nodes, liver, and ovaries
  - Signs and symptoms
    - Initially vague symptoms
      - Anorexia
      - Epigastric discomfort
      - Weight loss
      - Feeling of fullness after meals
    - Prognosis is poor
      - Diagnosed late because of vague symptoms
  - Risk factors
    - Male gender
    - Over 50 years of age
    - Race: Hispanic Americans, African-Americans, Native Americans, and Asian/Pacific Islanders more than in non-Hispanic whites
    - More common in Japan, China, Southern and Eastern Europe, and South and Central America than in the United States
    - *H. pylori* infection
    - History of mucosa-associated lymphoid tissue (MALT) lymphoma
    - High consumption of nitrate/nitrite in the diet (smoked foods, salted fish and meat, pickled vegetables)
    - Tobacco use
    - Overweight or obese
    - Previous stomach surgery
    - Pernicious anemia
    - Menetrier disease (hypertrophic gastropathy)
    - Type A blood
    - Inherited cancer syndromes (hereditary diffuse gastric cancer, Lynch syndrome, or hereditary nonpolyposis colorectal cancer, familial adenomatous polyposis, mutations of *BRCA1* and *BRCA2* genes, Li-Fraumeni syndrome, Peutz-Jeghers syndrome)
    - Family history (first-degree relatives) of stomach cancer
    - Adenomatous stomach polyps

- Epstein-Barr virus (EBV) infection
- Certain occupations (workers in coal, metal, and rubber industries)
- Common variable immune deficiency (CVID) liver cancer
  - Characteristics
    - Primary tumor is hepatocellular tumor.
    - Most often secondary tumors from metastatic cancer
  - Signs and symptoms of liver cancer
    - Anorexia
    - Vomiting
    - Fatigue
    - Weight loss
    - Hepatomegaly
    - Splenomegaly
    - Portal hypertension
  - Late diagnosis owing to vague symptoms
- Pancreatic cancer
  - Characteristics
    - Adenocarcinoma
      - Begins in epithelial cells in pancreatic ducts
    - Tumor at head of pancreas
      - Leads to obstruction of pancreatic enzymes
      - Obstruction of bile
        - Results in weight loss and jaundice
    - Tumor at the body or tail of pancreas
      - Remains asymptomatic
        - Until advances to
          - Liver
          - Stomach
          - Lymph nodes or posterior abdominal wall
          - Nerves
    - Pain increases as cancer spreads into the tissues
    - Mortality 95%
      - When diagnosed late
      - When cancer has spread to surrounding tissues
- Colorectal cancer
  - Second leading cause of cancer-related deaths in the United States
  - Characteristics
    - Polyps jut out of lumen of intestine.
      - Benign small clump of cells
    - Groups of polyps enlarge
      - Risk for malignant changes
    - Progression of tumor invasion
      - Intestinal wall
      - Mesentery
      - Spread to lymph nodes
      - Spread to the liver

- Signs and symptoms
  - Most patients asymptomatic until cancer has spread
  - Character of stool changes
    - Tumor in rectosigmoid colon (feces are solid)
      - Feeling of incomplete emptying
      - Vague abdominal cramping
      - Small flat "ribbons" of stool
    - Tumor in ascending colon (feces are liquid)
      - No obstruction
      - Feeling of fatigue
      - Weight loss
      - Iron-deficiency anemia
  - Bleeding may be present as occult blood or frank bleeding.
- Most deaths can be prevented by
  - Early diagnosis and treatment of polyps (precancerous lesions)
  - Early detection of malignancy
- Risk factors
  - Overweight or obese
  - Physical inactivity
  - Diet high in red meats and processed meats
  - Cooking meats at very high temperatures (frying, broiling, or grilling)
  - Smoking (long periods of time)
  - Moderate to heavy alcohol use
  - Over 50 years of age
  - Personal history of colorectal polyps (adenomatous) or colorectal cancer
  - Personal history of inflammatory bowel disease (ulcerative colitis or Crohn disease)
  - Family history (first-degree relative such as parent, sibling, or child) of colorectal cancer or adenomatous polyps
  - Inherited genetic mutations (e.g., Lynch syndrome/hereditary nonpolyposis colorectal cancer and familial adenomatous polyposis
  - African-Americans, Jews of Eastern European descent (Ashkenazi Jews)
  - Type 2 diabetes mellitus
  - Other possible risk factors include night shift work related to changes in levels of melatonin, previous radiation treatment for certain cancers (testicular and prostate).

Post-Gastrectomy Syndromes

- Dumping syndrome
  - May occur after gastric resection
    - Peptic ulcer disease
    - Surgery for gastric cancer
    - Bariatric surgery
  - Result of changes in structure of stomach and/or intestine
    - Results in
      - Loss of gastric capacity
      - Loss of emptying control into duodenum

- Characteristics
  - Early dumping syndrome
    - Rapid emptying of hypertonic GI contents to small intestine
      - 20 to 30 minutes after eating
      - Creates sudden shift of fluid from vasculature to intestine
        - Results in dehydration
        - Distention
        - Sense of fullness
        - Cramping
        - Nausea/vomiting
  - Late dumping syndrome
    - 1 to 3 hours after a meal
      - Results in weakness
      - Diaphoresis
      - Confusion
      - Hyperglycemia
        - Increased insulin release after carbohydrate meal

APPLICATION AND REVIEW

11. A client has had a gastric resection for the treatment of obesity. Which client statement would most concern the nurse?
    1. "I still always feel hungry even after I eat."
    2. "I don't like not eating what I want whenever I want."
    3. "I've developed some itching around the incision."
    4. "I usually get sweaty and weak about 2 hours after eating a meal."

12. Which client is at highest risk for developing colorectal cancer?
    1. A 42-year-old Caucasian client who has iron deficiency anemia
    2. A 36-year-old Asian client who smokes cigars several times per week
    3. A 72-year-old African-American client who consumes red meat daily
    4. An 82-year-old Native American client who reports drinking alcohol heavily for many years

13. What client statement may indicate the presence of a sign of colorectal cancer?
    1. "I've had hemorrhoids for years, but now they are bleeding."
    2. "This sounds strange, but my stool looks different now."
    3. "I lost 5 pounds over the past 3 months without really trying."
    4. "I eat a lot of red meat, especially burgers and steaks."

14. A client has been diagnosed with colorectal cancer that has invaded the mesentery layer. Which statement made by this client demonstrates an understanding of the progressive invasion process of this cancer?
    1. "Treatment will hopefully keep it from getting into the lymph nodes."
    2. "The biopsy is focused on whether the polyps are cancerous."
    3. "They are watching to see if it spreads to my intestinal wall."
    4. "The next place it could invade is my liver."

15. A client diagnosed with pancreatic cancer is reporting pain that is increasingly more difficult to manage. What statement by the client demonstrates an understanding of the consequence of the pain?
    1. "The cancer has blocked the passage of bile."
    2. "The tumor is located in the tail of my pancreas."
    3. "The cancer has invaded my liver and possibly my stomach."
    4. "The pain will lessen once they surgically remove my pancreas."
16. Which client statement would support a diagnosis of gastric cancer?
    1. "Both of my parents emigrated from Australia in the early 1950s."
    2. "We visited Iceland last year and plan to return someday."
    3. "I hunt and will smoke the meats I kill to eat."
    4. "I have irritable bowel syndrome."
17. Which initial sign or symptom of gastric cancer is the most unique to this form of cancer?
    1. Epigastric discomfort   3. Lack of appetite
    2. Post meal fullness   4. Weight loss
18. Which clients have a preexisting condition that is considered a risk factor for esophageal cancer? **Select all that apply.**
    1. A client who is an alcoholic
    2. A client who smokes tobacco
    3. A client with a high-fat dietary intake
    4. A client with a chronic fungal infection
    5. A client who is allergic to dairy products
19. The nurse is assessing a client at a community center. Which finding would be most suggestive of oral cancer?
    1. Bilateral white lesions on tongue
    2. History of alcohol abuse for 15 years
    3. Denies any mouth pain or soreness
    4. A 45-year-old male

See Answers on pages 376–378.

ANSWER KEY: REVIEW QUESTIONS

1. **3 A history of a peptic ulcer would trigger concerns about a reoccurrence of the lesion.**
   1 Iron deficiency anemia could trigger occult bleed, but it is not associated with pernicious anemia. **2** Although the bleeding can be the result of an anal fissure, the peptic ulcer is of greater concern. **4** Hemorrhoids would result in frank bleeding, not an occult bleed.
   Client Need: Physiological Adaptation; **Cognitive Level:** Analysis; **Nursing Process:** Analysis

2. **Answers: 2, 5.**
   2 Interference with bile flow into the intestine will lead to an increasing inability to tolerate fatty foods. **5** The gallbladder is in the upper right (mid-epigastric) quadrant of the abdomen, and when inflamed it will cause pain in this area.
   1 Diarrhea with melena is not associated with cholecystitis. Melena is tarry stools associated with upper GI bleeding; diarrhea is associated with increased intestinal motility. The unemulsified fat remains in the intestine for prolonged periods, and the result is an inhibition of stomach emptying with possible gas formation. **3** Coffee-ground emesis is indicative of gastric bleeding; it is not associated with cholecystitis. **4** Gnawing pain when the stomach is empty is associated with duodenal ulcers, not with cholecystitis
   Client Need: Physiological Adaptation; **Cognitive Level:** Applying; **Nursing Process:** Assessment

3. **Answers: 1, 3, 4, 5.**

   1 Vomiting is a sign of an intestinal obstruction. **3** Intestinal obstructions present with a specific type of pain. Asking the client to describe the sensation would help identify the presence of an obstruction. **4** An obstruction often results in the absence of a bowel movement. **5** Weakness is a sign of an intestinal obstruction.

   2 Dairy products do not trigger intestinal obstruction.

   Client Need: Physiological Adaptation; **Cognitive Level:** Applying; **Nursing Process:** Assessment

4. **2 Adhesions can be caused by previous surgeries, radiation, or infection.**

   1 Food allergies are not considered risks for intestinal adhesions. **3** Long-term antipsychotic medication therapy is not considered a risk for intestinal adhesions. **4** A history of GERD is not considered a risk for intestinal adhesions.

   Client Need: Physiological Adaptation; **Cognitive Level:** Applying; **Nursing Process:** Assessment

5. **3 Hemorrhoids and diverticulitis may result from chronic constipation.**

   1, 2, 4 These other options are assessment questions that focus on gathering information about constipation not of a complication of this elimination problem.

   Client Need: Physiological Adaptation; **Cognitive Level:** Applying; **Nursing Process:** Assessment

6. **2 At the second stage, if there is binge drinking there may be enough acute inflammation to caus iver failure.**

   1, 3 The first stage involves a build-up of fat in the liver cells creating a fatty liver. This stage is chara rized by an enlarged liver, but is usually asymptomatic and is reversed if alcohol intake is reduced. In the third stage, liver function is greatly reduced as fibrous tissue replaces normal liver tissue.

   Client Need: Physiological Adaptation; **Cognitive Level:** Applying; **Integrated Process:** Teaching and Lear ng

7. **2 Fast motility of contents through the GI tract results in diarrhea.**

   1, 4 Delayed motility of contents through GI tract results in constipation and bloating. **3** Hard stools are more likely a result of slow GI motility.

   Client Need: Physiological Adaptation; **Cognitive Level:** Understanding; **Integrated Process:** Teaching and Learning

8. **Answers: 2, 3, 4, 5.**

   2, 3, 4, 5 To confirm a diagnosis of IBS, food allergies, bacterial and parasitic infections, and lactose intolerance should first be ruled out as a cause of the symptomology.

   1 Anal fissure can cause constipation not diarrhea.

   Client Need: Physiological Adaptation; **Cognitive Level:** Understanding; **Integrated Process:** Teaching and Learning

9. **3 Barley is a grain that contains gluten and should be avoided.**

   1, 2, 4 Neither rice, corn, nor tapioca contain gluten.

   Client Need: Physiological Adaptation; **Cognitive Level:** Analysis; **Integrated Process:** Teaching and Learning

10. **3 Anemia is associated with Crohn disease owing to bleeding and chronic inflammation.**

    1 Peptic ulcers are associated with gastritis. **2** Dumping syndrome is associated with gastric resection surgery. **4** GERD is not associated with Crohn disease

    Client Need: Physiological Adaptation; **Cognitive Level:** Analysis; **Integrated Process:** Teaching and Learning

11. **4 Late dumping syndrome causes diaphoresis and weakness within 1 to 3 hours of eating a meal.**

    1 Feelings of hunger can be a psychological response. **2** Feeling regret about changing eating habits is common among clients having this surgery. **3** Itching around the incision is an expected finding.

    Client Need: Physiological Adaptation; **Cognitive Level:** Analysis; **Nursing Process:** Analysis

12. **3 This client has three risk factors for colorectal cancer: being over the age of 50 years, being an African-American, and consuming a diet that is high in red meat are all risk factors for colorectal cancer.**

    1 This client has no risk factors for colorectal cancer. **2** This client has one risk factor; smoking is a risk factor for colorectal cancer. **4** This client has two risk factors for colorectal cancer: age over 50 years and moderate to heavy alcohol consumption.

    Client Need: Physiological Adaptation; **Cognitive Level:** Applying; **Nursing Process:** Assessment

13. **2 A change in the character of stool is often the first sign of colorectal cancer.**
    1 Although the bleeding needs to be assessed and treated, it is not unusual for hemorrhoids to bleed; this is not related to colorectal cancer. **3** Although an unexplained weight loss needs additional assessment, numerous reasons are unrelated to colorectal cancer. **4** Eating red meat is a risk factor, not a sign of colorectal cancer.
    Client Need: Physiological Adaptation; **Cognitive Level:** Analysis; **Nursing Process:** Assessment

14. **1 After the invasion of the mesentery layer, colorectal cancer will spread to the lymph nodes.**
    2 Polyps are the original site of the cancer. **3** The intestinal wall is invaded prior to the mesentery layer. **4** The liver would indicate metastasis—invasion outside of the GI tract.
    Client Need: Physiological Adaptation; **Cognitive Level:** Analysis; **Nursing Process:** Evaluation

15. **3 Pancreatic cancer remains asymptomatic until the cancer spreads into surrounding tissue and organs.**
    1 The blockage of bile is not the primary source of pain, but rather of jaundice. **2** Location of the original tumor is not a primary factor in the degree of pain being experienced. **4** The degree of pain is less dependent on the pancreas than on the spread of the cancer.
    Client Need: Physiological Adaptation; **Cognitive Level:** Analysis; **Nursing Process:** Evaluation

16. **3 A diet high in smoked meats is a risk factor for gastric cancer.**
    1 No current research supports a connection between gastric cancer and the Australian population. **2** Although Iceland is considered a geographical risk area, likely from the dependence on smoked meats in the diet, a visit would not be considered a risk factor. **4** No current evidence supports a connection between gastric cancer and IBS.
    Client Need: Physiological Adaptation; **Cognitive Level:** Analysis; **Nursing Process:** Evaluation

17. **2 This form of cancer presents initially with a feeling of fullness after eating.**
    1 Epigastric pain is a vague symptom demonstrated with several forms of GI cancer. **3** Anorexia is a vague symptom demonstrated with several forms of GI cancer. **4** Weight loss is a vague symptom demonstrated with several forms of GI cancer and cancer in general.
    Client Need: Physiological Adaptation; **Cognitive Level:** Analysis; **Nursing Process:** Assessment

18. **Answers: 1, 2.**
    1, 2 Esophageal cancer is associated with chronic irrigation of that organ. Alcohol and tobacco use are recognized irritants associated with this form of cancer.
    3 A high-fat diet is not a risk associated with esophageal cancer, although a diet low in fruits and vegetables is a risk factor. **4** A chronic fungal infection is not a risk factor associated with esophageal cancer. **5** A dairy allergy is not a risk factor associated with esophageal cancer.
    Client Need: Physiological Adaptation; **Cognitive Level:** Applying; **Nursing Process:** Assessment

19. **White lesions located on the sides and/or floor of the mouth are common signs of oral cancer.**
    2 Although alcohol abuse is a risk factor, it is not a sign of possible oral cancer. **3** The classic lesions associated with oral cancer are painless. **4** Being over the age of 40 is considered a risk factor, but is not a sign of possible oral cancer.
    Client Need: Physiological Adaptation; **Cognitive Level:** Applying; **Nursing Process:** Assessment

Genitourinary System Disorders 18

OVERVIEW

- The genitourinary (GU) system consists of organs concerned with the production and excretion of urine (Fig. 18.1) and those concerned with reproduction.
- Renal function and urine formation depend on three basic processes
  - Glomerular filtration
  - Tubular reabsorption
  - Tubular secretion

Kidneys

- Two bean-shaped structures
  - Size of a fist
- Located retroperitoneally
  - Behind the peritoneum
  - Posterior abdominal wall
- Protected by the lower ribs
- Covered with a fibrous capsule and embedded in fat
  - Fascial
    - Renal fascia
  - Fatty
    - Perinephric fascia
  - True
    - Fibrous capsule
- Anatomic relations of the kidneys
  - Anterior
    - To the right kidney
      - Liver
      - Second part of the duodenum
      - Colon
    - To the left kidney
      - Stomach
      - Pancreas
      - Spleen
      - Jejunum
      - Descending colon
  - Posterior
    - Diaphragm
    - Quadratus lumborum
    - Psoas
    - Twelfth rib
    - Three nerves
      - Subcostal

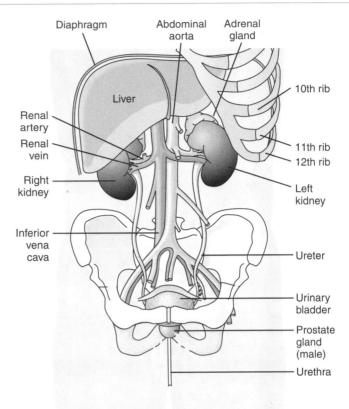

FIG. 18.1   **Structure of the urinary tract.** (From Banasik, J. L., & Copstead, L. C. [2019]. *Pathophysiology* [6th ed.]. St. Louis: Elsevier.)

- Iliohypogastric
- Ilioinguinal
- Medial
  - Hilum
    - A deep fissure containing the renal vessels, nerves, lymphatics, and the renal pelvis
  - To the left of kidney
    - Aorta
  - To the right of the kidney
    - Inferior vena cava
- Superior
  - Adrenal gland
- Inside each kidney
  - Cortex
    - Outer layer of the kidney
    - Glomeruli are located
  - Medulla
    - Inner section of tissue
    - Consist primarily of the tubules and collection ducts
    - The renal pelvis and calyces reside inside the medulla.

- Nephrons
  - Each kidney consists of over a million nephrons.
  - Functional units of the kidney
    - Must be maintained for effective renal function
- Renal corpuscle
  - Bowman capsule (glomerular capsule)
    - Blind end of the primal convoluted tubule
    - Consist of a network of capillaries called glomerulus (glomerular capillaries)
      - Form the filtration network for the blood
- Filtration
  - Fluids containing wastes, nutrients, electrolytes, and other dissolved substances pass from the blood into the tubules.
  - Protein and cells remain in the bloodstream.
  - As filtration pressure increases more filtrate forms and the result is an increase in urine production.
  - Tubules
    - The filtrate flows into the tubules.
      - Once filtrate has been processed, it is considered to be urine.
        - Urine is then transported through collecting ducts to the renal calyces and pelvis and then into the ureters.
    - Three parts of the tubules
      - Proximal convoluted tubule
      - Loop of Henle
      - Distal convoluted tubule
    - Process of the tubules
      - Reabsorption
        - Essential nutrients, water, and electrolytes are absorbed.
        - Proximal convoluted tubule
        - Active transport
          - Sodium ions
          - Requires carrier molecules and an energy source
        - Transport/tubular maximum
          - The limit on reabsorption
          - Glycosuria
            - Presence of glucose in urine
            - Maximum reabsorption is approximately 310 mg/min for glucose.
            - Indication of hyperglycemia
  - Osmosis
    - Water and electrolyte reabsorption
    - Loop of Henle and the distal convoluted tubule
    - Adjusted to the body's current needs
  - Hormones play major role in reabsorption of electrolytes and fluids.
    - Antidiuretic hormone (ADH)
      - Posterior pituitary
      - Controls water reabsorption by altering permeability of the distal convoluted tubule and collecting duct
    - Aldosterone
      - Secreted by adrenal cortex

- Controls sodium and water reabsorption by exchanging sodium ions for potassium or hydrogen ions in the distal convoluted tubule
  - Atrial natriuretic hormone
    - Heart hormone
    - Controls fluid balance by reducing sodium and fluid reabsorption in the kidneys
  - Secretion
    - Waste and electrolytes are removed.
  - Transpiration
    - Collecting ducts then transport the urine to the renal pelvis.
- Ureters
  - Urine is produced once the filtrate has been processed in tubules and collecting ducts.
  - Peristaltic movements encourage urine to flow to the urinary bladder.
  - Transitional epithelium
    - Lining of the renal pelvis, calyces, ureters, and bladder
    - Nonpermeable to water
      - Allows constant contact with urine without irritation.
- Bladder
  - Located retroperitoneally in pelvic cavity
  - Smooth muscle
  - Folds form an expandable sac
  - Opens to two ureters that bring urine in and out
    - Trigon of urinary bladder
      - Smooth triangular area in the internal urinary bladder
      - Formed from the two ureteric orifices and the internal urethral orifice
- Urethra
  - Female
    - 3 to 4 cm long
    - Opens onto the perineum anterior to the vagina and anus
    - Proximity promotes bladder infection
  - Male
    - Approximately 20 cm long
    - Passes through the penis
    - During orgasm, the sphincter closes off the flow of urine and instead allows semen to pass through the urethra.
- Micturition
  - Voiding of urine allowing the bladder to empty
  - Increased pressure from a distended bladder causes reflux stimulation.
  - Voluntary control of sphincters

Renal Arteries and Veins

- Kidneys process a large amount of blood at all times.
  - 20% to 25% of the cardiac output enters the renal arteries from the aorta.
- Hilum
  - Where blood enters and leaves the kidneys
  - No alternative blood flow supply available
    - Any obstruction of blood flow would cause necrosis and infarction.
  - Blood flow
    - Provides nourishment to renal tissues

- Summarizes blood flow (start to finish)
  - Renal artery → interloper artery → arcuate artery → interlobular artery → afforestation arteriole → glomerular capillaries → efferent arteriole → peritubular capillaries → interlobular vein → arcuate vein → interlobar vein → renal vein
- Glomerular filtration rate (GFR)
  - Pressure in the glomerular capillaries
    - Glomerular filtration pressure
  - Constriction or dilation of the arterioles; adjusts the amount of blood in the capillaries
  - Maintains normal filtration regardless of fluctuations in systemic blood pressure
  - Three factors control the degree of constriction.
    - Auto regulation
      - Local blood flow regulation despite changes in perfusion pressure
      - Adjustments in the diameter of the arterioles that are made in response to changes in the blood flow in the kidneys
      - Maintain normal filtration rate
    - Sympathetic nervous system (SNS)
      - When stimulated will increase vasoconstriction in both arterioles
    - Renin-angiotensin mechanism
      - Renin is secreted in the kidneys by juxtaglomerular cells in response to blood flow being reduced in the affront arteriole for any reason.
      - During enzyme reactions renin produces angiotensin I, this then passes through the lung and the angiotensin-converting enzyme (ACE) converts this to angiotensin II, which acts as a powerful systemic vasoconstrictor.
      - During a period of low blood flow to the kidneys (a drop in blood pressure) the SNS and the renin-angiotensin mechanisms are activated to restore the pressure and flow.

Urinary System Function

- Removal of metabolic waste
  - Nitrogenous
  - Acidic
- Fluid volume
  - Regulation of water
  - Regulation of electrolytes
- Blood pressure regulation
  - Strong correlation between kidney function and blood pressure
  - Blood pressure is frequently elevated in renal disease.
  - Renin-angiotensin-aldosterone system (RAAS)
    - Powerful systemic vasoconstrictor
    - Stimulates secretion of aldosterone
      - Increases sodium and fluid reabsorption
        - Increases blood volume, which increases blood pressure
    - During periods of low blood pressure, this system is activated to restore blood pressure to vital organs.
- Excretion
  - Drugs
  - Foreign materials
- Vitamin D conversion
  - Activation of vitamin D

- Vitamin D is a steroid hormone that is hydroxylated in the liver to form 25-hydroxy-cholecalciferol (25(OH)D3). Further hydroxylated in the proximal tubules.
- Essential vitamin for the mineralization of bones also promotes the absorption of calcium and phosphate.
- Acid–base balance
- Hormone synthesis

Diagnostic Tests

- Urinalysis
  - Tests of urine used for diagnostic purposes
    - Appearance
    - Concentration
    - Content
  - Can detect a wide range of disorders
    - Urinary tract infections (UTIs)
    - Kidney disease
    - Diabetes
  - Reference range
    - Color
      - Clear or straw-colored
        - Normal
      - Cloudy
        - Protein
        - Blood cells
        - Bacteria or pus
      - Dark
        - Hematuria
          - Blood
    - Urine pH
      - Normal range 4.5 to 8.0
  - Abnormal constituents
    - Microscopic hematuria
      - Small amount of blood in the urine
      - Indicative of infection, inflammation, or tumors in the urinary tract
    - Gross hematuria
      - Large amount of blood in the urine
      - Indicative of increased glomerular permeability or hemorrhage in the tract
    - Proteinuria
      - Protein (albumin) in the urine
      - Indicative of leakage of albumin or mixed plasma proteins into the filtrate caused by inflammation and increased glomerular permeability
    - Bacteriuria and pyuria
      - Bacteria and pus in the urine
      - Indicative of infection in the urinary tract
    - Urinary casts
      - Microscopic molds of the tubules
      - Indicative of inflammation of the kidney tubules

- Specific gravity
    - Ability of the tubules to concentrate the urine
    - Low specific gravity
        - Dilute urine
        - Indicative of renal failure
            - Assuming normal hydration limits
- Ketoacids
    - Glucose and ketones
    - Found in urine when diabetes mellitus is not well controlled
- Abnormal blood tests
    - Elevated blood urea nitrogen (BUN)
        - Failure to excrete nitrogen waste owing to increased GFR
    - Elevated serum creatinine
    - May warn of possible malfunction or failure of kidneys.
    - Metabolic acidosis (decreased serum pH and bicarbonate)
        - Decreased GFR and inability of tubules to control acid–base balance
    - Low hemoglobin (anemia)
        - Accumulated waste leads to decreased erythropoietin secretion and/or bone marrow depression.
    - Abnormal electrolyte balance
        - Dependent upon fluid balance; therefore may be subjective reflection of function.
    - Antistreptolysin (ASO) or antistreptokinase (ASK)
        - Antibody levels used for diagnosis of poststreptococcal glomerulonephritis
    - Kidney function levels
        - May aid in indicating cause of hypertension (HTN) (high blood pressure)
- Culture and sensitivity
    - Used to identify the specific, causative agent in urinary infection
        - Allows most appropriate drug treatment
- Clearance test
    - Used to assess GFR
    - Types
        - Creatinine
        - Insulin clearance
- Radiologic tests
    - Used to visualize structures and abnormalities of the urinary system
    - Types
        - Radionuclide imaging
        - Angiography
        - Ultrasound
        - Computed tomography (CT)
        - Magnetic resonance imaging (MRI)
        - Intravenous pyelography (IVP)
- Cystoscope
    - Used to visualize the lower urinary tract during kidney stone removal or biopsy
- Biopsy
    - Used to acquire tissue specimens that allow microscopic examination
        - Lesions in bladder or kidney

APPLICATION AND REVIEW

1. Which test result would be the best indicator that a transplanted kidney is functioning?
   1. Renal ultrasound
   2. Serum creatinine level
   3. White blood cell count (WBC)
   4. Serum potassium level

See Answers on pages 400–401.

Hormonal Influences

- Antidiuretic hormone
  - Arginine vasopressin
  - Produced by the hypothalamus and stored in the posterior pituitary gland
  - Released during change in concentration of blood or blood pressure
  - Helps kidneys regulate and balance the amount of water in the body
- Aldosterone
  - Mineralocorticoid
    - Steroid hormone
  - Produced in the adrenal gland
  - Helps regulate sodium and potassium levels in the body; this facilitates control of blood pressure and balance of fluids and electrolytes in the blood.
- RAAS
  - Powerful systemic vasoconstrictor
  - Stimulates secretion of aldosterone
  - Increases sodium and fluid reabsorption
    - Increases blood volume, which increases blood pressure
  - During periods of low blood pressure, this system is activated to restore blood pressure to vital organs.

Urinary Abnormalities

- Impaired elimination
  - Decreased flow or stasis of urine
  - Dysfunction may involve urethra, bladder, or ureters.
- Impaired renal function
  - Renal insufficiency; impaired kidney function in which kidneys fail to filter wastes from blood

Urinary Incontinence

- Stress incontinence
  - Increased intra-abdominal pressure forces urine through the sphincter
  - May occur during
    - Coughing
    - Laughing
    - Exercising
    - Lifting
  - Females are more susceptible to urinary incontinence as they age and/or after multiple pregnancies.
    - Urogenital diaphragm weakened

- Urge incontinence
  - Abnormal bladder contractions that lead to a sudden, intense urge to urinate, which results in involuntary loss of urine
  - Females are more susceptible
    - Weak bladder muscles, overactive bladder muscles, and nerve damage contribute.
      - Pregnancy
      - Childbirth
      - Menopause
- Reflex incontinence
  - Bladder muscle goes into an involuntary contraction, which causes urine leakage (typically large amount).
    - Occurs without warning or urge
  - Can be result of damage to the nerves that normally warn the brain the bladder is filling
- Overflow incontinence
  - Caused by an incomplete bladder sphincter
  - Elderly are more susceptible
    - Weakened debris or muscle prevents complete emptying of urine from the bladder.
      - Leads to incontinence and frequency of emptying
- Retention
  - Inability to completely empty the bladder of urine
  - May coincide with overflow incontinence
- Mixed incontinence
  - Combination of stress and urge incontinence—shares signs and symptoms of both.
- Functional incontinence
  - The individual is usually aware of the need to urinate, but because of one or more physical or mental reasons they are unable to get to a bathroom.
- Gross total incontinence
  - Continuous and total loss of urinary control
  - May be caused by a number of issues
    - Bladder fistula
    - Urethra injury
    - Ectopic ureter

Neurogenic Bladder

- Bladder may be spastic or flaccid.
- Results from interference with central nervous system (CNS) and autonomic nervous system control of the bladder emptying.
  - Frequently caused by spinal cord injuries (SCIs) or brain damage

Urinary Tract Infections

- Very common
  - An estimated 6 million Americans affected annually
  - Infection
    - Causative organisms
      - *Escherichia coli*
        - Resident flora in the intestine
        - Common causative agent of UTIs

- Other organisms associated with UTIs
  - *Klebsiella*
  - *Proteus*
  - *Enterobacteria*
  - *Citrobacter*
  - *Serratia*
  - *Pseudomonas*
  - *Enterococcus*
  - *Staphylococcus*
  - *Chlamydia*
  - *Mycoplasma*
- Most are ascending
  - Organisms in the perineal area travel up along the ominous mucosa in the urinary tract to the bladder and then along the ureters to the kidneys.
- Types
  - Cystitis and urethritis
    - Infections of the lower urinary tract
  - Pyelonephritis
    - Infection of the upper urinary tract
    - Can be result from blood-borne infection
- Etiology
  - Females
    - At greatest risk
    - Females have a shorter, wider urethra (compared to males).
    - Proximity to anus
    - Frequent irritation to tissues
      - Sexual activity
      - Baths
      - Use of feminine hygiene products
  - Elderly males with history of prostatic hypertrophy
    - Hypertrophy may lead to urine retention and bacteria build-up.
    - Infection of the prostate or testes is likely to extend to the urinary structures.
      - This is owing to shared structures between the male reproductive tract and the urinary tract.
  - Children with congenital abnormalities
    - Common where obstruction to flow or reflux is noted
  - Elderly
    - Increased risk factors
      - Incomplete emptying
      - Impaired blood supply to bladder
      - Immobility
      - Decreased fluid intake

Cystitis and Urethritis

- Cystitis
  - Inflammation of bladder wall
    - Red

- Swollen
- Ulcerated
- Urethritis
  - Inflammation of urethra
    - Red
    - Swollen
    - Ulcerated
- Signs and symptoms
  - Pain in lower abdomen
  - Dysuria
    - Painful urination
  - Urgency
    - Immediate urge to void
  - Nocturnal
    - Urination urge during sleep period
  - Systemic
    - Fever
    - Malaise
    - Leukocytosis
    - Nausea
  - Urine commonly appears cloudy and has an unpleasant odor.

Benign Prostatic Hyperplasia

- Enlarged prostate
- Two growth stages of prostate
  - During puberty
    - Prostate gland doubles in size
  - Begins at around 25 years of age and continues during most of a male's life
    - As males age the prostate may get larger
    - Benign prostatic hyperplasia (BPH) often occurs during this second growth phase
      - As the prostate enlarges it can cause pressure on the urethra.
      - Bladder wall thickens
      - Eventually the bladder may weaken and lose ability to completely empty the bladder of urine.
      - Urethra narrowing and urinary retention will result in many problems.
- Aging males
  - About 50% of males between 51 and 60 years of age have BPH.
  - Up to 90% of males over 80 years of age have BPH.

Polycystic Kidney Disease

- Inherited disorder
- Causes clusters of cysts to develop within kidneys, resulting in enlarged and dysfunctional kidneys
- Two types
  - Autosomal-dominant polycystic kidney disease (ADPKD)
    - Often develop signs and symptoms between 30 and 40 years of age
  - Autosomal-recessive polycystic kidney disease (ARPKD)
    - Less common
    - Signs and symptoms develop shortly after birth.

- Complications
  - High blood pressure
  - Loss of kidney function
  - Pregnancy complications
  - Heart valve abnormalities
  - Chronic pain
  - Colon problems

Nephrolithiasis

- Kidney stone caused by calculi
- Common condition with 200,000 cases in the United States each year
  - An estimated 5% of adults in the United States
- Signs and symptoms
  - Sudden onset of pain originating in the flank area, radiating inferiorly and anteriorly
    - Caused by dilation, stretching, and spasm
  - Nausea and vomiting
  - Hematuria
  - Individuals with small, nonobstructing stones may present asymptomatically or experience mild signs and symptoms.
- Etiology
  - More common in males
  - Caucasians at greater risk

Hydronephrosis

- Excessive fluid in kidneys caused by backup of urine
- Presents secondary to a complication of calculus, tumors, scar tissue in the kidney or ureter, and untreated prostatic enlargement
- Signs and symptoms
  - Typically asymptomatic
  - Mild flank pain may be noted as the renal capsule is distended.
  - Development of infections would cause other signs and symptoms to arise.

Pyelonephritis

- Infection which extends from the ureter into the kidney(s)
  - Ascending infection involving the renal pelvis and medullary tissues
- May involve one or both kidneys
  - Bilateral obstruction commonly owing to acute kidney injury (AKI)
- Severe infections
  - May compromise renal artery and , which would obstruct urine flow to the ureter
- Recurrent infections
  - Can lead to fibrous scar tissue forming over calyx
    - Loss of tubule function
    - Hydronephrosis
- Signs and symptoms
  - Dysuria
    - Caused by infections being present in kidneys and bladder
  - Pain
    - Usually presents as dull, aching pain in lower back flank area

Glomerulonephritis (Acute Poststreptococcal Glomerulonephritis)

- Glomerulus is formed by the invagination of a ball of capillaries into the Bowman capsule.
- Nephrotic syndrome
  - Characterized by massive loss of protein, which leads to various complications
  - Secondary to many renal diseases and a variety of systemic disorders
    - Systemic lupus erythematosus
    - Exposure to toxins or drugs
  - Pathophysiology
    - Not well established, but the following sequence develops
      - Abnormality in glomerular capillaries and increased permeability that allows large amounts of plasma protein (albumin) to escape into the filtrate
      - This leads to hypoalbuminemia and decreased plasma osmotic pressure, resulting in generalized edema.
      - Blood pressure may remain low owing to hypovolemia or it may be elevated depending on angiotensin II levels.
      - Decrease in blood volume causes an increase in aldosterone secretion that results in severe edema.
      - Hyperlipidemia (high levels of lipids in blood) and lipiduria (high levels of lipids in the urine), which is a possible correlation of the response of the liver to heavy protein loss
  - Signs and symptoms
    - Anasarca
      - Significant edema causing weight gain
    - Pallor
    - Ascites
    - Breathing difficulties
      - Pleural effusion
    - Hindered activity owing to excessive edema
    - Skin breakdown
    - Urinalysis
      - Proteinuria
      - Lipiduria
      - Casts
        - Fatty
        - Epithelial
        - Hyaline
- Nephritic syndrome
  - Characterized by hematuria, oliguria, and hypertension; does have some proteinuria
  - Pathophysiology
    - Often caused by an immune response owing to infection or other disease
      - Common causes in adults
        - Goodpasture syndrome
        - Abdominal access
        - Hepatitis B or C
        - Infective endocarditis
        - Viral disease
          - Mononucleosis

○ Measles

○ Mumps

- Signs and symptoms
  - Oliguria
    - Low urine output
  - Anuria
    - Low urine output
    - Defined as less than 50 mL urine output per day
  - Hypertension
  - Fluid retention
    - Facial edema
  - Hematuria
    - Micro- or macroscopic
  - Uremia
    - High levels of waste products in the blood
  - Proteinuria
    - Protein in the urine

APPLICATION AND REVIEW

2. What is the fundamental characteristic of nephrotic syndrome?
   1. Massive plasma protein loss
   2. Exposure to specific toxins
   3. Decrease in serum hemoglobin
   4. Increased renal capillary permeability
3. What renal condition results in a backup of urine caused by excessive fluid in the kidneys?
   1. Pyelonephritis
   2. Nephrolithiasis
   3. Hydronephrosis
   4. Polycystic kidney disease (PKD)
4. Which client is at greatest risk for developing nephrolithiasis?
   1. A Caucasian male client
   2. A postmenopausal female client
   3. An African-American female client
   4. A male client with a history of tobacco use
5. The nurse is caring for a female client with PKD. Which complications may occur in a client with PKD? **Select all that apply.**
   1. Pregnancy complications
   2. Hypertension
   3. Heart valve dysfunction
   4. Chronic pain
   5. Gastroesophageal reflux disease (GERD)
6. What percentage of males experience signs and symptoms associated with benign prostatic hyperplasia (BPH) by the age of 80 years?
   1. 60%
   2. 70%
   3. 80%
   4. 90%

See Answers on pages 400–401.

Acute Kidney Injury

- Occurs when the kidneys suddenly stop filtering waste from the blood
  - Causes dangerous levels of wastes to accumulate
    - Can develop over a few hours or days

- Involves both kidneys
- Signs and symptoms
  - Rapid development
  - Uremia
    - Clinical signs and symptoms that arise when metabolic waste accumulates in the blood
  - Decreased urine output
  - Edema
    - Caused by fluid retention
  - Shortness of breath
  - Fatigue
  - Nausea/vomiting
  - Seizures/coma in severe cases
- Etiology
  - Primary problem causing reduced blood flow to kidneys
  - Inflammation and necrosis of tubules may cause obstruction and backup.
    - Leads to reduced GFR, oliguria, or anuria
  - Circulatory shock or heart failure, which is severe and prolonged
  - Shock associated with burns
    - Damaged erythrocytes break down in the circulation, the hemoglobin released can accumulate in the renal tubules causing obstruction.
      - Hemoglobin is toxic to tubule epithelium; causes necrosis.
  - Crush injuries
    - Myoglobin release is similar to that of hemoglobin; causes inflammation and necrosis to tubules.
  - Sepsis
  - Nephrotoxins
    - Drugs
    - Chemicals
    - Toxins
  - Mechanical obstructions
    - Tumors
    - Blood clots
- Diagnosis, types, and causes of AKI (named for their location within renal system)
  - Prerenal conditions
    - Condition
      - Inadequate blood circulation to the kidneys, which leaves them unable to filter blood properly
    - Causes
      - Hypovolemia
        - Ineffective circulating volume
        - Dehydration, hemorrhage, burns
      - Cardiac failure
      - Liver failure
      - Shock
      - Renal artery stenosis or emboli
      - ACE inhibitors and nonsteroidal anti-inflammatory drugs (NSAIDs)
        - Impair renal autoregulation mechanisms

- History
  - Weight loss
  - Thirst
  - Volume loss
    - Diuretics
    - Surgery
  - Ineffective circulating volume
- Findings
  - Signs of dehydration
    - Hypovolemia
    - Hypotension
    - Increased heart rate
    - Decreased jugular venous pulse
- Urinalysis
  - Increased urine osmolality; high specific gravity
  - Decreased urine sodium and fractional expressed sodium
  - Increased urine serum creatinine
- Intrinsic (intrarenal) conditions
  - Conditions
    - Failure that is not caused by prerenal or postrenal factors
    - Involves damage and/or injury to both kidneys
    - Accounts for 40% of AKI cases
  - Causes
    - Acute tubular necrosis
      - Ischemia
      - Drug toxicity
        - Antibiotics
          - Acyclovir
          - Roscarnet
        - Chemotherapy
          - Cisplatin
          - Ifosfamide
        - Radiocontrast dyes
          - Used during imaging procedures
      - Toxins
        - Rhabdomyolysis
          - Intoxication
          - Traumatic crush injury
          - Seizure
        - Hypercalcemia
    - Glomerular disease
    - Acute interstitial nephritis
      - Drugs
      - Infections
      - Multiple myeloma
    - Vascular disease
  - History
    - Prior abnormal urinalysis

- Exposure to toxic agents
- New medications
- Hypertension
  - Findings
    - Hypertension
    - Skin lesions and vasculitis
  - Urinalysis
    - Proteinuria
    - Hematuria
    - Pyuria
    - Casts
    - Rental tubular epithelial cells in urine
- Postrenal conditions
  - Condition
    - Acute obstruction which affects normal flow of urine out of kidneys. This obstruction causes backup in the nephrons and causes them to shut down.
  - Causes
    - Bladder overflow obstruction
      - Urethral strictures
      - Benign prostate hypertrophy
    - Tumor
      - Prostate
      - Bladder
      - Gynecologic malignancy (females)
    - Stone
      - Bilateral
    - Retroperitoneal fibrosis
      - Causing obstruction
  - History
    - Renal colic
    - Frequency, hesitancy
    - Nocturia
  - Findings
    - Distended bladder
    - Enlarged prostate (men)
  - Urinalysis
    - Crystalluria
      - Renal calculus
- Phases of AKI
  - Asymptomatic
    - Precipitating event
      - Kidney blockage
      - Decreased cardiac output
  - Oliguric
    - Elevated BUN and serum creatinine levels
    - Urine-specific gravity levels
      - Decreased
        - Prerenal causes

- ▪ Normal
  - ○ Intrarenal causes
- ▪ Hyperkalemia
- ▪ Decreased GFR and creatinine clearance
- ▪ Possibly decreased serum sodium
- ▪ Hypocalcemia
- ▪ Hyperphosphatemia
- Diuretic
  - BUN levels remain elevated, but gradually decrease.
  - Continued low creatinine clearance
  - Improving GFR
  - Hypokalemia
  - Hyponatremia
  - Hypovolemia
- Recovery
  - Increased GFR
  - Stabilization in BUN
  - Serum creatinine levels toward normal
  - Complete recovery may take 1 to 2 years.

Chronic Kidney Disease

- Chronic glomerulonephritis causes CKD as a result of progressive nephron loss.
- Gradual loss of kidney function over time
- As the disease progresses, the kidney shrinks.
  - Cortical thinning
  - Granular scarring
- Glomerulosclerosis
  - Scarring of the glomerulus
  - Histologic hallmark of CKD
- Signs and symptoms
  - Early stages (Table 18.1)
    - ▪ Often asymptomatic
  - Later stages (see Table 18.1)
    - ▪ Signs and symptoms develop as disease progresses.
      - ▪ Waste products accumulate.
    - ▪ Erythropoietin/vitamin D production is reduced.
    - ▪ Hypertension
    - ▪ Edema
      - ▪ Salt and water retention
    - ▪ Anemia
    - ▪ Nausea, vomiting, and diarrhea
    - ▪ Gastrointestinal bleeding
    - ▪ Itching
    - ▪ Lethargy
    - ▪ Polyuria and nocturnal
      - ▪ Paresthesias as a result of polyneuropathy
    - ▪ Altered mental status
      - ▪ Most common during terminal stage of disease

TABLE 18.1	Stages of Chronic Kidney Disease	
Stage	**Description**	**Signs/Symptoms**
I	Normal kidney function Normal or high GFR (>90 mL/min)	*Usually none* Hypertension common
II	Mild kidney damage, mild reduction in GFR (60–89 mL/min)	*Subtle* Hypertension Increasing creatinine and urea levels
III	Moderate kidney damage GFR 30–59 mL/min	*Mild* As above
IV	Severe kidney damage GFR 15–29 mL/min	Moderate As above Erythropoietin deficiency anemia Hyperphosphatemia Increased triglycerides Metabolic acidosis Hyperkalemia Salt/water retention
V	End-stage kidney disease Established kidney failure GFR <15 mL/min	*Severe* As above

GFR, Glomerular filtration rate.
From Huether, S. E., McCance, K. L., Brashers, V. L., & Rote, S. R. (2017). *Understanding pathophysiology* (6th ed.). St. Louis: Elsevier.

- Etiology
  - Intrinsic renal
    - Glomerulonephritis
    - Chronic pyelonephritis
    - PKD
    - Bladder or urethral obstruction
    - Interstitial nephritis
    - Myeloma
    - Amyloid
    - Alport syndrome
    - Renal vascular disease
  - Systemic (extrarenal)
    - Hypertension
    - Diabetes mellitus
    - Heart failure
    - Gout
    - Renovascular disease
    - Vasculitis
  - Drugs
    - Penicillamine
    - Cyclosporine
    - Analgesics

APPLICATION AND REVIEW

7. A client is admitted with severe acute kidney injury (AKI). Which clinical manifestations would the nurse expect? **Select all that apply.**
   1. Seizures
   2. Flank pain
   3. Shortness of breath
   4. Low urine output
   5. Swelling of lower extremities

8. Which client is at risk for developing AKI? **Select all that apply.**
   1. A client diagnosed with PKD
   2. A client diagnosed with sepsis associated with pneumonia
   3. A client who received third-degree burns over 15% of the body
   4. A client experiencing circulatory shock resulting from blood loss
   5. A client who received crushing injuries to the pelvis and both legs

9. What is the cause of the uremia associated with acute renal injury?
   1. Retention of fluids
   2. Chronic hypertension
   3. Accumulation of waste in the blood
   4. Obstruction of urinary flow out of the kidneys

10. What assessment finding suggests the client is in the oliguric phase of AKI?
   1. Decreased serum calcium levels
   2. Near normal serum creatinine levels
   3. Increased glomerulus filtration rate (GFR)
   4. Gradual decreasing blood urea nitrogen (BUN) level

11. A severely burned client is at risk for AKI because of red blood cell damage. What mechanism causes damage to the kidneys?
   1. Initiation of the inflammatory process
   2. Surge of myoglobin into the blood
   3. Obstruction of the renal tubules
   4. Acceleration of clot formation

12. Which medical diagnoses are associated with chronic kidney disease (CKD)? **Select all that apply.**
   1. Gout
   2. PKD
   3. Urethral obstruction
   4. Chronic hypotension
   5. Renal vascular disease

See Answers on pages 400–401.

Wilms Tumor (Nephroblastoma)

- Rare kidney tumor primarily affecting children
  - Most common type of kidney cancer in children
    - 9 of 10 (makes up 9 of 10 kidney cancers in children)
  - Unilateral tumor
    - Only 5% of children will have bilateral disease.
  - Commonly affects children 3 to 4 years of age; much less common after 5 years of age.
  - More common in African-Americans compared to Caucasians; less common in Asians.
  - More common in females than males.
  - Types of Wilms tumor
    - Favorable histology
      - Less aggressive

- Cancer cells do not look quite normal; however, there is no anaplasia.
    - Unfavorable histology (anaplastic Wilms tumor)
        - Anaplastic cells
            - Poor cellular differentiation
            - Cells vary significantly and the cell nuclei tend to be very large and distorted.
            - The greater the anaplastic the tumor is, the harder it is to treat/cure.
    - Signs and symptoms
        - Abdominal pain
        - Constipation
        - Nausea/vomiting
        - Fever
        - Loss of appetite
        - Weakness/fatigue
        - Hematuria
        - High blood pressure

Renal Cell Carcinoma

- Adenocarcinoma of the kidney
- Malignant cancer cells are found in the lining of the tubules in the kidney.
- Signs and symptoms
    - Early stage
        - Typically asymptomatic
            - Typically diagnosis is made in one-third of cases after disease has progressed and metastasized to other areas (liver, lungs, bone, or CNS).
        - Painless hematuria
            - Gross or microscopic
    - Later stage
        - Flank pain
        - Palpable mass
        - Unplanned and unexplained weight loss
        - Anemia
        - Paraneoplastic syndromes
            - Hypercalcemia
                - Increased parathyroid hormone
            - Cushing syndrome
                - Increased adrenocorticotropic hormone
- Etiology
    - Commonly in males
    - More frequent in smokers
    - Very rarely in individuals 45 years of age and younger
    - 5-year survival rate
        - Stage I
            - 95%
        - Stage IV
            - 23%

APPLICATION AND REVIEW

13. Which assessment findings support a client's diagnosis of later stage renal carcinoma? **Select all that apply.**
    1. Anemia
    2. Flank pain
    3. Weight loss
    4. Gross hematuria
    5. Microscopic hematuria
14. Which client is at greatest risk for the development of a Wilms tumor?
    1. A 3-year-old African-American client
    2. A 13-year-old client with a history of asthma
    3. A 35-year-old client who started smoking at age 15
    4. A 50-year-old client with a history of type 2 diabetes

See Answers on pages 400–401.

ANSWER KEY: REVIEW QUESTIONS

1. **2 Serum creatinine concentration measures the kidney's ability to excrete metabolic wastes. Creatinine, a nitrogenous product of protein breakdown, is increased with renal insufficiency.**

   1 A renal ultrasound is more valuable for assessing structure than function. **3** WBC count does not measure kidney function; WBCs usually are depressed because of immunosuppressive therapy to prevent rejection. **4** A serum potassium level would be increased with renal failure, but would not be as specific to renal function as the serum creatinine.

   Client Need: Physiological Adaptation; **Cognitive Level:** Applying; **Nursing Process:** Analysis

2. **1 Nephrotic syndrome is characterized by a massive loss of protein, which leads to various complications.**

   2 Exposure to toxins can trigger the loss of protein, but is not a characteristic of nephrotic syndrome. **3** Increased serum hemoglobin is not a characteristic of nephrotic syndrome. **4** Increased capillary permeability allows for the characteristic loss of plasma protein.

   Client Need: Physiological Adaptation; **Cognitive Level:** Understanding; **Integrated Process:** Teaching and Learning

3. **4 Hydronephrosis is excessive fluid in kidneys owing to backup of urine.**

   1 Pyelonephritis is an infection that extends from the ureter into the kidney(s). **2** Nephrolithiasis is a condition where calculi form kidney stones. **4** PKD causes clusters of cysts to develop within kidneys, resulting in enlarged and dysfunctional kidneys.

   Client Need: Physiological Adaptation; **Cognitive Level:** Understanding; **Integrated Process:** Teaching and Learning

4. **1 Nephrolithiasis (or kidney stones caused by calculi) are more common in Caucasian males.**

   2 Nephrolithiasis are more common in Caucasian males. **3** Nephrolithiasis are more common in Caucasian males. **4** Although more common in males, tobacco use is not an identified risk factor for nephrolithiasis.

   Client Need: Physiological Adaptation; **Cognitive Level:** Applying; **Nursing Process:** Assessment

5. **Answers: 1, 2, 3, 4**

   1 PKD can result in pregnancy complications. **2** PKD can result in hypertension. **3** PKD can result in heart valve abnormalities. **4** PKD can result in chronic pain.

   5 PKD is not associated with GERD.

   Client Need: Physiological Adaptation; **Cognitive Level:** Analysis; **Nursing Process:** Planning

6. **4 By the age of 80, up to 90% of the male population has signs and symptoms associated with BPH.**

   1, 2, 3 These values do not reflect the percentage of the male population aged 80 and older who have signs and symptoms associated with BPH.

   Client Need: Physiological Adaptation; **Cognitive Level:** Understanding; **Integrated Process:** Teaching and Learning

7. **2 Flank pain occurs with acute pyelonephritis or renal calculi not AKI.**

   1 Seizures can occur in severe cases of AKI. **3** Shortness of breath is a classic sign of AKI. **4** A decrease in urinary output is a classic sign of AKI. **5** Edema is an expected sign of AKI.

   Client Need: Physiological Adaptation; **Cognitive Level:** Analysis; **Nursing Process:** Evaluation

8. **Answers: 2, 3, 4, 5**

   2 Sepsis can trigger AKI because of the resulting effect on blood circulation. **3** Burns severe enough to produce shock can trigger AKI because of the resulting effect on blood circulation. **4** Circulatory shock and the resulting effect on blood circulation can trigger AKI. **5** Crushing injuries and the resulting effect on blood circulation can trigger AKI.

   1 PKD is associated with CKD.

   Client Need: Physiological Adaptation; **Cognitive Level:** Applying; **Nursing Process:** Assessment

9. **3 Uremia is associated with a collection of clinical symptoms that arise when metabolic waste accumulates in the blood.**

   1 Edema is a result of fluid retention. **2** Chronic hypertension can ultimately affect blood flow to the kidneys, but is not directly associated with uremia. **4** Urine flow from the kidneys is not directly associated with uremia.

   Client Need: Physiological Adaptation; **Cognitive Level:** Understanding; **Integrated Process:** Teaching and Learning

10. **1 Hypocalcemia occurs in the oliguric phase of AKI.**

    2 Normal or near normal serum creatinine levels are associated with the recovery phase of AKI. **3** An increasing glomerular filtration rate is associated with the recovery phase of AKI. **4** Decreasing BUN is associated with the diuretic phase of AKI.

    Client Need: Physiological Adaptation; **Cognitive Level:** Applying; **Nursing Process:** Assessment

11. **3 When damaged erythrocytes (red blood cells) break down in the circulation, the hemoglobin released can accumulate in the tubules causing obstruction.**

    1, 2 Myoglobin resulting from muscle injury is released into the blood, causing inflammation. **4** Natural clot formation is not directly affected by erythrocyte damage.

    Client Need: Physiological Adaptation; **Cognitive Level:** Analysis; **Integrated Process:** Teaching and learning

12. **Answers: 1, 2, 3, 5**

    1 Gout is an extrarenal cause of CKD. **2** PKD is an intrinsic renal cause of CKD. **3** A urethral obstruction is an intrinsic cause of CKD. **5** Renal vascular disease is an intrinsic cause of CKD.

    4 Hypertension is considered an extrarenal cause of CKD.

    Client Need: Physiological Adaptation; **Cognitive Level:** Applying; **Nursing Process:** Analysis

13. **Answers: 1, 2, 3**

    1, 2, 3 Later stage signs and symptoms of renal carcinoma include anemia, flank pain, and weight loss. **4** Gross hematuria is seen in early-stage renal carcinoma. **5** Microscopic hematuria is seen in early-stage renal carcinoma.

    Client Need: Physiological Adaptation; **Cognitive Level:** Understanding; **Nursing Process:** Assessment

14. **1 Wilms tumor is a rare kidney tumor primarily affecting children; most commonly diagnosed between ages 3 to 4 years; Wilms tumor is more common in African-Americans than in Caucasians.**

    2, 3, 4 Neither asthma, smoking, nor diabetes is considered a risk factor for a Wilms tumor.

    Client Need: Physiological Adaptation; **Cognitive Level:** Applying; **Nursing Process:** Assessment

19 Female Reproductive System Disorders

OVERVIEW

- Ovaries
  - Female gonads
    - Produce the ova that is released each month during the reproductive years between menarche (onset) and menopause (end) of menses
  - Two ovaries are held, suspended by ligaments, one on each side of the uterus.
  - Ovaries supply estrogen and progesterone on a cyclic basis (Table 19.1).
- Fallopian tubes (oviducts)
  - Originate near top of uterus
    - Under fundus
  - Each tube curves up and out, ending at the ovary.
    - End portion has fimbriae, which draw the released ovum into the tube; the ovum is then moved toward the uterus.
- Uterus
  - Muscular sac where a fertilized ovum would be implanted and developed
  - Uterine wall is made up of three layers.
    - Parietal peritoneum
      - Outer layer
    - Myometrium
      - Thick, middle layer of smooth muscle
    - Inner endometrium
      - Functional layer
        - Responsible for hormones during the menstrual cycle
      - Underlying basal layer
        - Responsible or regeneration of the endometrium after menses
- Vagina
  - Entryway to the reproductive tract
  - Muscular, distensible canal extending upward from the vulva to the cervix
  - Lined with mucosal membrane and falls in rugae (folds)
    - This structure allows for expansion during intercourse or childbirth.
- External genitalia (vulva)
  - Made up of
    - Mons pubis
      - Adipose tissue and hair coving the symphysis pubis
    - Labia
      - Labia minora
        - Outer fold
      - Labia minora
        - Inner area
      - Protect orifices
    - Clitoris
      - Small projection of erectile tissue located anterior to the urethra

TABLE 19.1	Principal Female Reproductive Hormones	
Hormone	**Target Organs**	**Significant Actions**
Estrogen	Multiple sites through-out body, including reproductive struc-tures, bone, fat, and muscle tissues	Development of reproductive organs during puberty Development of secondary sex characteristics, including breast maturation, widening of pelvis, and distribution of fat and muscle tissues in a distinctively female pattern Cyclic preparation of endometrium for implantation of an ovum
Progesterone	Primarily uterus and breasts	Cyclic preparation and maintenance of endometrium for implantation of an ovum Stimulation of development of breast lobes and alveoli
Follicle-stimulating hormone	Ovary	Stimulates ovarian follicle development; with luteinizing hormone, stimulates secretion of estrogen and ovulation
Luteinizing hormone	Ovary	Stimulates final development of ovarian follicle, process of ovulation, and development of corpus luteum

From Banasik, J. L., & Copstead, L. C. (2019). *Pathophysiology* (6th ed.). St. Louis: Elsevier.

- Vaginal orifice
  - Entryway to reproductive tract
- Mammary glands
  - Milk-producing gland in females
  - Located in the breast overlying the pectoralis major muscles

Menstrual Cycle

- Consists of the hormonal secretions, release of ova, and associated endometrial changes females experience
- Occurs in a cyclic pattern during reproductive years
- Average cycle is 28 days
  - Range of 21 to 45 days is considered normal.
  - Some females experience irregular cycles.

Menstrual Phases

- Menstruation (menses)
  - Sloughing of the endometrial tissue
  - Occurs when implantation of the ovum has not occurred
- Endometrial proliferation
  - Increasing follicle-stimulating hormone (FSH) is secreted by the anterior pituitary gland.
  - Maturing follicle secretes estrogen, causing proliferation.
    - Thickening of the functional layer of the endometrium
  - As luteinizing hormone (LH) levels increase, ovulation takes place with release of the mature ovum.
  - LH then converts the ovarian follicle into the corpus luteum.
    - Increases progesterone production
  - Progesterone increases the development of endometrial blood vessels and glycogen-secreting glands to prepare for implantation of a fertilized ovum.
- Secretory
  - If fertilization does not occur, estrogen and progesterone levels drop.

- Corpus luteum and endometrial degeneration
- Results in menstruation
  - Also begins another cycle

Menstrual Disorders

- Amenorrhea
  - Absence of menstruation
  - May be primary or secondary
    - Primary
      - Menarche has never occurred.
      - May be owing to genetic disorders or congenital defects
        - Genetic disorders
          - Turner syndrome
            - Chromosome abnormality in which ovaries do not function properly
        - Congenital defects
          - Congenital defects affecting the hypothalamus, central nervous system (CNS), or pituitary
          - Congenital absences of the uterus and uterine hypoplasia
            - Infantile uterus
    - Secondary
      - Cessation of menstruation in a female who previously experienced cycles
      - Commonly results from an impediment in the hypothalamic-pituitary axis
        - Hypothalamus may be suppressed by several conditions.
          - Tumors
          - Sudden weight loss
          - Stress
          - Eating disorders
            - Low body fat
      - Systemic factors may also cause secondary amenorrhea
        - Anemia
        - Chemotherapy
- Dysmenorrhea
  - Painful menstruation
    - Pain significantly interrupts normal activities.
    - Pain is related to the excessive release of prostaglandin during endometrial shedding.
  - Pain develops 24 to 48 hours prior to onset of menses.
  - May be primary or secondary
    - Primary
      - No organic foundation
      - Develops when ovulation commences
    - Secondary
      - Results from pelvic disorders
        - Endometriosis
        - Uterine polyps or tumors
        - Pelvic inflammatory disease (PID)
  - May be accompanied by other signs and symptoms
    - Nausea

- Vomiting
- Headache
- Dizziness
- In many cases dysmenorrhea may be relieved after childbirth.
- Bleeding abnormalities
  - Mcnorrhagia
    - Increased amount and duration of flow
  - Metrorrhagia
    - Bleeding between cycles
  - Polymenorrhea
    - Short cycles
      - Less than 3 weeks
  - Oligomenorrhea
    - Long cycles
      - More than 6 weeks
- Premenstrual syndrome (PMS)
  - Begins about a week before onset of menses and ends with the onset of menses
  - Hormonal factors could contribute.
  - Signs and symptoms
    - Weight gain
    - Breast tenderness
    - Abdominal distention
      - Bloating
    - Irritability
    - Emotional lability
    - Sleep disturbances
    - Depression
    - Headache
    - Fatigue
  - Premenstrual dystrophic syndrome
    - A more severe form of PMS
- Menopause
  - Natural biological process marking the end of female menstrual cycles.
    - Function of the ovaries cease
  - Diagnosis
    - After 12 months without a menstrual period
  - Average onset age is 51 years of age
  - After menopause estrogen and progesterone hormones levels drop significantly.
  - Signs and symptoms
    - Irregular periods
    - Hot flashes
    - Sleeping difficulties
    - Night sweats
    - Mood changes
      - Irritability
- Uterine prolapse
  - Descent of the cervix or uterus into the vagina

- Classifications
  - First degree
    - Cervix drops into the vagina.
  - Second degree
    - Cervix lies at the opening of the vagina and the body of the uterus is in the vagina.
  - Third degree (procidentia)
    - Uterus and cervix protrude through the vaginal orfice.
- Signs and symptoms
  - Early stages
    - May be asymptomatic
  - Advanced stages
    - Discomfort
    - Heaviness in vagina
    - Irritation
    - Infection
- Ovarian cyst
  - Multiple, small, fluid-filled sacs
  - Located under the serosa covering the ovary
  - Most commonly follicular and corpus luteum cysts
  - Develops unilaterally in both ruptured and unruptured follicles
  - Lasts about 8 to 12 weeks, then disappear without complications
  - Signs and symptoms (large cysts)
    - Discomfort
    - Urinary retention
    - Menstrual irregularities
    - Bleeding
      - May cause more serious inflammation in the peritoneal vanity.
      - Requires surgery
    - Torsion of the ovary
- Polycystic ovary syndrome (PCOS)
  - Imbalance of reproductive hormones
    - Affects ovaries
      - Egg may not develop as it should or it may not be released during ovulation as it should be.
  - Enlarged ovaries with small cysts on outer edge
  - Commonly in females during reproductive age
    - Affects 1 in 10 females
    - One of the most common causes of female infertility
  - Etiology
    - Obesity
    - Inherited factor
      - Increased risk if individual has mother, sister, or aunt with PCOS
  - Signs and symptoms
    - Irregular periods
      - Infertility
      - Development of cysts in the ovaries
    - Hirsutism
      - Excess hair on face, chin, or parts of the body where men usually have hair.

- Acne
- Thinning hair
  - Male pattern baldness
- Weight gain
  - Difficulty losing weight
- Darkening of skin
  - Commonly along crease lines (groin, under breast)
- Skin tags
  - Excess flaps of skin in armpit and/or neck area

Candidiasis

- Form of vaginitis
- Yeast infection
  - Candida albicans
- Not sexually transmitted
  - Opportunistic superficial infection of mucous membranes or skin
- Etiology
  - Following antibiotic therapy
    - Creates more alkaline pH and upsets the normal flora balances
  - Decreased resistance
    - Immune-deficiency states
  - Increased glycogen or glucose levels in the secretions
    - Pregnancy
    - Use of oral contraceptives
    - Diabetes
  - Signs and symptoms
    - Red and swollen prurience mucous membranes
    - Thick, white curd-like discharge
    - White patches on vaginal wall
    - Dysuria
      - Painful urination
    - Dyspareunia
      - Painful intercourse

Endometriosis

- Presence of endometrial tissue outside the uterus
  - Tissue may be present on outer structures.
    - Ovaries
    - Ligaments
    - Colon
    - Lungs
      - Rare
- Responds to cyclic hormone variations
  - Grows during proliferation and secretory phases of menstrual cycle, then degenerating, shedding, and bleeding
- No exit point for blood
  - Blood irritates tissue.

- Causes local inflammation and pain
- Eventually causes development of fibrous tissue at the site.
- Involved structures may develop adhesions and obstructions over time.
- Diagnosis is confirmed by laparoscopy.
- Signs and symptoms
  - Dysmenorrhea
    - Painful menstruation
  - Dyspareunia
    - Painful intercourse
    - Occurs when vagina and ligaments are affected by adhesions
      - Infertility
      - Pain
      - Dyschezia
        - Pain upon defecation
      - Constipation
      - Abnormal vaginal bleeding
      - If implants are located within the pelvis they may cause an asymptomatic pelvic mass having irregular, movable nodules and a fixed, retroverted uterus.

Fibroids (Leiomyoma)

- Benign tumor of the myometrium
- Cause is unknown.
- Common in females during reproductive years
  - Occur in more than 30% of females
  - Greater in Asian and African American women
- Classified by location
  - Intramural
    - In the uterine wall
  - Submucosal
    - Beneath the endometrium
  - Subserosal
    - Under the serosa
- Signs and symptoms
  - Commonly asymptomatic until they are large enough to be palpated
  - Large tumor symptoms
    - Abnormal bleeding
    - Causes pressure on adjacent structures
      - Urinary frequency
      - Constipation
      - Heavy sensation in lower abdomen
    - May interfere with implantation of the fertilized ovum or the course of pregnancy

Fibrocystic Breast Disease; (Benign Breast Disease; Fibrocystic Change)

- Broad range of breast lesions
- Presence of nodules or masses in the breast tissue that change during the menstrual cycle in response to fluctuating hormone levels
  - Particularly estrogen

- Connective breast tissue eventually is replaced by dense fibrous tissue.
- Three categories
  - Nonproliferation lesions
    - Mircocysts and fibroadenomas
    - Not considered precancerous
      - Benign tumors
  - Proliferation lesions without atypia
    - No atypical cells
    - Risk of developing breast cancer in this group increases if there is a family history.
  - Atypical hyperplasia
    - Proliferative changes with atypical cells
    - Increased risk with family history
    - Requires monitoring
    - Breast biopsy may be needed to determine benign from malignant cells.
- Signs and symptoms
  - Occur before menstruation
  - Heavy, painful, and tender breast

Mastitis

- Two types
  - Lactation (puerperal) mastitis
    - Common condition affecting breastfeeding women
      - Approximately 1 in 10 females affected
  - Periductal mastitis
    - Occurs in nonbreastfeeding women
    - Caused by cracked or pierced nipple, which allows bacteria to get into the milk ducts, therefore causing infection
- Signs and symptoms
  - Breast swelling
  - Redness
  - Tenderness
  - Warm/hot to touch
  - Body aches
  - Fever
  - Chills
  - Fatigue

Pelvic Inflammatory Disease

- Infection of the reproductive tract
  - Fallopian tubes and ovaries
- Many types of bacteria can cause PID
  - Polymicrobial
    - Involving several causative bacteria
  - Most commonly (from sexually transmitted diseases [STDs])
    - Gonorrhea
    - Chlamydia
  - May also be caused by bacteria found in the vagina
    - Not always from sexual intercourse

- Condition includes
  - Cervicitis endometritis
    - Uterus
  - Salpingitis
  - Oophoritis
- May be acute or chronic
  - Acute
    - Comes on suddenly
    - More severe symptoms
  - Chronic
    - Low-grade infection
    - Milder symptoms
- Can cause scarring to fallopian tubes and permanent damage to female reproductive organs
  - Most common cause of infertility and ectopic pregnancy
- Etiology
  - Bacteria
    - Gonorrhea
    - Chlamydiosia
    - Bactericides
    - *Gardnerella vaginalis*
    - Group B streptococci
    - *Escherichia coli*
    - Pseudomonas
    - *Haemophilus influenzae*
    - Enterococcus
  - Prior episodes
    - Commonly presenting with few symptoms
      - Precedes the development of PID
  - During or immediately following menses
    - Endometrium is more vulnerable
  - Insertion of an intrauterine device (IUD) or other contaminated instrument
    - Instruments and devices are likely to traumatize the tissue or perforate the wall, leading to inflammation and/or infection.
- Signs and symptoms
  - Lower abdominal pain
    - Characterized by a steady pain that increases with walking
  - Purulent discharge
  - Dysuria
    - Discomfort, pain, and/or burning during urination
  - Fever
  - Leukocytosis
    - Elevated white blood cell (WBC) count
  - Peritonitis
    - Inflammation of the peritoneum

Breast Cancer

- Malignant tumors commonly develop in the upper outer quadrant of the breast.
  - In approximately half of the cases

- Central portion of the breast is the next most common location for development.
- Most tumors are unilateral.
  - Bilateral primary tumors may develop, but are not as common.
- Several types of breast carcinomas
  - Most commonly arise from cells of the ductal epithelium
    - Infiltrates surrounding tissue and commonly adheres to skin, causing dimpling
    - Tumor is fixed.
      - Adheres to muscle or fascia of the chest wall
- Malignant cells spread at an early stage.
  - First spread to the nearby lymph nodes
- Upper outer quadrant and central breast area tumors spread to the auxiliary lymph nodes.
  - Several nodes are commonly affected by the time of diagnosis.
- Widespread dissemination may follow.
  - May metastasize to the lungs, brain, bone, and liver
- Grading
  - Tumor cells are graded based on the degree of differentiation or anaplasia.
  - Grades
    - Grade 1
      - Well differentiated
      - Usually slow-growing
    - Grade 2
      - Moderately differentiated
      - Growing faster
    - Grade 3
      - Poorly differentiated
      - Fast-growing
- Staging
  - Based on the size of the primary tumor, the involvement of lymph nodes, and the presence of metastasis
- Etiology
  - Females more than 50 years of age
  - Strong genetic predisposition
    - *BRCA-1* and *BRCA-2*
  - Hormones
    - Exposure to high estrogen levels
      - Long period of regular menstrual cycles
        - An early menarche to late menopause
      - Nulliparity
        - Female that has not borne offspring
      - Delay of first pregnancy
      - Exogenous estrogen in oral contraceptives
  - Fibrocystic disease with atypical hyperplasia
  - Prior carcinoma in the uterus or in the other breast
  - Exposure of the chest to radiation
    - Primarily in younger women
  - Lifestyle choices
    - Lack of exercise
    - Smoking

- High-fat diet
- Signs and symptoms
  - Initial sign is single, small, hard, painless nodule.
  - Mass is freely movable in the early stage; will become fixed later.
  - As mass becomes more advanced other symptoms will appear.
    - Dimpling of skin
    - Retraction of or discharge from the nipple
    - Change in breast contour

APPLICATION AND REVIEW

1. What is the classic symptom of endometriosis?
   1. Amenorrhea
   2. Dysmenorrhea
   3. Uterine fibroids
   4. Iron deficiency anemia
2. What lifestyle choices will the nurse suggest when discussing the reduction of breast cancer risks? **Select all that apply.**
   1. Incorporating exercise into a weekly routine
   2. Reducing the consumption of fried foods
   3. Wearing a well-fitted bra regularly
   4. Taking a multiple vitamin daily
   5. Avoiding tobacco smoking
3. Which assessment findings support the diagnosis of advanced breast cancer? **Select all that apply.**
   1. Discharge reported from right nipple
   2. Dimpling noted on breast tissue lateral of left nipple.
   3. A painless nodule palpated in the area of the left axilla
   4. Left breast is observed to be slightly larger than right breast
   5. A fixed lump palpated in the right upper quadrant of right breast

See Answers on pages 421–423.

Cervical Cancer

- The Centers for Disease Control and Prevention (CDC) defines cervical carcinoma as an STD.
- Majority of cervical carcinomas arise from squamous cells.
- Early changes in cervical epithelial tissue consist of dysplasia.
  - Abnormal cells within a tissue
- Usually occurs at the junction of the columnar cells with the squamous epithelial cells of the external so of the cervix
  - The transformation zone
- Grades
  - Cervical intraepithelial neoplasia
    - Graded from I to III
      - Based on the amount of dysplasia and the degree of cell differentiation
      - Stage 0
        - Represents carcinoma in situ
      - Stage I
        - Cancer restricted to the cervix
      - State II
        - Further spread to surrounding tissue

- Stage III
  - Advanced spreading
- Time span from mild dysplasia to carcinoma in situ may be 10 years; this presents many opportunities to be detected in the early stage.
- Carcinoma in situ
  - Noninvasive stage, to be followed by the invasive stage
- Invasive carcinoma
  - Varying characteristics
  - Protruding modular mass
  - Ulceration
  - Infiltrating the wall
- Etiology
  - Strongly linked to oncogenic STDs
  - Herpes simplex virus type 2 (HSV-2)
    - Human papilloma virus (HPV) strains 16, 18, 31, 34, and 45
  - High risk factors
    - Multiple sexual partners
    - Promiscuous partners
    - Sexual intercourse during early teen years
    - History of STDs
    - Smoking
- Prevention
  - Vaccine
    - Gardasil
      - Covers several HPV strands
        - HPV-6
        - HPV-11
        - HPV-16
        - HPV-18
      - Recommended for girls before adolescence
- Signs and symptoms
  - Early stage
    - Asymptomatic
  - Invasive stage
    - Slight bleeding/spotty
    - Watery discharge
    - Anemia
    - Weight loss

Endometrial Cancer (Uterine Cancer)

- Leiomyosarcomas
  - Uterine cancers derived from connective tissue or muscle
  - Have poor prognosis
  - Frequently have metastasized to lungs by the time of diagnosis
- Adenocarcinomas
  - Majority of endometrial carcinomas
  - Arising from glandular epithelium
  - Excessive estrogen stimulation is a major factor.

- Slow-growing tumor, may infiltrate the uterine wall
- Staging
  - Based on the degree of localization
    - Stage I
      - Tumors are confined to the body of the uterus.
      - Five-year survival rate is 99%.
    - Stage II
      - Tumor is limited to the uterus and cervix.
      - Five-year survival rate is 80%.
    - Stage III
      - Tumor has spread outside the uterus; however, remains within the true pelvis.
      - Five-year survival rate is 60%.
    - State IV
      - Tumor has spread to the lymph nodes and distant organs.
      - Five-year survival rate is 32%.
- Grade
  - Graded from 1, indicating well-differentiated cells, to grade 3, indicating poorly differentiated cells
- Etiology
  - Common in women more than 40 years of age
    - Majority of cases between 55 and 65 years age range
  - Hormonal factors
  - Estrogen therapy postmenopause
  - Birth control pills
  - Tamoxifen
  - Number of menstrual cycles (over a lifetime)
  - Pregnancy
  - Certain ovarian tumors
  - Polycystic ovarian syndrome
  - Diet and exercise
  - Diabetics
  - Family history
  - Having been diagnosed with breast or ovarian cancer in the past
  - Having been diagnosed with endometrial hyperplasia in the past
  - Treatment with radiation therapy to the pelvis to treat another cancer
- Symptoms
  - Early signs
    - Painless vaginal spotting or bleeding
  - Late signs
    - Palpable mass
    - Discomfort/pressure in lower abdomen
    - Bleeding after intercourse
- Treatment
  - Surgery in combination with radiation is recommended treatment.
  - Chemotherapy is used in later stages.

Ovarian Cancer

- Considered a silent tumor
  - Only 25% diagnosed in the early stage
- Different types vary in virulence.
  - Serous
    - Accounts for the majority of cases
  - Mutinous
  - Endometriosis tumors
- Etiology
  - More than 55 years of age
    - Two-thirds of women diagnosed
  - Genetic factors
  - Being overweight or obese
  - Having children later or never having full-term pregnancy
  - Taking hormone therapy after menopause
  - Having a family history of ovarian cancer, breast cancer, or colorectal cancer
  - Having family cancer syndrome
  - About 5% to 10% of ovarian cancers are part of family cancer syndromes resulting from inherited mutations.
  - Hereditary breast and ovarian cancer syndrome
  - Inherited mutations in the genes BRCA1 and BRCA2
  - PTEN tumor hamartoma syndrome
  - Also known as Cowden disease
  - Primarily affected with thyroid problems, thyroid cancer, and breast cancer
  - Hereditary nonpolyposis colon cancer
  - Women with this syndrome have a very high risk of colon cancer and have an increased risk of developing cancer of the uterus and ovarian cancer.
  - Peutz-Jeghers syndrome
  - Rare genetic disorder
  - Develop polyps in the stomach and intestine; usually during teenage years
  - MUTYH-associated polyposis
  - Individuals develop polyps in the colon and small intestine and have a high risk of colon cancer.
  - Having been diagnosed with breast cancer
  - Smoking and alcohol use
- Symptoms
  - Early signs
    - Feeling of fullness/bloating
    - Indigestion
    - Frequent urination
    - Back pain
    - Pain with sexual intercourse
  - Late signs
    - Large mass

APPLICATION AND REVIEW

4. A nurse is assessing a client who is experiencing postmenopausal bleeding. The tentative diagnosis is endometrial cancer. Which findings in the client's history are risk factors associated with endometrial cancer? **Select all that apply.**
   1. Obesity
   2. Multiparity
   3. Cigarette smoking
   4. Early onset of menopause
   5. Previous hormone replacement therapy

5. Which client is at **highest** risk for ovarian cancer?
   1. A 55- year-old client who is postmenopausal
   2. A 20-year-old client with a family history of ovarian cancer
   3. A 62-year-old client reporting back pain
   4. A 40-year-old client experiencing recurrent indigestion

6. Which diagnostic finding would support a 60% survival rate for a client with uterine cancer?
   1. Tumors confined to within the true pelvis
   2. Cervix and uterus are sites of tumor spread
   3. Tumors are found only in the uterus
   4. Tumor has spread to lymph nodes

7. Which chronic health issues increase a female's risk for developing uterine cancer? **Select all that apply.**
   1. Asthma
   2. Diabetes
   3. Hypertension
   4. Cystic fibrosis
   5. Osteoporosis

8. What statement, if made by the nurse, demonstrates an understanding of the term "dysplasia" when used to describe the results of a client's cervical cell biopsy?
   1. "This means that cancer treatment will be prescribed very soon."
   2. "The term doesn't relate to the risk of developing cancer."
   3. "There are signs of precancerous cellular change."
   4. "The client has signs of advanced staged cancer."

9. A client with stage I cervical cancer asks the nurse to explain the diagnosis. Which is the best response by the nurse?
   1. "There are four stages, and this means it could be much worse."
   2. "The cancer cells are found only in your cervix and that's a favorable sign."
   3. "It's a really good cancer diagnosis since the cancer cells haven't spread at all."
   4. "There are cancer cells in tissue surrounding your cervix so chemotherapy will be prescribed."

10. What assessment findings would indicate that a client is at high risk for developing cervical cancer? **Select all that apply.**
    1. Has a 1½ pack a day smoking habit
    2. Became sexually active at age 13 years
    3. Being treated for genital warts
    4. Has given birth to two live babies
    5. Is 30 years old

11. What statement, if made by the nurse, indicates an understanding of the signs and symptoms of cervical cancer that have been identified in its early stage?
    1. "It often begins with a watery discharge."
    2. "There are no signs or symptoms present."
    3. "Feeling unusually tired is a common symptom."
    4. "A classic sign is slight vaginal bleeding between periods."

See Answers on pages 421–423.

Sexually Transmitted Diseases (Table 19.2)

- STDs encompass a broad range of infectious diseases that are spread by sexual contact.

TABLE 19.2 Sexually Transmitted Diseases

Infection	Cause	Signs	Complications	Treatment/Cure
Chlamydia	Chlamydia *Chlamydia trachomatis*	Mild dysuria and discharge or asymptomatic	Arthritis females—pelvic inflammatory disease and infertility Neonates—conjunctivitis and pneumonia	Antimicrobial therapy (e.g., azithromycin) Retest for eradication
Gonorrhea	Bacterium *Neisseria gonorrhoeae*	Dysuria and discharge Mild or asymptomatic in women	Arthritis Male—prostatitis and epididymitis Female—pelvic inflammatory disease and infertility Neonates—conjunctivitis	Antibacterial drugs (penicillin or ceftriaxone + doxycycline) Some drug-resistant strains Retest for eradication
Syphilis	Bacterium *Treponeno pallidum*	Primary syphilis—painless ulcer or chancre at site of entry Secondary syphilis—rash, fever, headache	Tertiary syphilis—gumma, neurosyphilis, or cardiovascular system damage Congenital syphilis in child	Penicillin G—long-acting Retest for eradication
Genital herpes	Virus Herpes simplex 2	Vesicles and ulcers	Recurs Meningitis Fetus/neonate damage	No cure Antiviral drug (e.g., oral acyclovir) reduces activity and shedding
Genital warts	Virus Human papillomavirus	Soft gray mass or polyp	None	Can be removed, but rarely cured
Trichomoniasis	Protozoa *Trichomonas vaginalis*	Asymptomatic, or women may have discharge and dysuria	None	Antimicrobial drugs (e.g., metronidazole)

From Hubert, R. J., & VanMeter, K. C. (2018). *Gould's pathophysiology for the health professions* (6th ed.). Philadelphia: Saunders.

- Incidence of STDs has increased in recent years.
  - Factors contributing to an increase in STDs
    - Increased participation in premarital sex
    - Increased divorce rate
    - Increased number of sexual partners
    - Decreased protective measures
- Concerns about STDs
  - Immunity against recurrent infections is not achieved; therefore recurrence is common.
  - Careful testing and diagnosis to uncover the presence of secondary infections are necessary.
    - More than one STD may be present.
  - STDs may present as asymptomatic, particularly in women, thus promoting the spread of infection.
  - Viral STDs have no cure.
    - Herpes
    - Human immunodeficiency virus (HIV)
  - Drug-resistant microorganisms are becoming more common; this increases the inherent risks associated with STDs.
  - Infections can be transmitted from mother to newborn.
    - Results in congenital defects, disability, or death for child
  - Sexual partners of an infected individual may be difficult to trace, notify, and treat.
  - Protective measures (condoms) are often not used (or used improperly) in high-risk situations.

Bacterial Sexually Transmitted Diseases

- Chlamydial infection
  - One of the most common STDs
    - Leading cause of PID
  - Pathogen is *Chlamydia trachomatis*.
    - Gram-negative obligate intracellular parasite
    - Requires a host cell to reproduce
- Invade the epithelial tissue of the urogenital tract causing inflammation
- Signs and symptoms
  - Females
    - Asymptomatic until PID develops
- Gonorrhea
  - Caused by *Neisseria gonorrhoeae*
    - Gram-negative aerobic diplococcus (gonococcus)
    - Many strands have become resistant to penicillin and tetracycline.
  - Uses pili to attach to the epithelial cells then damage the mucosa.
    - Causes an inflammatory reaction and formation of a purulent exudate
- Signs and symptoms
  - Females
    - Frequently asymptomatic
    - PID frequently follows the infection
- Syphilis
  - Causative organism is *Treponema pallidum*
    - Anaerobic spirochete

- Systemic infection that consist of four stages
  - Primary stage
    - Presence of chancre
      - Painless, firm, ulcerated nodule that develops at the point of contact on the skin or mucosa about 3 weeks after exposure
    - Asymptomatic
  - Second stage
    - Chancre heals (several weeks) later; by this time the organisms have entered the general circulation.
    - If left untreated, the second stage of infections begins with widespread symmetric rash.
      - Rash is commonly maculopapular and reddish.
      - Mucous patches may appear on the tongue.
      - Rash disappears spontaneously in a few weeks.
  - Latent stage
    - This stage may persist for years.
    - Occasionally the skin lesions may reappear.
    - Person remains asymptomatic, although serologic evidence of the disease remains.
  - Tertiary syphilis
    - May develop in some untreated patients
    - Gumma
      - Typical lesion of this stage
        - Area of necrosis and fibrosis
      - Bone gummas
        - Leads to destruction and pathologic fractures
      - Liver gummas
        - Manifest as nodules similar to those of cirrhosis
      - Cardiovascular system
        - Frequently affected by gummas
        - Damage to the arterial wall
        - Development of aortic aneurysms
- Neurosyphilis
  - Damage to the CNS
    - Dementia
    - Blindness
    - Motor disabilities
      - Tabes dorsalis

Viral Sexually Transmitted Diseases

- Infection cannot be eradicated.
  - Antiviral agents reduce the severity of the acute stage of infection.
- HIV-acquired immunodeficiency syndrome (AIDS)
  - HIV
  - AIDS
  - Interferes with the body's ability to fight infections
- Herpes genitalis
  - HSV

- Usually caused by HSV-2
  - Can result from HSV-1
- Causes lesions
  - Tingling and burning sensation followed by appearance of lesion
  - Vesicle ruptures after several days resulting in painful, ulcerated area.
- Signs and symptoms
  - Acute
    - Fever
    - Headache
    - Lymphadenopathy
  - Latent stage
    - Virus migrates along the dermatologist to the dorsal sacral root ganglion.
  - Cervical cancer commonly develops in women with genital herpes.
- HPV—condylomata acuminata (genital warts)
  - Circular, double-stranded virus
  - Several types of HPV can affect the genital tract.
    - Many of these types can lead to cervical cancer.
  - Incubation period can be up to 6 months.
    - During this time the virus is asymptomatic.
  - Signs and symptoms
    - Condylomata (warts)
      - Vary in appearance
        - Soft, fleshy projections
          - Cauliflower-like masses
        - Flat lesions
        - Small pointed masses

Parasitic Sexually Transmitted Disease

- Trichomoniasis
  - Caused by *Trichomoniasis vaginalis*
    - Anaerobic flagellated protozoan
  - Localized infection caused by parasite
  - Signs and symptoms
    - Females
      - Infections may be subclinical and flare up as the microbial balance of the vagina shifts.
      - Active infection/flare up
        - Copious yellowish, foul-smelling discharge
        - Inflammation
        - Itching of the mucosa

APPLICATION AND REVIEW

12. Which statement, if made by a female client, is most suggestive of a trichomoniasis infection?
    1. "My vagina itches."
    2. "I get very bad cramps during my period."
    3. "I've developed this foul-smelling yellow discharge."
    4. "My period has been late for the last several months."

13. What information will the nurse include when discussing genital herpes with a client? **Select all that apply**.
    1. The warts can resemble tiny cauliflowers.
    2. The infection is caused by a parasite.
    3. Incubation can take up to 6 months after exposure.
    4. The virus presents no symptoms until fully developed.
    5. Genital herpes is a risk factor associated with cervical cancer.

14. What statement, if made by a client diagnosed with syphilis, indicates the second stage of the disease process?
    1. "It been several years since I was exposed."
    2. "I came to get something for this red rash I have."
    3. "I'm concerned about these hard nodules on my thigh."
    4. "My primary provider says I may have tertiary syphilis."

15. What assessment finding is the nurse likely to obtain from a female client suspected of having developed gonorrhea?
    1. Purulent discharge noted
    2. Mucous patches present on tongue
    3. Client reports having yellow discharge
    4. Client reports being asymptomatic at present

16. Which statements, if made by a young adult, suggest an increased risk for developing a sexually transmitted disease (STD)? **Select all that apply**.
    1. "I enjoy sex, and I don't feel guilty about feeling that way."
    2. "I have had three different sexual partners in the last 2 months."
    3. "I've heard it's pretty easy to treat sexual infections these days."
    4. "I know it's important to use protection, but I don't always insist on it."
    5. "I know several people who have gotten sexually transmitted infections."

See Answers on pages 421–423.

ANSWER KEY: REVIEW QUESTIONS

1. **2 A classic symptom of endometriosis is dysmenorrhea—painful menstruation.**
   1 Menstruation is not absent (amenorrhea); it is painful. **3** Endometriosis can cause scarring but not fibroid formation. **4** Endometriosis does not generally cause bleeding so it is not associated iron deficiency anemia.
   Client Need: Physiological Adaptation; **Cognitive Level:** Understanding; **Nursing Process:** Assessment

2. **Answers: 1, 2, 5.**
   1 Lack of regular exercise is considered a risk factor for breast cancer. **2** A high-fat diet is considered a risk factor for breast cancer. **5** Tobacco smoking is considered a risk factor for breast cancer.
   3 Although not inappropriate, providing breast support is not considered an action that will minimize the risk of breast cancer. **4** Vitamin deficiency is not considered a strong risk factor for breast cancer.
   Client Need: Physiological Adaptation; **Cognitive Level:** Applying; **Nursing Process:** Implementing

3. **Answers: 1, 2, 5.**
   1 Advanced breast cancer presents with discharge from an affected nipple. **2** Advanced breast cancer presents with dimpling of skin on the affected nipple. **5** Advanced breast cancer presents with a fixed nodule.
   3 Initial signs of breast cancer include a small, hard, painless nodule. **4** It is not unusual that a woman's breasts may differ in size.
   Client Need: Physiological Adaptation; **Cognitive Level:** Applying; **Nursing Process:** Assessment

4. **Answers: 1, 5.**

   1 Obesity is a risk factor for endometrial cancer because adipose cells store estrogen; the extent of exposure to estrogen is the most significant risk factor. **5** Endometrial cancer has a relationship to the exposure to estrogen.

   2 Nulliparity, not multiparity, is a risk factor for endometrial cancer because of the increased exposure to estrogen. **3** Cigarette smoking is not identified as a risk factor for endometrial cancer. **4** Late, not early, onset of menopause is a risk factor for endometrial cancer because of the increased exposure to estrogen.

   Client Need: Physiological Adaptation; **Cognitive Level:** Applying; **Nursing Process:** Assessment

5. **2 A family history of ovarian cancer is the greatest risk factor.**

   1 Age over 55 is a risk factor, but not as specific as a genetic risk. **3** Although back pain is a possible sign of ovarian cancer, there are many other possible causes for the pain. **4** Although indigestion is a possible sign of ovarian cancer, there are many other possible causes.

   Client Need: Physiological Adaptation; **Cognitive Level:** Analysis; **Nursing Process:** Assessment

6. **1 Stage III: tumor has spread to outside the uterus and cervix but is contained within the true pelvis, which projects a 5-year survival rate of 60%.**

   2 Stage II: tumor is limited to the uterus and the cervix, which projects a 5-year survival rate of 80%. **3** Stage I: tumor is confined to the uterus, which projects a 5-year survival rate of 99%. **4** Stage IV: tumor has spread to lymph nodes and distant organs, which projects a 5-year survival rate of 32%.

   Client Need: Physiological Adaptation; **Cognitive Level:** Applying; **Nursing Process:** Assessment

7. **Answers: 2, 3.**

   2, 3 Diabetes and hypertension are recognized risk factors for the development of uterine cancer.

   1, 4, 5 Neither asthma, cystic fibrosis, nor osteoporosis are known to be risk factors for uterine cancer.

   Client Need: Physiological Adaptation; **Cognitive Level:** Analysis; **Nursing Process:** Assessment

8. **3 Early changes in cervical epithelial tissue are referred to as dysplasia. These abnormal cells within a tissue can result in cancer cells.**

   1 Dysplasia is not a cancer indicator, but rather a possible precancerous state. **2, 4** The term dysplasia refers to cells that could be precancerous.

   Client Need: Physiological Adaptation; **Cognitive Level:** Analysis; **Integrated Process:** Teaching and Learning.

9. **2 Stage I cancer remains in the organ of origin; in this case the cervix.**

   1 Explaining the number of stages fails to provide the client with any relevant information and lacks empathy. **3** Stage 0 represents carcinoma in situ; the cancer remains in its original site of origin and shows no spreading. **4** Stage II shows significant spread of cancer cells deep into the surrounding tissue.

   Client Need: Physiological Adaptation; **Cognitive Level:** Analysis; **Integrated Process:** Teaching and Learning.

10. **Answers: 1, 2, 3.**

    1 Smoking increases the risk of cervical cancer. **2** Being sexually active in the early teen years increases the risk of cervical cancer. **3** A history of an STD increases the risk of cervical cancer.

    4 Multiple births is not associated with an increased risk for cervical cancer. **5** Age is not generally considered a risk factor for cervical cancer.

    Client Need: Physiological Adaptation; **Cognitive Level:** Applying; **Nursing Process:** Assessment

11. **2 The early stage of cervical cancer is asymptomatic.**

    1, 3, 4 Watery discharge, anemia-related tiredness, and spotty bleeding are all noted when the cancer has advanced to the invasive, later stages of the disease process.

    Client Need: Physiological Adaptation; **Cognitive Level:** Applying; **Nursing Process:** Assessment

12. **3 Trichomoniasis presents with a foul-smelling yellow discharge.**

    1 Although trichomoniasis presents with vaginal itching, many sexually transmitted infections present with itching as well. **2** Period-related cramping is not associated with trichomoniasis. **4** Abnormal periods are not associated with trichomoniasis.

    Client Need: Physiological Adaptation; **Cognitive Level:** Analysis; **Nursing Process:** Assessment

13. **Answers: 1, 3, 4, 5.**

    1 The warts can be flat, pointed, or cauliflower-like in appearance. **3** Genital herpes has an incubation period of up to 6 months. **4** During incubation, the virus is asymptomatic. **5** Many types of these viruses can lead to cervical cancer.

    2 Genital herpes is a viral infection not parasitic.
    Client Need: Physiological Adaptation; **Cognitive Level:** Applying; **Nursing Process:** Planning

14. **2 The second stage of syphilis presents with a rash that is reddish and maculopapular.**

    1 The latent stage of the disease process occurs years after exposure to the bacteria. **3** The primary stage is when the lesions (chancre) are noted. **4** Tertiary syphilis develops in untreated patients.
    Client Need: Physiological Adaptation; **Cognitive Level:** Analysis; **Nursing Process:** Assessment

15. **4 Gonorrhea is frequently asymptomatic in females, but frequent pelvic infections are noted.**

    1 Purulent discharge is noted in male clients diagnosed with gonorrhea. **2** Mucous patches on the tongue are associated with second stage syphilis. **3** A yellow discharge is associated with trichomoniasis.
    Client Need: Physiological Adaptation; **Cognitive Level:** Applying; **Nursing Process:** Assessment

16. **Answers: 2, 4.**

    2 This is a statement of fact concerning the client's sexual practices. An increased number of sexual partners does increase the risk of developing an STD. **4** This is a statement of fact concerning the client's sexual practices. Unprotected sex does increase the risk of developing an STD.

    1 This is a statement of the client's feelings, but not of personal sexual practices. **3** This is a statement that identifies the client's level of understanding, but not of personal sexual practices. **5** This statement does not identify any of the client's sexual practices.
    Client Need: Physiological Adaptation; **Cognitive Level:** Analysis; **Nursing Process:** Evaluation

20 Male Reproductive System Disorders

MALE REPRODUCTIVE SYSTEM DISORDERS

Structure and Function (Fig. 20.1)

- The male gonads (testes)
  - Are contained in the scrotum sac outside the abdominal cavity
  - Are suspended by spermatic cord
  - Produce sperm
  - Produce testosterone, a sex hormone
- Scrotal sac
  - Has a skin layer continuous with the perineal area
  - Has an inner layer of muscle and fascia
  - The covering of the scrotal sac is loose; the ridges of the folds are called rugae.
  - The two testes in the scrotum are divided by a septum.
  - Each testis has an attached epididymis.
    - Enclosed in tunica vaginalis
      - Double-walled membrane with fluid between layers
  - The spermatic cord of the testes contains
    - Arteries
    - Veins
    - Lymphatics
- Testes
  - Positioned outside abdominal cavity for temperature regulation
    - Optimal temperature for sperm production
      - 1º to 2º C (2º to 3º F) below normal body temperature
      - With a decrease in environmental temperature, scrotal muscle draws testes closer to the body.
      - With an increase in environmental temperature, scrotal muscle relaxes to let testes move away from the body.
  - In the third trimester, the fetal testes descend into the scrotum from the inguinal canal.
    - After testes descend, the inguinal canal closes.
  - During puberty, the testes mature.
    - Gonadotropins are secreted by adenohypophysis.
    - Testes produce sperm and testosterone.
- Male reproductive system includes
  - Extensive duct system connected to accessory glands and structures
    - These structures form and transport semen preparatory for ejaculation from the penis during intercourse.
- Spermatogenesis
  - Continuous production of spermatozoa
  - The process takes 60 to 70 days.

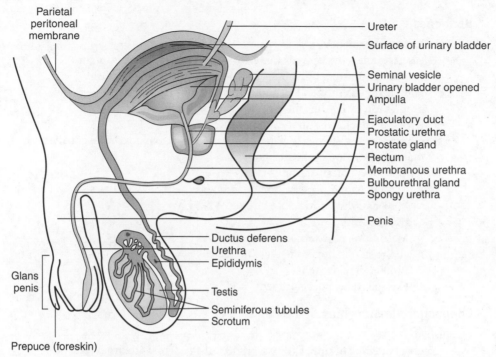

Parietal peritoneal membrane

Ureter
Surface of urinary bladder
Seminal vesicle
Urinary bladder opened
Ampulla
Ejaculatory duct
Prostatic urethra
Prostate gland
Rectum
Membranous urethra
Bulbourethral gland
Spongy urethra
Penis
Ductus deferens
Urethra
Epididymis
Testis
Seminiferous tubules
Scrotum
Glans penis
Prepuce (foreskin)

FIG. 20.1 **Anatomy of the male reproductive system.** (From Hubert R. J., & VanMeter, K. C. [2018]. *Gould's pathophysiology for the health professions* [6th ed.]. Philadelphia: Saunders.)

- Testes contain many lobules.
- Each lobule has seminiferous tubules, "sperm factories."
- Sperm travel into the epididymis to mature, through the efferent ducts.
- Through peristaltic movements in the epididymis
  - Sperm move to the ductus deferens (vas deferens) and then to the ampulla.
  - Motile sperm can be stored for several weeks.
  - Vasectomy (method of birth control) includes the blocking of the passage of sperm through the cutting/obstruction of the vas deferens.
- Semen
  - Formed at time of release
  - Fluid contains many substances from other accessory structures.
    - Seminal vesicles behind the bladder provide a secretion containing fructose to nourish sperm.
    - Prostate gland encircles the urethra (at base of bladder); it provides an alkaline fluid.
      - Optimizes pH at 6 for fertilization
      - Vaginal secretions and other sperm containing fluids are acidic.
    - Bulbourethral glands (Cowper glands) located at base of penis
      - Secrete an alkaline mucus
      - Neutralize any residual urine in urethra
  - Semen consists primarily of fluid
    - Each ejaculation is 2 to 5 mL with 100 to 200 million sperm

Hormones

- Gonadotropic hormones
  - Released by adenohypophysis (anterior pituitary gland) and contain
    - Follicle-stimulating hormone (FSH) that starts spermatogenesis
    - Luteinizing-hormone (LH, interstitial cell-stimulating hormone) invokes testosterone production by Leydig (interstitial) cells in the testes.
- Testosterone is vital for maturation of sperm.
  - Serum levels of testosterone impart a negative feedback loop to control gonadotropin secretions.
    - Males do not have cyclic hormones.
  - Other purposes of testosterone
    - Development and preservation of secondary sex characteristics
      - Male hair distribution
      - Deeper voice
      - Maturation of external male genitalia
    - Anabolic steroid hormone that stimulates
      - Protein development
      - Skeletal muscle development

Congenital Abnormalities of the Penis

- Epispadias
  - Urethral opening of upper (dorsal) aspect of the penis, proximal to glans
  - If the defect extends proximal and affects the urinary sphincter
    - Incontinence of urine can occur.
    - Infection can result from stricture of opening.
  - Exstrophy of the bladder (bladder forms outside abdominal wall) is often associated with epispadias.
- Hypospadias
  - Urethral opening on the ventral (under) area of the penis
  - Proximal opening is most severe and is associated with chordee (ventral curvature of penis).
  - Other abnormalities associated with hypospadias
    - Cryptorchidism

Disorders of the Penis

- Phimosis and paraphimosis
  - Foreskin or prepuce is too tight.
  - Phimosis: foreskin cannot be retracted over glans.
  - Paraphimosis: foreskin is retracted and cannot be moved to cover glans.
  - Both situations can result in penile pathologic conditions.
  - In infancy, the inability to retract the foreskin is normal, which is owing to congenital adhesions.
  - After age 3 the adhesions separate naturally.
  - Phimosis can occur at any age.
    - Owing to poor hygiene and chronic infection
    - Chronic balanoposthitis (inflammation of glans and prepuce) predisposes males with diabetes to phimosis in later years of life.
    - Primarily uncircumcised males
      - Can occur in circumcised males with excessive skin remaining

- Signs and symptoms
  - Edema
  - Erythema
  - Tenderness or pain of the prepuce
  - Purulent discharge
  - Inability to retract foreskin
- Complications
  - Phimosis: higher incidence of penile carcinoma in uncircumcised males (but could be caused by chronic infections)
  - Paraphimosis: retracted foreskin can constrict penis and cause edema of the glans, if it cannot be retracted manually
    - Surgery is needed to prevent necrosis of glans caused by constricted blood vessels.
    - Severe restriction can impair urinary output and requires emergency surgery to release the constriction.
- Peyronie disease (bent nail syndrome)
  - Fibrotic, condition of the penis
  - Stiffening of the fascia of the corpora cavernosa
  - Different degrees of curvature of the penis
  - Variability in sexual function
  - Prevalence approximately 9% of male population, but underdiagnosed
  - Onset is middle-aged men.
  - Signs and symptoms
    - Painful erection
    - Painful intercourse for each partner
    - Erection distal to the area has poor involvement with an erection.
    - No pain when penis is relaxed.
  - Cause
    - Unknown etiology
    - May be owing to local inflammatory reaction resulting in decreased oxygen and resulting fibrosis and calcification
    - Peyronie disease is associated with
      - A flexion deformity of toes or finger, shortening or fibrosis of plantar or palmar fascia
      - Diabetes
      - Keloid tendency
      - Beta-blocker medication
- Priapism
  - Unusual prolonged penile erection lasting more than 4 hours without sexual stimulation
  - Most cases have unknown causes, but the remaining 40% are related to the following conditions
    - Spinal cord trauma
    - Sickle cell disease
    - Leukemia
    - Pelvic tumors or infections
    - Penile trauma
    - Cocaine utilization
    - For erectile dysfunction, intracavernous (base of penis) injection therapy
  - Two corpora cavernosa in the erect penis are filled with blood and painful to touch.

- Vascular congestion assumed to be caused by venous obstruction
- Continued erection for days results in edema, fibrosis, and erectile dysfunction.
- Erectile dysfunction occurs in more than half the prolonged cases.

APPLICATION AND REVIEW

1. What outcome does Peyronie disease have on sexual functioning?
   1. Painful erection
   2. Decreased sexual desire
   3. Ineffective sperm motility
   4. Insufficient testosterone production.

See Answers on pages 445–447.

Penile Cancers

- Penile cancer
  - Most common squamous cell carcinoma
  - Begins as small, ulceration on the glans or foreskin
  - Will grow to involve the entire penile shaft
  - Incidence is rare; 1 in 100,000 men in the United States, but 10% of cancers in African and South American men.
  - In the United States, four of five cases involve men over the age of 55 years.
  - Risk increases with
    - Prior infection with human papillomavirus (HPV)
      - Smoking
      - Psoriasis treated with medication psoralen and ultraviolet (UV) light
      - Circumcision at birth reduces risk by 50%.
      - History of phimosis or acquired immunodeficiency syndrome (AIDS)
  - Signs and symptoms
    - White plaque involving the meatus
    - Inflamed areas of Paget disease
    - Ulcerative lesions involve the glans.
    - Large, scaly growths of Buschke-Lowenstein tumor
    - Red plaque with encrustations
    - Pain and bleeding are late signs.
    - Genital wart (condylomata)
    - HPV infection
  - Diagnosis
    - Ultrasound
    - Computed tomography (CT)
    - Magnetic resonance imaging (MRI)
    - Fine needle aspiration of lymph nodes
    - Penile cancer stages: stage 0 (carcinoma in situ), stage I, stage II, stage III, stage IV
  - Extensive lesions have a poor prognosis and can be associated with metastases.
    - Metastatic sites are frequently the regional and iliac nodes.
  - Untreated can result in death within 2 years

Disorders of the Urethra

- Urethritis
  - Inflammatory activity that involves the urethra
  - Without concurrent bladder infection

- Organism associated with infection
  - *Neisseria gonorrhoeae*
  - *Chlamydia trachomatis*
  - *Ureaplasma urealyticum*
  - Less common, mycobacteria
    - Parasites (*Trichomonas vaginalis*)
    - Viruses (herpes simplex virus [HSV])
- Causes
  - Can be associated with post-urologic procedure
  - Insertion of foreign bodies into urethra
  - Anatomic differences
  - Trauma
  - Non-infectious urethritis is rare.
  - Ingestion of wood alcohol, ethyl alcohol, or turpentine
  - Associated with Reiter syndrome (reactive arthritis)
- Signs and symptoms
  - Urethral burning, itching, and tingling
  - Urinary symptoms
    - Dysuria
    - Frequency
    - Urgency
    - Purulent discharge or clear mucus from urethra
- Diagnosis
  - Detection of organisms (*N. gonorrhoeae* and *C. tachomatis)* in first void urine
- Urethral stricture
  - Narrowing of urethra by fibrotic tissue owing to scarring
  - Scars can be congenital.
  - Other factors
    - Untreated urethral infections (long-term use of indwelling urinary catheters)
    - Post trauma (pelvic fracture)
    - Post urologic instrumentation
    - Post hypospadias surgery
- Complications
  - Prostatitis and infection to urinary stasis
  - Prolonged obstruction can lead to hydronephrosis and renal failure.
  - Chronic strictures can result in urethral fistulas and periurethral abscesses.
  - Diagnosis
    - History and physical examination
    - Urinary flow rates
    - Voiding cystourethrogram
    - Urethroscopy
    - Biopsy

Alterations of Sexual Maturation

- Sexual maturity (puberty)
  - Characteristics of puberty in males
    - Development of secondary sexual characteristics
    - Rapid growth

- Ability to reproduce
- Congenital or endocrine disorders can accelerate or retard sexual maturation.
  - Delayed puberty: occurs late
  - Precocious puberty: occurs early
- Onset of puberty has remained steady for boys, ages 14 to 14.5 years.
- Delayed puberty is not showing clinical signs by age 14 years.
- Possible causes of delayed puberty
  - Chronic conditions
    - Lung disease
    - Renal failure
    - Cystic fibrosis
  - Other causes of delayed puberty
    - Disruption of the human gonadal function (HPG) owing to various etiologies
- Diagnostic tests
  - Comprehensive physical examination
  - Medical history
  - Family history
  - Laboratory analysis
    - X-ray for bone age
    - Thyroid function measurements
    - Prolactin, adrenal, and gonadal steroid blood levels
    - Radioimmunoassay of plasma gonadotropins
    - Rule out systemic disorders
  - High gonadotropin levels-follow with karyotype
    - Rule out genetic causes
  - Low gonadotropin levels: follow with skull film
    - Computed tomography
    - Magnetic resonance imaging
    - Rule out pituitary or other central nervous system (CNS) tumors or infiltrates.

Disorders of the Testes and Scrotum

- Cryptorchidism (undescended testis)
  - One or both testes fails to descend into the scrotum during the latter part of pregnancy.
  - Testis may stay in the abdominal cavity or stop the descent in the inguinal canal.
  - Ectopic testis is an abnormal position outside the scrotum.
  - Causes
    - Possible hormonal abnormalities
    - Short spermatic cord
    - Small inguinal ring
  - With prolonged arrest of descent
    - Seminiferous tubules degenerate.
    - Spermatogenesis is disrupted.
    - Increased risk for testicular cancer
- Hydrocele, spermatocele, and varicocele
  - Hydrocele
    - Between layers of the tunica vaginalis, there is excessive accumulation of fluid.
    - Can occur on one side or both (bilaterally)
    - Use of light (transillumination) to visualize

- During birth, a congenital defect can occur that allows peritoneal fluid into the scrotum; this is absorbed over time.
- If after descent of the testes the proximal portion of the processus vaginalis (peritoneal membrane) remains open, the scrotum will fill with fluid during the day and subside at night.
- Commonly in an infant, a loop of intestine will pass through the abdominal opening.
  - Resulting hernia can become an intestinal obstruction.
- Acquired hydrocele is common in adulthood and results from a scrotal injury, tumor, infection, or unknown etiology.
  - Accumulation of large amounts of fluid can reduce blood supply to testes.
  - Aspiration of fluid may be required.

- Spermatocele
  - A cyst develops between the testis and epididymis (outside the tunica vaginalis).
  - The cyst is filled with fluid and sperm.
  - Can be related to an abnormality of the tubules
- Varicocele
  - Distended vein in the spermatic cord
  - Often located on the left side
  - Often develops after puberty, from a lock of valves in the veins
    - Blood backflows, pressure increases in the vein
    - Can be mild and relieved by scrotal support
    - Extensive varicocele is tender or painful.
    - Can result in infertility owing to impaired blood flow to testes and subsequent spermatogenesis
- Torsion of the testis
  - Testes twist on the spermatic cord.
  - Compression of the arteries and veins
  - Ischemia develops.
  - Scrotal swelling
  - Swift treatment includes restoring blood flow to testes manually and surgically.
  - During puberty, it can occur after trauma and spontaneously.
- Orchitis
  - Acute infection of the testes
  - Usually associated with systemic infection or concurrent epididymitis
  - Occasionally noninfectious response to a granulomatous response to spermatozoa in middle-aged men
  - Cause
    - Infectious organism reaches the testes through the blood or lymphatic system, or ascent from the epididymis, vas deferens, or urethra.
    - Post mumps infection in postpubertal males, 3 to 4 days after parotitis onset
  - Signs and symptoms
    - High fever (>104° F or 40° C)
    - Bilateral or unilateral erythema, edema, and tenderness of scrotum
    - Noted prostration
    - Hydrocele can occur.
    - Urinary symptoms
    - Atrophy and irreversible damage to spermatogenesis can result in 30% of affected testes.

- Cryptorchidism
  - Associated with mal descent
  - Testis strays from normal path of descent.
  - Cause
    - Multifactorial
      - Genetic
      - Maternal
      - Environment
  - Normally occurs as an isolated disorder.
    - May be caused by an abnormal connection at the distal end of the gubernaculum
      - Leads to gonad in an unusual position
      - Often at superficial inguinal site
  - Signs and symptoms
    - Testes remain in abdomen.
    - Found in palpation of scrotum in newborn
    - Occurs in 3% of full-term newborns and decreases to 0.8% to 1.2% by first year of life
    - Significant increase with low-birth-weight infants
      - Infant weighing less than 2000 g, incidence is 7.7%
      - Infant weighing 2000 to 2500 g, incidence is 2.5%
      - Infant weighing 2500 g or greater, incidence is 1.41%
    - Commonly associated with vasal or epididymal abnormalities
      - Impacts one-third to two-thirds of newborns with cryptorchidism
  - Diagnosis
    - Absence of one or both testes in the scrotum
    - Atrophic scrotum on affected side
    - If undescended testes is in a compromised position, severe pain may be present.
    - Ultrasonography, CT, or MRI can be used to locate nonpalpable testis.
    - Testicular cancer is a potential complication.
      - Chance of testicular cancer is 35 to 50 times greater for a man with a history of cryptorchidism.
  - Treatment
    - Surgical intervention prior to 1 year of age, testes located and moved surgically (orchiopexy)
    - Administration of GnRH or human chorionic gonadotropin (hCG) that can be a catalyst for the normal descent of the testes.
    - Surgical removal of the testes (orchiectomy) in adults.

Inflammation and Infections

- Prostatitis
  - The National Institute of Health (NIH) recognizes four categories
    - Category 1—acute bacterial prostatitis
      - Acute bacterial infection of the prostate that is associated with generalized signs of infection and a positive urine culture
    - Category 2—chronic bacterial prostatitis
      - Chronic bacterial infection; the bacteria are detected in the purulent prostatic fluid. Also, the bacteria present are likely the reason for recurrent urinary tract infections in men.
    - Category 3—nonbacterial prostatitis or chronic pelvic pain syndrome (CPPS)

- No pathogenic bacteria are specific to the prostate, including expressed prostatic fluids or after prostate massage urinalysis.
  - Category 3a—inflammatory CPPS where white blood cells are localized to the prostate
  - Category 3b—noninflammatory
  - Category 4—asymptomatic prostatitis
    - White blood cells and bacteria are localized to the prostate but individuals show no symptoms.
- Prostate protected from ascending infection by
  - Intact mucus membranes
  - Flushing action of ejaculation, urination
  - Prostate secretions contain antimicrobial factors.
  - Close proximity to the urinary tract increases the chance of infection.
  - Nonbacterial prostatitis and pain (prostatodynia) have unknown cause.
- Pathophysiology
  - Enlarged gland is soft with palpation.
  - Urinalysis contains microorganisms, pus, and leukocytes.
  - Expressed prostatic secretions also contain organisms.
    - Painful process and can spread infection
  - Nonbacterial prostatitis
    - Urinalysis and secretions contain leukocytes.
    - Prostate is not enlarged.
  - Chronic prostatitis
    - Prostate irregular in shape
    - Firm from fibrous tissue
- Prostatitis is usually accompanied by a urinary tract infection (UTI).
  - Symptoms of a UTI include urinary frequency, urgency, and dysuria.
  - Can include inflammation of the epididymis and testes
- Etiology
  - Ascending infection primarily caused by *Escherichia coli* or other organisms
    - Pseudomonas
    - Proteus
    - Enterobacter
    - Klebsiella
    - Serratia
    - *Streptococcus faecalis*
- Occurrence
  - Young men with UTI caused by coliform bacteria from intestine
  - Older men with benign prostatic hypertrophy
  - Associated with sexually transmitted disease
  - From instruments, such as catheterization
  - From the blood stream (hematogenous spread)
- Signs and symptoms
  - Dysuria
  - Chills and fever (acute infections)
  - Low back pain
  - Severe inflammation may enlarge the prostate and obstruct urine flow.
    - Decrease in urinary stream
    - Hesitancy with urination

- Incomplete bladder emptying
- Nocturia
- Frequency in urination
- Systemic signs and symptoms
  - Fever
  - Malaise
  - Anorexia
  - Muscle aching
- Nonbacterial prostatitis includes urinary symptoms intermittently, but systemic signs are lessened.
- Balanitis
  - Fungal infection transmitted during sexual activity to the glans penis
  - *Candida albicans* is the causative type of fungus.
  - Most often affects uncircumcised males
  - Signs and symptoms
    - Penile vesicles
    - Later burning and itching patches
  - Diagnosis
    - Positive identification of the fungus candida

Tumors

- Benign prostatic hypertrophy (BPH) (Fig. 20.2)
  - Frequently affects older men
    - Approximately 50% of men over 65 years of age have some degree of BPH.

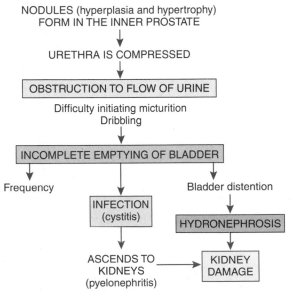

BENIGN PROSTATIC HYPERTROPHY (BPH)

NODULES (hyperplasia and hypertrophy)
FORM IN THE INNER PROSTATE

↓

URETHRA IS COMPRESSED

↓

OBSTRUCTION TO FLOW OF URINE

Difficulty initiating micturition
Dribbling

↓

INCOMPLETE EMPTYING OF BLADDER

Frequency   INFECTION   Bladder distention
                   (cystitis)
                                     HYDRONEPHROSIS

ASCENDS TO ——————→ KIDNEY
KIDNEYS   DAMAGE
(pyelonephritis)

FIG. 20.2 **Complications of benign prostatic hypertrophy.** (From Hubert, R. J., & VanMeter, K. C. [2018]. *Gould's pathophysiology for the health professions* [6th ed.]. Philadelphia: Saunders.)

- The prostatic tissue enlarges with nodules that encircle the urethra.
  - Compression of urethra causes variable amount of urinary obstruction.
- Cause of hyperplasia (enlargement of prostate)
  - Owing to aging, possibly imbalance of estrogen and testosterone
  - No correlation between BPH and cancer of the prostate has been determined.
- Diagnosis
  - Rectal examination finding is enlarged prostate.
  - Often accompanied by urinary tract infections owing to incomplete emptying of the bladder
  - Other findings may include
    - Distended bladder
    - Dilated ureters
    - Hydronephrosis
    - Renal damage
- Signs and symptoms
  - Obstruction of urine
    - Hesitancy
    - Dribbling
    - Lessened urine stream
  - Incomplete bladder emptying
    - Frequency
    - Nocturia
    - Recurring urinary tract infections
- Cancer of the prostate
  - Pathophysiology
    - Tumors (adenocarcinomas) occur near the surface of the gland.
    - More than one focus of neoplastic cells may be present.
    - Degree of cellular differentiation varies
      - Undifferentiated (anaplastic) cells grow and spread faster, and are aggressive.
    - Prostate cancer can invade regional tissues, lymph nodes, urethra, and bone.
    - Early identification with screening improves survival rates.
      - Localized cancer tumor has 100% survival rate.
      - Regional spread of tumor has 89% survival rate.
      - Distant metastases to bone or organs has 27% survival rate.
  - Etiology
    - Inherited mutations account for 5% to 10% of prostatic cancers.
      - *HPC1* gene is distinguished as the cause of these cancers.
    - High androgen levels (intrinsic or extrinsic)
    - Increased insulin-like growth factor
    - Recurrent prostatitis
    - Prostate cancer is common in North America and Europe, but not in countries in the Far East.
    - Higher incidence in African-Americans than Caucasians
    - Testosterone receptors identified in cancer cells of prostate
  - Signs and symptoms
    - Rectal examinations can detect a hard nodule in the periphery of the prostate, often the posterior lobe.

- Growth of the tumor causes obstruction of urine and associated symptoms.
  - Hesitancy with urination
  - Decreased urine stream
  - Urinary frequency
  - Bladder infection (cystitis)
- Diagnostic tests
  - Serum markers are elevated when cancer is present.
    - Prostate-specific antigen (PSA)
      - Elevated with BPH or infection
      - Not diagnostic by itself, but can monitor effectiveness of treatment
    - Prostatic acid phosphatase
    - Can use serum markers to monitor treatment progress
    - Testing is recommended over age 50 for all men, and after age 45 for men with risk factors.
    - Ultrasonography used with a probe and biopsy to validate disease
      - Bone scans
      - Monoclonal antibody scans
    - Tri-fold criteria for diagnosis
      - Elevated PSA
      - Abnormal digital rectal examination
      - Biopsy results (Gleason scale is a numeric score based on the proportion of abnormal cells in the biopsy specimen.)
  - Recommended diet for patients with prostate cancer as a result of epidemiologic studies
    - Reduce total fat in intake, including saturated fat; red meat and dairy products have all been correlated with an increased risk of prostate cancer.
  - Obesity has been associated with aggressive prostate cancer.
  - High body mass index (BMI) is linked to a worse outcome and more aggressive disease.
  - Excessive carbohydrate diet or a calorie dense diet has been associated with an increased risk of prostate cancer.
  - A high-fat diet can increase oxidative stress, androgen, and reactive oxygen species (ROS).
  - Monounsaturated fats may help lower the risk of prostate cancer.
  - After consumption of processed meat containing nitrites and heme iron present in large amounts of red meat, carcinogenic nitrosamines are formed.
  - The Western diet of increased omega-6 versus omega-3 ratios has been linked to a proinflammatory state.
  - Heterocyclic amines and aromatic hydrocarbons are carcinogenic and are produced when meat is cooked at high temperature.
  - Vitamin E is considered a benefit for cancer prevention in both in vitro and in vivo animal studies.
  - Selenium is a trace mineral present in plant and animal products. There has been a reported 50% reduction in risk for developing prostate cancer with a diet high in selenium.
  - The isoflavones in soy appear to have anticancer properties, including hindering cell proliferation, antiogenesis, and reducing the PSA androgen receptor levels.
  - Lycopene found in tomatoes or tomato products appears to reduce PSA levels in men with benign prostatic hyperplasia, although there is not enough evidence to support this finding.

- Cruciferous vegetables, such as broccoli, Brussels sprouts, Chinese cabbage, and so forth, may be protective against prostate cancer. Cruciforms contain phytochemicals that have anticancer properties.
- Cancer of testes
  - Benign tumors are rare.
  - Malignant tumors arise from germ cells.
  - Low but increasing incidence in men
    - Men age 15 to 35 years
    - Approximately 1 in 263 men will be affected.
  - Etiology unknown
    - Most frequent solid tumor found in young men
      - Recommend monthly self-examination of testes.
  - Pathophysiology
    - Testicular cancer can occur from
      - One type of cell
        - Seminoma
      - Mixed cells from different sources
        - Teratoma
          - Mixture of dissimilar germ cells
      - Testicular neoplasms (abnormal growth of tissue)
        - Spread during the early stages
          - Choriocarcinoma
      - Remaining localized for an extended time period
        - Seminomas
  - Testicular tumors, when spreading, follow a predictable pattern.
  - In common iliac and para-aortic lymph nodes
  - Disperse to mediastinal and supraclavicular lymph nodes
  - Cancer cells metastasize through the blood to organs
    - Lungs
    - Liver
    - Bone
    - Brain
  - Cancer staging system is based on
    - Primary tumor
    - Degree of lymph node involvement
      - Retroperitoneal
    - Presence of distal metastases
  - Etiology
    - Genetic pattern
      - Switch from chromosome 12
      - Possible association with infection or trauma
      - Failure of descent of testes (mal descent) is a predisposing risk factor.
  - Signs and symptoms
    - Painless, firm masses on one side (unilateral)
    - Testes enlarged or heavy
    - Dull ache or pain in lower abdomen

- Inflammation may result in development of
  - Hydrocele
  - Epididymitis
- Gynecomastia may appear.
  - Enlargement of breast caused by hormones secreted by tumor
- Diagnostic tests
  - Ultrasound
  - CT (scan)
  - Lymphangiography
  - Presence of tumor markers (AFP, hCG)
  - Surgical removal of mass identified with diagnostic imaging
    - Biopsy not recommended, owing to the potential to spread cancer.

APPLICATION AND REVIEW

2. A client with testicular cancer should be monitored closely for metastases to which organs? **Select all that apply.**
   1. Lungs
   2. Liver
   3. Bone
   4. Brain
   5. Kidneys

3. Which client statements support a diagnosis of testicular cancer? **Select all that apply.**
   1. "My testicles feel heavy."
   2. "I've been diagnosed with gynecomastia."
   3. "I have this dull ache in my lower abdomen."
   4. "We can't get pregnant, and I think it's my fault."
   5. "I found a small, firm knot on the side of my scrotum."

4. Which diagnostic tests are done to confirm the presence of testicular cancer? **Select all that apply.**
   1. Biopsy
   2. CT scan
   3. Ultrasound
   4. Lymphangiography
   5. Blood test to confirm tumor markers

5. What is the survival rate for localized prostate cancer?
   1. 40%
   2. 60%
   3. 80%
   4. 100%

6. A client diagnosed with benign prostatic hypertrophy (BPH) asks the nurse, "How high are my odds of this developing into cancer?" Which response by the nurse is best?
   1. "You seem concerned about dying from cancer."
   2. "There is no research that connects BPH with prostatic cancer."
   3. "Close monitoring will identify cancer early if that should occur."
   4. "If you don't have a family history of prostatic cancer, your risk is low."

7. Which assessment findings would confirm the diagnosis of cryptorchidism?
   1. A cyst develops between the testis and epididymis
   2. Testes have failed to descend from the abdomen
   3. Vein distension in the spermatic cord
   4. Extreme tenderness of the scrotum

See Answers on pages 445–447.

Sexual Dysfunction

- Impairment to any of the normal sexual responses: erection, emission, and ejaculation
- More than half of the cases in men over age 50 years is owing to organic causes, such as
  - Vascular
  - Endocrine
  - Neurologic
  - Chronic disease (renal and diabetes)
  - Penile disease or trauma
  - Iatrogenic factors (surgery or medication)
- Vascular disorders can prevent erection.
  - Arterial disease interrupts or lessens circulation to the penis.
  - Lower blood low prevents engorgement of corpora cavernosa and corpus spongiosum.
  - Endocrine disorders
    - Reduce testosterone
      - Affect sexual function
      - Diminished libido
      - Cause may be inadequate secretion of gonadotropins owing to
        - Pituitary dysfunction
        - Hyperprolactinemia
      - Feminizing tumors and estrogen therapy
  - Neurologic disorders
    - Interfere with sympathetic, parasympathetic, and CNS mechanisms needed for erection, emission, and ejaculation
    - Spinal cord injury or tumor
      - Upper motor neuron lesions
        - Reflexogenic erection is possible, but not emission and ejaculation.
      - Lower motor neuron lesions
        - Prevent erection
    - Multiple sclerosis
    - Disorders that cause peripheral neuropathies
      - Diabetes
    - Causes peripheral vascular and neurologic pathology that results in erectile dysfunction
      - Chronic kidney disease
      - More than half the men undergoing dialysis have decreased testosterone levels, autonomic neuropathy, advancing vascular disease, polypharmacy, worsening renal disease, and psychological stress.
- Priapism causes fibrosis to erectile tissue within the corpora cavernosa, impairing erection.
- Peyronie disease causes intercourse to be painful.
- Penile trauma can disrupt the arteries and nerves, and damage erectile tissue.
- Iatrogenic factors (drugs and surgery) can potentially cause erectile dysfunction.
  - Radical pelvic floor surgery
  - Radical prostatectomy
  - Prostatectomy: transurethral, suprapubic, or retropubic
  - Aortoiliac surgery (potential to damage nerves)
  - Retroperitoneal lymphadenectomy

- Sympathectomy can result in loss of ejaculation.
  - Medications can cause a decrease in sexual desire, erectile ability, or ejaculatory ability.
    - Antihypertensives
    - Antidepressants
    - Antihistamine
    - Antispasmodics
    - Sedative
    - Barbiturate
    - Diuretics
    - Sex hormone preparations
    - Narcotics
    - Psychoactive medication
    - Alcohol can induce neuropathy or increase estrogens owing to hepatic dysfunction.
    - Marijuana depresses testosterone.
    - Cigarette smoking can result in vasoconstriction and venous leakage.
- Diagnostic tests
  - Techniques to determine penile blood flow (Doppler and arteriography)
    - Erectile tissue anatomy
    - Nervous system function
    - Nocturnal emission (erection/emission at night)
    - Corpora cavernosography
    - Rapid eye movement (REM) and non-REM sleep

Impairment of Sperm Production and Quality

- Spermatogenesis is a process in men requiring
  - FSH and LH secreted by the pituitary
  - Testosterone secreted by the Leydig cells (located between the tubules)
  - Sertoli cells (located within the seminiferous tubules), secretion of
    - Androgen-binding protein
    - Growth factors
    - Inhibin B
    - Peptides
  - Without sufficient testosterone levels, spermatogenesis is impaired.
  - Inhibin B is a marker of competence of Sertoli cells and therefore spermatogenesis.
  - Lower levels of inhibin B have been associated with
    - Azoospermia
    - Testicular disorders
    - Infertility
  - Genetic disorders
    - Klinefelter syndrome
    - Myotonic dystrophy
    - Testicular trauma
  - Other conditions that can reduce spermatogenesis
    - Systemic illness
    - Renal failure
    - Hepatic disease
    - Sickle cell disease

- Exposure to gonadotoxins (chemotherapy, radiation)
- Varicocele
- Cryptorchidism
- Fertility is also affected when spermatogenesis is normal, but sperm are not.
  - Produced in sufficient quantities
  - Chromosomally abnormal
    - Caused by external variables and genetic factors
    - Radiation and toxic matter
  - Morphologically abnormal
  - Normal sperm count averages 50 to 100 million sperm per milliliter of semen.
  - Minimum sperm count for fertility is 20 million sperm per milliliter of semen.
- Sperm motility
  - Important aspect impacting fertility
  - Sperm motility can be affected by chemicals in the sperm's surroundings.
  - Variables that can alter sperm motility
    - Prostatic dysfunction
    - Excessive semen viscosity
    - Presence of drugs/toxins in the semen
    - Presence of antisperm antibodies
    - Estimated antisperm antibodies are present in 3% to 7% of infertile males.
      - Antisperm antibodies can develop owing to
        - Epididymitis
        - Inflammation of the genitourinary tract
        - Testicular injury or torsion
        - Previous vasectomy or biopsy
        - Cryptorchidism
    - Antisperm antibodies work in two ways.
      - Cytotoxic antibodies that attack sperm and reduce sperm count
      - Sperm-immobilizing antibodies that impair sperm motility
      - By reducing motility, the sperm are unable to traverse the endocervical canal.
- Male evaluation of infertility includes
  - Thorough history, physical, and imaging for varicocele
  - Two semen analyses
  - Serum levels of FSH, LH, testosterone, and prolactin, as needed
  - Semen and urethral cultures
  - Serum analysis of monoclonal antibody for white blood cells
  - Immunobead monoclonal antibody test
  - Testing of semen activity postcoital
  - Sperm penetration analysis
  - Inhibin B assays and possibly a testicular biopsy
  - Imaging studies (vasogram, transrectal ultrasound), as needed
- In infertility situations, the male is responsible for 50% of the cases of the infertility.
- Treatment for male infertility depends on the cause and removal of negative factors.
  - Avoidance of toxins and radiation
  - Androgens, human gonadotropins, and antiestrogens may intensify spermatogenesis.
  - Semen can be changed to improve sperm motility.
  - With antisperm antibodies, sperm can be obtained, diluted/concentrated, and washed to remove the antibodies, and implanted with artificial insemination.

APPLICATION AND REVIEW

8. What diagnostic testing should the nurse discuss with a male being treated for infertility issues? **Select all that apply**.
   1. Semen analysis
   2. Urethral culture
   3. Inhibin B assay
   4. Prostate-specific antigen (PSA)
   5. Sperm penetration analysis

9. A couple is seeking treatment for infertility. The male states, "It is usually women who have problems with fertility." Which is the best response by the nurse?
   1. "Let's wait to see what the testing shows before we assign responsibility."
   2. "Research shows that infertility issues are shared equally by males and females."
   3. "It's difficult for anyone to deal with the fact that they may be unable to conceive a child."
   4. "It is important that you both engage in mental health counseling to help deal with infertility."

10. What factors contribute to impaired sperm motility? **Select all that apply**.
    1. Prostatic dysfunction
    2. A protein-deficient diet
    3. Increased semen viscosity
    4. Presence of certain drugs in the semen
    5. Existing inflammation of the genitourinary tract

11. Which client's sperm count is at the minimal level to support conception?
    1. 10 million sperm per milliliter of semen
    2. 20 million sperm per milliliter of semen
    3. 40 million sperm per milliliter of semen
    4. 60 million sperm per milliliter of semen

12. What diagnostic testing should the nurse discuss with a male being treated for sexual dysfunction issues? **Select all that apply**.
    1. REM and non-REM sleep cycles
    2. Nervous system function
    3. Erectile tissue anatomy
    4. Endocrine function
    5. Urinary function

13. Which hormone has the most impact on the process of spermatogenesis?
    1. Follicle-stimulating hormone (FSH)
    2. Luteinizing hormone (LH)
    3. Testosterone
    4. Growth

14. Which clients may develop decreased male sexual performance and desire? **Select all that apply**.
    1. A client taking medications for insomnia
    2. A client taking medications for depression
    3. A client taking medications for hypotension
    4. A client taking medications for seasonal allergies
    5. A client taking medications for irritable bowel syndrome

15. The recreational use of what substance can affect sexual performance by depressing the effect of testosterone?
    1. Alcohol
    2. Tobacco
    3. Marijuana
    4. Cocaine

16. Which client is at risk for the development of peripheral neuropathy that can have a negative impact on sexual function?
    1. A client diagnosed with hypotension
    2. A client diagnosed with type 2 diabetes mellitus
    3. A client who experienced a spinal cord injury
    4. A client who experienced pituitary dysfunction

See Answers on pages 445–447.

Disorders of Male Breast

- Gynecomastia
  - Overdevelopment of male breast tissue
  - Most of masses in male breast are gynecomastia, which affects 32% to 40% of the male population.
  - Incidence highest among adolescents and males older that age 50 years
  - Unilateral affected, it is usually the left breast.
  - Causes
    - Hormonal alterations
    - Idiopathic or caused by systemic disorders, drugs, or neoplasm
    - Imbalance of estrogen/testosterone
    - Elevated estrogen levels and testosterone levels normal
      - Tumor-induced cases of hyperestrogenism
    - Testosterone levels low and estrogen levels are normal
      - Example of hypergonadism
    - Changes in breast-tissue responsiveness to hormonal stimulation
      - Increased reaction to estrogen
      - Decreased reaction to androgen
    - Estrogen-testosterone imbalances are often seen with
      - Hypogonadism
      - Klinefelter syndrome
      - Testicular neoplasms
      - Hormonal induced-gynecomastia is usually bilateral.
    - Pubertal gynecomastia is self-limiting.
      - Goes away in 4 to 6 months
    - Senescent gynecomastia regresses in 6 to 12 months.
    - Systematic disorders of gynecomastia can alter estrogen and testosterone balance owing to
      - Obesity
      - Cirrhosis of the liver
      - Infectious hepatitis
      - Chronic kidney disease
      - Chronic obstructive lung disease (COPD)
      - Hyperthyroidism
      - Tuberculosis
      - Chronic malnutrition
    - Gynecomastia occurs in men receiving estrogen therapy for
      - Prostatic carcinoma
      - Preparation for a sex change operation

- Other drugs that can cause gynecomastia
  - Digitalis
  - Cimetidine
  - Spironolactone
  - Reserpine
  - Thiazide
  - Isoniazid
  - Ergotamine
  - Tricyclic antidepressants
  - Amphetamines
  - Vincristine
  - Busulfan
  - 5-alpha reductase inhibitors for BPH increase risk
- Malignancies of the testes, adrenals, or liver can also alter balance of estrogen to testosterone.
- Pituitary adenomas and lung cancer have been associated with gynecomastia.
- Diagnosis
  - Based of physical examination
  - Health history
  - Medication review
- Male breast cancer (MBC)
  - Incidence is rare.
  - Less than 1% of all male cancers
  - Highest rate in Israel: 1.24 per 100,000
  - Lowest rate in Thailand: 0.16 male and 18.0 female
  - Mean age of diagnosis is 60 to 70 years of age.
- Risk factors
  - Radiation exposure
  - Estrogen administration
  - Diseases associated with hyperestrogenism
    - Cirrhosis
    - Klinefelter syndrome
  - Increased rate in males with a family history of female breast cancer
  - Increased rate in males with *BRCA2* gene mutations
  - Similar to females, infiltrating ductal cancer is the most common type.
  - Intraductal cancer, inflammatory carcinoma, and Paget disease are diagnosed in the nipple.
  - Pattern of metastasis is similar to women.
- Diagnosis
  - Confirmed by biopsy
- Prognosis
  - Poor because men usually delay treatment until the disease is at advanced stages of progression
  - Mean age of diagnosis is 60 to 70 years of age.
  - Most male breast cancer is estrogen positive.

APPLICATION AND REVIEW

17. What explanation about the cause should the nurse provide to a 20-year-old male who has developed gynecomastia?
    1. Puberty-induced enlargement of male breasts
    2. Unilateral overdevelopment of male breast tissue
    3. Inflammation of the tissue comprising the male breast
    4. Temporary swelling of the breast area caused by a hormone imbalance
18. What information concerning outcome should the nurse provide the client demonstrating senescent gynecomastia?
    1. Surgery will be required to reduce breasts.
    2. The breasts will reduce in size in 6 to 12 months.
    3. The condition, although permanent, is not a serious health threat.
    4. The condition needs to be monitored to manage cancer risks.
19. What history situation serves as a risk factor for male breast cancer?
    1. Female family members diagnosed with breast cancer
    2. Extended personal use of inhaled tobacco products
    3. Moderate alcohol use lasting more than 10 years
    4. Being treated for chronic hypertension
20. Which clients should be screened regularly for gynecomastia? **Select all that apply**.
    1. A male client who is obese
    2. A male client with hypothyroidism
    3. A male client with cirrhosis of the liver
    4. A male client with chronic kidney disease
    5. A male client with chronic obstructive lung disease (COPD)

See Answers on pages 445–447.

ANSWER KEY: REVIEW QUESTIONS

1. **1** Peyronie disease is the development of fibrous scar tissue inside the penis that causes curved, painful erections.
   2, 3, 4 Peyronie disease does not affect sexual desire, sperm motility, or testosterone production.
   Client Need: Physiological Adaptation; **Cognitive Level:** Applying; **Integrated Process:** Teaching and Learning
2. **Answers: 1, 2, 3, 4.**
   1, 2, 3, 4 Testicular cancer cells metastasize through the blood system to the lungs, liver, bone, and brain.
   5 The kidneys are not a usual site for testicular cancer metastases.
   Client Need: Physiological Adaptation; **Cognitive Level:** Applying; **Integrated Process:** Teaching and Learning
3. **Answers: 1, 2, 3, 5.**
   1 Signs and symptoms of testicular cancer include the enlargement of the testes. **2** Gynecomastia can occur because of hormonal effects on the breast tissue. **3** A dull ache or pain in the lower abdomen is a classic symptom of testicular cancer. **5** A painless, firm mass is a classic sigh of testicular cancer.
   4 Infertility is not associated with testicular cancer.
   Client Need: Physiological Adaptation; **Cognitive Level:** Analysis; **Nursing Process:** Assessment
4. **Answers: 2, 3, 4, 5.**
   2, 3, 4, 5 Diagnostic tests to confirm the diagnosis of testicular cancer include CT scan, ultrasound, lymphangiography, and confirmation of AFP and hCG tumor markers.

1 Biopsy not recommended owing to the potential to spread cancer.
Client Need: Physiological Adaptation; **Cognitive Level:** Understanding; **Integrated Process:** Teaching and Learning

5. **4 Early identification and treatment result in 100% survival rate for localized prostate cancer tumors.**

   1, 2, 3 These percentages do not reflect the survival rate for localized prostate cancer tumors when the disease is identified and treated early.
   Client Need: Physiological Adaptation; **Cognitive Level:** Understanding; **Integrated Process:** Teaching and Learning

6. **2 No correlation between BPH and cancer of the prostate has been determined.**

   1 Although encouraging the client to express fears, the immediate concern can be addressed by providing the client with the knowledge that BPH is not a risk factor for prostate cancer. **3** Because of no correlation between BPH and prostate cancer, this statement is not helpful in managing the client's fears. **4** This statement does not address the concern of BPH being a risk for prostate cancer, but rather a risk factor for prostate cancer itself.
   Client Need: Physiological Adaptation; **Cognitive Level:** Analysis; **Nursing Process:** Implementation

7. **2 Cryptorchidism occurs when the testes fail to descend from the abdomen.**

   1 A spermatocele occurs when a cyst develops between the testis and the epididymis. **3** Varicocele results in distention of the spermatic cord's veins. **4** Orchitis presents with tenderness of the scrotum.
   Client Need: Physiological Adaptation; **Cognitive Level:** Applying; **Nursing Process:** Assessment

8. **Answer: 1, 2, 3, 5.**

   1, 2, 3, 5 Male evaluation of infertility includes semen analysis, urethral culture, inhibin B assay, and sperm penetration analysis.

   4 PSA is used to assist in the diagnosis of prostate cancer.
   Client Need: Physiological Adaptation; **Cognitive Level:** Understanding; **Integrated Process:** Teaching and Learning

9. **2 In infertility situations, the male is responsible for 50% of the cases of infertility.**

   1 Although the statement tends not to assign blame, it does not clearly state the known facts related to infertility. **3** Although the statement is true, it does not clearly state the known facts related to infertility. **4** Although the statement is true, it does not clearly state the known facts related to infertility.
   Client Need: Physiological Adaptation; **Cognitive Level:** Analysis; **Integrated Process:** Teaching and Learning

10. **Answers: 1, 3, 4, 5.**

    1, 3, 4, 5 Variables that can alter sperm motility include the conditions identified in these options.

    2 A diet lacking protein is not associated with sperm motility.
    Client Need: Physiological Adaptation; **Cognitive Level:** Understanding; **Integrated Process:** Teaching and Learning

11. **2 Minimum sperm count for fertility is 20 million sperm per milliliter of semen.**

    1 A 10 million sperm per milliliter of semen is too low to support conception. **3** 40 million sperm per milliliter of semen is below average, but can support conception. **4** 60 million sperm per milliliter of semen is within the normal sperm count (50 to 100 million) and should support conception.
    Client Need: Physiological Adaptation; **Cognitive Level:** Understanding; **Integrated Process:** Teaching and Learning

12. **Answers: 1, 2, 3, 4.**

    1, 2, 3, 4 Assessment for male sexual dysfunction should include the foci presented in these options.

    5 Urinary function is not usually a source of sexual dysfunction.
    Client Need: Physiological Adaptation; **Cognitive Level:** Understanding; **Integrated Process:** Teaching and Learning

13. **3 Without sufficient testosterone levels, spermatogenesis is impaired.**

    1, 2, 4 Although spermatogenesis requires all the hormones mentioned, a testosterone deficiency has the most impact.
    Client Need: Physiological Adaptation; **Cognitive Level:** Understanding; **Integrated Process:** Teaching and Learning

14. **Answers: 1, 2, 4, 5.**

    1 Sedatives prescribed to treat insomnia can affect male sexual performance and desire. **2** Antidepressants prescribed to treat depression can affect male sexual performance and desire. **4** Antihistamines prescribed to treat seasonal allergies can affect male sexual performance and desire. **5** Antispasmodics prescribed to treat irritable bowel syndrome can affect male sexual performance and desire.

3 Antihypertensives prescribed to treat hypertension can affect male sexual performance and desire.
Client Need: Physiological Adaptation; **Cognitive Level:** Applying; **Nursing Process:** Assessment

15. **3 Marijuana is known to depress testosterone.**

    1 Alcohol's effect on sexual function is related to induced neuropathy. **2** Tobacco use results in vasoconstriction. **4** Cocaine affects sperm motility.
    Client Need: Physiological Adaptation; **Cognitive Level:** Applying; **Integrated Process:** Teaching and Learning

16. **2 Peripheral neuropathies often result from the pathology associated with diabetes.**

    1 Hypotension interferes with the circulation needed to create sufficient blood engorgement to create and sustain an erection. **3** Depending on its location, a spinal cord injury can affect erection, emission, and ejaculation because of impaired neuron functioning. **4** Pituitary dysfunction affects secretion of gonadotropins, but does not cause peripheral neuropathy.
    Client Need: Physiological Adaptation; **Cognitive Level:** Applying; **Nursing Process:** Assessment

17. **2 Gynecomastia is the overdevelopment of male breast tissue found unilaterally in the left beast.**

    1 Although there is a pubertal form of gynecomastia, it self-resolves in 4 to 6 months. **3** Inflammation is not involved in gynecomastia. **4** Gynecomastia is not a temporary swelling of breast tissue.
    Client Need: Physiological Adaptation; **Cognitive Level:** Applying; **Integrated Process:** Teaching and Learning

18. **2 Senescent gynecomastia regresses in 6 to 12 months.**

    1 Surgery is not required for the management of senescent gynecomastia. **3** This statement does not address the expected reduction in breast size. **4** Senescent gynecomastia is not known to be associated with breast cancer, but can mask signs of cancer.
    Client Need: Physiological Adaptation; **Cognitive Level:** Applying; **Integrated Process:** Teaching and Learning

19. **1 Breast cancer rates are higher in men with a familial history of female breast cancer.**

    2, 3, 4 Tobacco, alcohol, and hypertension have not been associated with the development of breast cancer in males.
    Client Need: Physiological Adaptation; **Cognitive Level:** Applying; **Nursing Process:** Assessment

20. **Answers: 1, 3, 4, 5.**

    1, 3, 4, 5 The alteration of estrogen and testosterone caused by obesity, cirrhosis of the liver, chronic kidney disease, and COPD contributes to gynecomastia development.

    2 Hyperthyroidism is a risk factor for the development of gynecomastia.
    Client Need: Physiological Adaptation; **Cognitive Level:** Applying; **Nursing Process:** Assessment

Bibliography

Adkison, L. R. (2012). Mechanism of inheritance. In *Elsevier's integrated review: Genetics* (2nd ed., pp. 28–45). Philadelphia: Elsevier.

American Academy of Allergy, Asthma, and Immunology. (2017). *Primary immunodeficiency diseases.* https://www.aaaai.org/conditions-and-treatments/conditions-dictionary/primary-immunodeficiency-diseases.

American College of Cardiology. (2017). New ACC/AHA high blood pressure guidelines lower definition of hypertension. http://www.acc.org/latest-in-cardiology/articles/2017/11/08/11/47/mon-5pm-bp-guideline-aha-2017.

Bartels, C. M., & Daniel Muller. (2017). *Systemic lupus erythematosus.* (2017). In Diamond, H. S. (Ed). *MedScape.* https://emedicine.medscape.com/article/332244-overview.

Berkowitz, A. (2007). *Clinical pathophysiology made ridiculously simple.* MedMaster: Miami, FL.

Cancer.gov. (2015). *Staging.* https://www.cancer.gov/about-cancer/diagnosis-staging/staging.

Centers for Disease Control and Prevention. (2017). *HIV/AIDS.* https://www.cdc.gov/hiv/default.html

Hubert, R.J., VanMeter, K.C. (2018). *Gould's pathophysiology for the health professions* (6th ed.). Philadelphia: Saunders.

Huether, S.E., & McCance, K.L. (2016). *Understanding pathophysiology* (6th ed.). St. Louis: Mosby.

Jarvis, C. J. (2016). *Physical examination & health assessment* (7th ed.). St. Louis: Elsevier.

Jones, T. L. (2012). *Crash course: Renal and urinary systems* (4th ed.). Edinburgh: Mosby.

Jorde, L. B., Carey, J. C., & Bamshad, M. J. (2010). Medical genetics. In *Medical genetics* (4th ed., pp.1–4). St. Louis: Elsevier.

Lewis, S. L., Bucher, L., Heitkemper, M. M., Harding, M. M., Kwong, J., & Roberts, D. (2017). *Medical-surgical nursing: Assessment and management of clinical problems* (10th ed.). St. Louis: Mosby.

Mahan, L. K., Raymond, J. L., & Escott-Stymp, S. (2012). Nutrition in eating disorders. In *Krause's food and the nutrition care process* (13th ed., pp. 489–493). Philadelphia: Saunders.

McCance, K. L., & Huether, S. E. (2019). *Pathophysiology: The biologic basis for disease in adults and children* (8th ed.). St. Louis: Elsevier.

National Cancer Institute. (2013). *Tumor grade.* https://www.cancer.gov/about-cancer/diagnosis-staging/prognosis/tumor-grade-fact-sheet#q2.

VanMeter, K. C., & Hubert, R. J. (2014). *Pathophysiology for the health professions.* St. Louis: Elsevier.